The Sex Education Debates

The Sex Education Debates

NANCY KENDALL

The University of Chicago Press
Chicago and London

Nancy Kendall is assistant professor of educational policy studies at the University of Wisconsin–Madison.

The University of Chicago Press, Chicago 60637
The University of Chicago Press, Ltd., London
© 2013 by The University of Chicago
All rights reserved. Published 2013.
Printed in the United States of America

22 21 20 19 18 17 16 15 14 13   1 2 3 4 5

ISBN-13: 978-0-226-92227-0 (cloth)
ISBN-13: 978-0-226-92228-7 (paper)
ISBN-13: 978-0-226-92229-4 (e-book)
ISBN-10: 0-226-92227-8 (cloth)
ISBN-10: 0-226-92228-6 (paper)
ISBN-10: 0-226-92229-4 (e-book)

Library of Congress Cataloging-in-Publication Data
Kendall, Nancy.
    The sex education debates / Nancy Kendall.
        p.   cm.
    Includes bibliographical references and index.
    ISBN-13: 978-0-226-92227-0 (alk. paper)
    ISBN-10: 0-226-92227-8 (alk. paper)
    ISBN-13: 978-0-226-92228-7 (pbk. : alk. paper)
    ISBN-10: 0-226-92228-6 (pbk. : alk. paper) [etc.]
    1. Sex instruction—United States.   2. Sex instruction for teenagers—United
States.   3. Sex instruction—Government policy—United States.   4. Sex
instruction for teenagers—Government policy—United States.   I. Title.
HQ57.5.A3K465 2012
613.9071—dc23   2012005112

♾ This paper meets the requirements of ansi/niso z39.48-1992
(Permanence of Paper).

Contents

To Tomas, Gabriel, and Cecilia
To the teachers and students who let me sit and learn with them
And to my Aunt Phyllis. We miss you.

Acknowledgments

This book would not exist without the love and support of my family. Tomas, Gabriel, and Cecilia have lived with this book for years now and dealt with its demands with equanimity and love. It is dedicated to them. My mother, father, and sisters have listened to me whine, slogged through chapters, helped me to improve the book and my writing process, told me they loved me, and assuaged guilt as needed. K. J. provided unending moral support and an occasional kick in the pants. Peggie Hansen made writing and parenting possible. Sharon Goldfarb kept me charged, Febe Chale kept me laughing, and the cousins reminded me how much fun life can be. My deepest thanks to each of them. It takes a village, as they say, and they have been mine.

This book was made possible by a ten-year program called the Sexuality Research Fellowship, led by Dr. Diane diMauro and funded by the Ford Foundation. The Fellowship provided the time, money, and colleagues necessary to conduct comparative ethnographic research on sex education—resources that are extremely difficult to find. I thank the Ford Foundation for their support; Dr. diMauro provided visionary leadership, Dr. Amy Stambach provided collegial mentoring, and my co-recipients provided the intense conversations and friendships necessary to keep trying to get into schools and get talking to people about sex education in the United States.

Each research setting was made possible by generous individuals and institutions who opened their doors for me to conduct ethnography on a subject no school was particularly excited to host. I am grateful for and humbled by their willingness to let me join them to learn about sex education in classroom settings. Particular thanks to GOG and BC in this regard. Thank you to each teacher, administrator, parent, activist, advocate, policy maker, and service provider who set aside time to speak with me. Special thanks to the schools and teachers referred to in the book as Teton High and Ms. Jeffries, Mr. Lauder, and Mr. Dean; Jefferson High and Come On In!; and Fontaine High and Mrs. Shane and Mr. Kelly. And the deepest of thanks to the students whom I was able to interview, and who, through their passion and concern, provided essential insights into the consequences of sex education for students' health, identities, well-being, and sense of belonging in schools and society.

Ray McDermott, Buddy Peshkin, George Spinder, and Elliot Eisner taught me about the kind of ethnographer I wanted to be. My graduate students waited patiently for me to resurface, and my colleagues in EPS and UW–Madison's African Studies, Development Studies, Gender and Women's Studies, Global Health Institute, and FACES provided a wonderfully interdisciplinary and intellectually stimulating environment in which to write. Special thanks to Adam, Aili, Amita, Amy, Bill, Chiqui, Christine, Claire, Dan, Doug, Fely, Fran, Francoise, Gay, Hilary, John, Lesley, Liz, Lora, Mark, Mariamne, Mary, Michael, Mimi, Nancy, Patrice, Peter, Sara, Shawn, Stacey, Tom, and Tricia for creating communities of both scholarship and care. Shirley Miske, Lori diPrete-Brown, and Zikani Kaunda have role modeled how to be professional, loving, and incredibly good at one's work; I hope to get there someday.

Patricia Burch, Colette Chabbott, Amita Chudgar, Katie Elliott, Andrew Epstein, Kristy Kelly, Cris Mayo, Paula McAvoy, John Meyer, Erin Murphy-Graham, Elizabeth Palmerson, Jen Sandler, and Donna Stonecipher all read parts or all of the manuscript and provided essential insights into how to improve the arguments I am trying to make. Thank you so much. Special thanks for their insights to Chloe O'Gara on chapters 4, 5, and 10; Carl Kendall on chapter 7; Colette Chabbott on chapter 8; Jen Sandler on chapter 9; and Cris Mayo on chapter 11. Of course, all mistakes and failures of insight are mine! I gratefully acknowledge Nicolette Pawlowski's energy, passion for truly comprehensive sexuality education, and help with RefWorks.

Kristin Cheney, Diane diMauro, Jessica Fields, Gil Herdt, Cris Mayo, Sameena Mulla, Terry Stein, Deb Tolman, and Wanda Pillow each gave me an opportunity to think through this research in new ways, with new audiences. Thanks to them for helping me expand my understanding of the many ways that sexuality education may be consequential in youth's lives.

The two blind reviewers of the book provided incredibly rich and thorough feedback that strengthened the book significantly and led me in new analytic directions. Elizabeth Branch Dyson's support as editor has been unfailing and irreplaceable. I would have given up early on without her enthusiasm, kindness, critical eye, and willingness to answer my interminable questions.

Introduction

The Battle over Sex Education in the United States

The statistics are grim: the United States has the highest rates of adolescent and unwanted pregnancies among industrialized countries, one in three girls will become pregnant before the age of twenty, and four out of every one hundred girls will give birth to a baby before they are twenty years old (CDC 2010b). Sexually transmitted infection (STI) rates among US teens are some of the highest in the industrialized world, and one in four adolescents between the ages of fourteen and nineteen has already been diagnosed with an STI (Forhan et al. 2009).

In response to these realities, there has been a sea change in public support for school-based sex education. In the 1980s, the HIV/AIDS epidemic and rising teen pregnancy and STI rates led to political and grassroots advocacy for school involvement in sex education. Since that time, the vast majority of public schools have begun offering some form of sex education to their students (Kaiser Family Foundation 2000), and the vast majority of parents and teachers say they approve of this change (National Public Radio, Kaiser Family Foundation, and Kennedy School of Government 2004).

Beyond this broad approval, however, public discussion indicates that there is little agreement about what forms of sex education should be taught in schools. Should students be taught about contraception? Abortion? Sexual identity? Should they learn relationship skills? Practice refusal skills? Teach each other about sex? Practice putting condoms on cucumbers?

The content of sex education programs has become a key battlefield in the so-called culture wars,[1] and sex education has been cast in terms of two diametrically opposed positions. On one side are Abstinence Only Until Marriage education (AOUME) proponents, who support the belief that sex is private and sacred and that abstinence is the only morally correct option for unmarried people. On the other side are Comprehensive Sexuality education (CSE) proponents, who believe that sex is a natural act and that people are empowered by receiving complete and correct information they can use to improve their sexual decision-making and, by extension, their health (Luker 2006).

This divide shapes the legal, political, media, research, resource, and curricular debates that occur throughout the country, producing a highly contentious and shifting policy arena that involves some of the most important actors and institutions in Americans' daily lives: families, friends, religious institutions, schools, government actors, and the media. Over the past decade, a tension has built between those policy makers who favor AOUME approaches, and the general public and sex education researchers, who tend to favor some type of abstinence-emphasizing CSE (e.g., Bleakley, Hennessy, and Fishbein 2006). The policy makers seem to be winning: in 1988, one in fifty teachers who taught sex education reported that they were required by school, district, or state officials to teach abstinence-only approaches; by 1999, this figure was one in four (Dailard 2001). Between 1996 and 2010, the federal government provided over $1.5 billion to fund AOUME activities throughout the United States, but provided no resources to fund school-based CSE activities until 2010 (SIECUS 2010).

There is recent and uneven movement away from the trend of federal and state policy makers supporting AOUME approaches. A mounting body of scientific evidence indicating the limited success of AOUME programs in meeting their stated goals has led to recent federal cuts to AOUME funding (Landau 2010), and new federal funding may support abstinence-based CSE programs.[2] An increasing number of state governments have stopped accepting federal AOUME funding and have passed legislation declaring that sex education curricula must present "medically accurate" information—a strike at AOUME curricula, which are often charged with misrepresenting sexual health and contraceptive facts (e.g., United States House of Representatives, Committee on Government Reform 2004). Recent positive evaluations of abstinence-based (not AOUME) programs have generated interest in mixed abstinence-based and CSE programming, potentially tailored to specific student populations. At the same moment, however, some states are returning to stricter AOUME policies after adopting more CSE-supportive policies.[3]

Caught in the middle of these debates and policy shifts, public school teachers, parents, students, and administrators are trying to navigate the highly charged terrain of talking with kids about sex in a public institution. I decided to write this book because I have become increasingly concerned with the growing divide between teens' daily experiences with sex and sexuality and adults' school-based efforts to inform and regulate these experiences. The debates about school-based sex education have made it harder for schools to be responsive to students' concerns and needs, have often negatively affected student, teacher, and community relations, and have played a key role in reshaping our national commonsense notions of who has the right to influence decisions about what happens in public schools. The issues surrounding school-based sex education are thus twofold: what adults try to teach teens about sex, and what lessons students, teachers, district officials, and parents learn about their roles, rights, and responsibilities in shaping public institutions like schools. On both fronts, I will argue, school-based sex education is not serving us well.

The ethnographic research on which this book is based was conducted in schools, communities, and districts in five states in the United States. In examining the voices and actions of teachers, students, parents, district officials, and sex education instructors, activists, and advocates, the book reveals some disturbing trends concerning both the formal lessons students are learning about "the facts" of sex and sexuality, and the hidden lessons that students and teachers are learning about equity, social relations and expectations, and democratic participation and processes.

Consequences Matter

Sex education is important in and of itself, but also because it reflects and influences central facets of our society and democracy. The evidence from this study suggests that (1) school-based sex education, as currently conceptualized and practiced, is not doing a lot of good for students, schools, or communities; (2) in order to improve sex education and students' experience of it, we need to better understand the full range of consequences, intended and unintended, of different sex education approaches; and (3) by paying more attention to sex education practices and consequences, instead of just policies and official outcomes, we can shift the debates about and daily experiences that constitute school-based sex education and civic engagement in public schools. If we reframe the sex education debate from one of official policies to one of sociopolitical consequences, then rather than AOUME and CSE supporters sparring over how to best decrease pregnancy and STI rates through formal programming interventions, we could focus on how students, teachers, parents, schools, and communities interact around these issues. These patterns of interaction would serve as a basis to determine how school-based sex education experiences can support physically, emotionally, socially, politically, and economically healthier teens, as well as more engaged and more democratically inclined students and community members.

The premise of this work is that understanding the range of intended and unintended consequences of sex education practices on US public schools and students is a necessary springboard to improving sex education. To that end, this book argues for a shift in our national conversations away from a focus on the official policies (such as federal AOUME definitions), content (the formal curriculum in a school), and official outcomes (such as reported changes in STI rates) of sex education and toward a focus on the sociopolitical consequences of sex education. These consequences include the lessons students and parents learn about themselves as sexual and social beings, about how we as a country make decisions and talk about sex in public institutions, about critical thinking, about broader school and social mores and values, and about appropriate forms of civic engagement with public institutions.

What Is School-Based Sex Education, Anyway?

Current debates and research concerning the effectiveness of different school-based sex education[4] approaches are important because they reveal some of the key ideological assumptions underlying AOUME and CSE approaches—assumptions that largely account for the unintended, inequitable, and undemocratic consequences that I observed resulting from sex education programs in public schools. The section below describes the kinds of sex education approaches I observed and lays out in broad strokes the central ideological concerns of each. It also defines terms used throughout the book, many of which are contentious and used in a variety of ways in sex education literatures.

ABSTINENCE ONLY UNTIL MARRIAGE EDUCATION (AOUME) AND THE NEW CHRISTIAN RIGHT

AOUME approaches are based on a moral framework that derives from a particular interpretation of biblical and contemporary Christian texts. Many of the people and organizations involved in the national AOUME movement, and most of the popular AOUME curricula, come from the New Christian Right, a term I use to denote a heterogeneous group of socially conservative evangelical Christian people and organizations that seek to shape the social and political cultures of the United States through direct involvement in political, legal, and social movements and activism.

Since its inception in the 1970s, individuals and institutions of the New Christian Right have been more or less unified in their approaches to engaging the secular world and their calls for a reconstruction of American culture and society based on God's authority, as transmitted through and reflected in the "traditional family" (Liebman and Wuthnow 1983). The movement operates within a religious framework that makes particular claims about biblical truth and its connection to patriotism and national morality (Rose 1989). Although not all members of the New Christian Right are in agreement on all issues, central components of this ideological framework include the idea that the nuclear family is the basic unit of identity, community, and nation, that the male is the head of the family and adults have authority over children, that these hierarchies are biblically ordained and necessary to the social order, that sex is a sacred act that should be kept private and within marriage, that sex that occurs outside of marriage is socially destructive, and that when sinful behavior is widespread, the sinner, society, and nation all suffer.

AOUME proponents believe that teaching students these values will help restore the country's morality and cure "social ills" including homosexuality, single-parent families, and the STI epidemic.[5] As such, although the recipient of school-based AOUME is the student, conceptually the nuclear family is the primary unit of social analysis and importance in AOUME approaches. Moreover, although proponents often draw on public health rationales to argue for AOUME approaches, for members of the New Christian Right, AOUME is not fundamentally (public) health education but moral education.

The federal role in defining AOUME

The federal government played a key role in the first decade of the twenty-first century in defining which programs would qualify for federal AOUME funding through what are commonly called the federal A-H guidelines. These guidelines emphasize the core AOUME beliefs that abstinence before marriage is the only morally acceptable and healthy behavioral option for teens, and that sex outside of marriage has negative implications for individuals and society. Abstinence programs that do not specifically embody these moral prescriptions are not eligible to receive federal AOUME funding.[6]

In 1996[7] large-scale federal support for AOUME created a new funding mechanism for individuals and organizations to develop, market, and profit from AOUME materials and programs (Pruitt 2007). States' capacity to fund AOUME advocacy organizations and to provide free AOUME services to schools, community groups, and religious institutions was dramatically expanded. To access these federal resources, organizations had to standardize their programs in terms of both the A-H guidelines and federal rules concerning the separation of church and state. Federal involvement thus narrowed the range of AOUME curricula and programs implemented in public schools to a portion of all existing AOUME curricula. In this study, when I talk about AOUME curricula and programs, I am referring only to those programs that have or could have been implemented in public schools with federal AOUME funding. A number of AOUME curricula and programs have two versions: one for use in churches and by families, and one for use in public schools. This book refers to only the second version.

COMPREHENSIVE SEXUALITY EDUCATION (CSE)

Comprehensive Sexuality Education (CSE) is less clearly defined than AOUME. There is no official definition tied to federal resources or monitoring processes, and the actors and institutions involved in creating curricula and programs have historically been more ideologically and disciplinarily diverse than those in the AOUME movement. CSE definitions come into being for various reasons: for example, some are developed in response to AOUME approaches and claim to positively address topics (such as contraception, abortion, and sexual identity) that AOUME programs do not. Others, often crafted by individuals and organizations that have been involved in CSE for decades, reflect institutional mandates (for example, to serve Latin@ youth or improve teenage girls' reproductive health). The latter include frameworks developed by groups such as the Sexuality Information and Education Council of the United States (SIECUS) and Planned Parenthood, curricula developed by groups such as the Unitarian Church, and compendia of best-practice programs and curricula put together by sex educators, community leaders, and others.[8] CSE programs range from those that strongly emphasize the benefits of abstinence but provide extensive facts about contraceptive devices to programs designed to support adolescents' positive exploration of their own sexuality. Still other programs focus on building self-esteem or exploring sexual identity and identity-based bullying.

CSE programs implemented in public schools generally understand sex and sexuality to be natural aspects of individuals, each of whom has the right to explore and represent their sexuality as they see fit so long as they do not impinge on others' right to do the same. Most CSE supporters view themselves first and foremost as providing scientifically "complete and correct" information to adolescents, who are thereby empowered to make better individual decisions about their sexual behavior and health. In practice, however, as McKay (1998) points out, these ideals of rational individual agency, scientific rationality, and political liberalism combine to create a set of assumptions about what "healthy sexuality" looks like that is more constrained than might be imagined. CSE supporters claim that their approaches are based on scientific evidence and a rational public-health model, and therefore do *not* constitute morality education. However, like AOUME models, CSE models are shaped by embedded assumptions about what constitutes "good" individual decision-making and "good" sexual behavior and relations.

ABSTINENCE-AND . . .

The rhetoric in the sex education debates often makes it seem that there only exist AOUME and CSE approaches. In fact, between these approaches lies a vast (and expanding) range of programs that are often classified as "abstinence," "abstinence-plus," "abstinence-based," or "abstinence-centered" programs.

A growing number of researchers and policy makers view "abstinence-and" approaches as efforts to combine the strengths of AOUME and CSE approaches into a new formulation that emphasizes abstinence as the healthiest and best alternative for adolescents, but that does not present sex-negative messages and provides more information about topics like contraception than traditional AOUME approaches, do. Pruitt describes the difference between AOUME and "abstinence-and" approaches as follows:

> Abstinence-only essentially tells youth not to have sex and is unconcerned for those who don't take the directive. Abstinence-plus tells kids to remain abstinent but allows for those who don't listen. That allowance means that sometimes abstinence-plus programs teach about contraception. Abstinence-plus programs, by the way, usually do not meet the letter of the law as stated in the A-H definition. (Pruitt 2007, 3)

Pruitt's definition reveals some of the assumptions underlying "abstinence-and" approaches: a strong desire to have teens refrain from sex, but also a recognition that if teens do have sex, it is better that they have safer sex. As AOUME programs do not, and conceptually cannot, engage with the idea of "safer sex"—to them, abstinence is the only safe *moral* option for unmarried people—"abstinence-and" approaches represent a real ideological departure from AOUME approaches. It is often less clear how to conceptualize the difference between CSE programs and "abstinence-and" programs, as most mainstream CSE programs emphasize abstinence as the best option for teens. Both "abstinence-and" and many CSE programs thus align with models of teen sexual health, desire, responsibility, rights, and action that discourage or even stigmatize teen sexual activity and exploration of sexuality; as such, these programs are a real departure from sex-positive CSE models.

Politics and the Sex Education Debate

The current AOUME-to-CSE spectrum appears at first glance to map easily onto a politically "conservative" to "liberal" ideological spectrum. A number of researchers have argued, however, that political and sexual spectra are related but do not fully overlap (e.g., Luker 2006; McKay 1998), and that in some cases, radicals on either end of the political spectrum may be more similar to one another in their sexual ideologies than to moderates (Pruitt 2007). Similarly, my research indicates that it is not possible to simply categorize AOUME programs or supporters as socially and politically "conservative" and CSE programs and supporters as socially and politically "liberal." For example, teachers most often combined discourses, activities, and approaches that would usually be categorized as either "liberal" or "conservative" in their classroom sex education activities. Likewise, common aspects of AOUME programs, such as their understanding of people's sexuality as fundamentally relational, may be seen as more "progressive" than CSE programs' common assumption that sexuality and sexual decision-making is entirely individualized.

In other words, the "sex education debates" oversimplify and dichotomize the complex ideas and positions that people and institutions hold concerning sex education. They obscure how profoundly interrelated and important the ideological assumptions of programs, their implementers, and the context—the informal curriculum of school and classroom environment—are to how students experience and respond to learning about sex and sexuality in schools. My research design allowed me to examine similarities and differences within and across programs and schools, and in so doing revealed some of the ways that official policy and curricula come together in schools and classrooms to shape lived consequences for teachers and students. Lived consequences matter most for our understanding of what sex education programs do in and for schools and students because, unlike the official outcomes, they reveal the intended *and* unintended consequences of sex education: the effects on pregnancy rates and also whether a program fails to engage with students' daily lives and needs; the STI rates and the consequences of school-based sex education on relations among school and community members.

Sex Education in This Book

This book is divided into two sections. The first section describes the rationale for and limitations of the methods used for this study. It then gives a brief overview of (1) sex education research and methods and (2) sex education policy structures around the country and in the settings where I conducted research (chapter 2). The remainder of the first section takes the reader into schools, classrooms, and sex educator trainings in Florida (chapter 3), Wyoming (chapter 4), Wisconsin (chapter 5), and California (chapter 6).[9] Each of these chapters has two goals: to provide an ethnographic overview of the particular sex education programs and schools I observed, and to present a microanalysis of the interactions among students, teachers, parents, administrators, and community organizations that shaped sex education practices in each setting. This microanalysis reveals how the ideological assumptions of curricula, teachers, and students interacted in each setting to shape complex, sometimes contradictory, and often inequitable, sex education practices.

The first section of the book reveals the high level of variation in sex education practices and consequences between and within states, schools, and classrooms. The policy-as-practice analytic framework that I employ, described in chapter 2, helps to develop a clear understanding of the constellations of forces—from official policies, to geography, to political movements, to local histories, to individual experiences—that shape sex education in different places. Part 1 highlights the importance of understanding how official sex-education policies are taken up by actors and institutions (that is, how these policies are "localized" through daily practices), and the centrality of students' and teachers' relationships in determining sex education practices. In particular, these chapters reveal the significant constraints that many sex education teachers felt in presenting sex education. Their discomfort stemmed from their own beliefs, their perceptions of community pressures, and school policies. These chapters also reveal students' sense that formal sex education curricula failed to connect with their concerns or experiences; it was instead shaped by adults' interactions and concerns. Beyond the official curriculum, students spoke passionately about their experiences of a "hidden curriculum" about sexuality: one that reflected an adult fear of teen sexuality, that often reinforced sexist, racist, and heteronormative messages, and that silenced students' voices in curricular and school decision-making processes. In other words, students felt that current sex education approaches exemplify what Sharon Stephens identifies as "the high price children must pay when their bodies and minds become the terrain for adult battles" (Stephens 1995, vii).

In part 2 of the book, I build off of the microanalyses of classroom- and school-level interactions to examine four key macrosocial consequences of current sex-education approaches: inequitable and disempowering conceptions of adolescent reproductive health and fertility (chapter 7), the reinscription of "traditional" gender norms (chapter 8), the denial or scientific rationalization of LGBTQ sexual identities (chapter 9), and the official silence about and commodification of rape and sexual violence (chapter 10). Each of these chapters draws on an analysis of popular AOUME and CSE curricula and the data collected in the states to explore similarities and differences among CSE and AOUME approaches.

The conclusion of the book (chapter 11) describes the political consequences of current sex education approaches and debates, and examines what they demonstrate about "democracy in action" in US schools and public institutions. The chapter argues for a reconceptualization of the goals, daily practices, and measures of success used to judge sex education. It outlines an alternate framework for student, teacher, and community involvement in sex education policy-making that centers students' needs, desires, concerns, and experiences as sexual beings, social actors, and citizens-in-training. The framework acknowledges the health, social, economic, and moral implications of sex education, but argues that the implications of sex education as citizenship education, often ignored in current evidence-based decision-making frameworks, might be the most important ones to consider.

Sex Education Research and Policies

The Research We Have

There are hundreds of surveys about and program evaluations of sex education. These studies have been used to argue for wildly different understandings of how people feel about sex education and what its effects are on teen sexual health. Generally, surveys whose questions follow scientific best practices show widespread support among adults and teens for CSE programming that emphasizes the benefits of abstinence,[1] but these results are used to very different ends by CSE and AOUME advocates.[2]

Most sex education outcome studies measure whether a particular curriculum or program affects a small set of student health and behavioral outcomes (e.g., Kirby 1985, 1991, 1997, 2001; Trenholm et al. 2007). Very few studies have systematically examined other outcomes, including the emotional, social, psychological, or spiritual effects of sex education programs on individuals; peer-group effects; effects on school-community or teacher-student relations; or the interactions among sex education programs and broader social, economic, political, and cultural processes. This means that we know very little about the unofficial or unintended consequences of sex education programs and approaches.

Reviews of scientific studies that examine the officially intended health outcomes of sex education programs indicate that most sex education curricula and programs—AOUME, "abstinence-and," and CSE—have either no effect or only a small effect on measures of behavioral and sexual health outcomes (e.g., Hedman, Larsen, and Bohnenblust 2008; Zimmerman et al. 2008). A few programs (e.g., Kirby 2007) have shown greater effects for a subpopulation (for example, girls but not boys), and some have shown an initially significant effect on, for example, delaying sexual initiation, but these effects tend to disappear over six months to two years.[3] A very good sex education program—and in terms of official outcomes, almost all of the effective programs are CSE programs—may decrease reported pregnancy rates by 30 percent, delay sexual initiation by one year, or increase reported condom use by 12 percent (Suellentrop 2009). These are important and significant results. But, as Suellentrop and the National Campaign to Prevent Teen and Unwanted Pregnancy explain,

> Because teen pregnancy has many causes, and because even effective programs do not eliminate the problem, it is unreasonable to expect any single curriculum or community program to make a serious dent in the problem on its own. Making true and lasting progress in preventing teen pregnancy requires a combination of community programs and broader efforts to influence values and popular culture, to engage parents and schools, to change the economic incentives that teens face, and more. (Suellentrop 2009, 7)

Our limited knowledge about the consequences of existing sex education programs and their practical implementation in schools limits our capacity to improve such programs, not only in terms of officially intended health outcomes, but more broadly in terms of the social, political, and relational outcomes we desire for all students and schools. And because of the focus on program evaluation, we understand even less about the lessons students learn about sex and sexuality in schools but outside of the official sex education classroom.

The Research We Need

While adult battles about sex education most often refer to formal curricular materials or things teachers say in sex education classes, surveys of students, ethnographic research, and legal challenges filed by students about sexuality and schooling most often relate to the "hidden" sex education curriculum. This includes speech, norms, and practices in all of the students' classrooms, school cafeterias, locker rooms, dances, nurse's offices, libraries, principals' offices, and so forth. The hidden curriculum might include teachers monitoring the way girls and boys dress, physical and verbal abuse directed by teachers and students toward sexual- and gender-identity norm-breaking students, teacher and student responses to such abuse, debates over whether students should be allowed to form after-school Gay-Straight Alliances (GSAs), and peer pressure to adhere to particular sexual norms. For students, in other words, the "sex education curriculum" has always been larger than just the formal curriculum upon which so many adults are focused, and the consequences of students' school-based experiences of sexuality have always been greater than the short list of behavioral and medical outcomes upon which current sex-education debates are focused. We know very little, however, about the hidden sexuality curriculum.

We also know very little about how sex education affects schools as institutions: how districts and schools select the programs and curricula they will use or what effects this process has on community-school relations, how the size and makeup of classes influences teachers' comfort and practices, how teachers' sense of parental and community support for sex education affects their classroom conversations and use of curricular materials, and so forth.

These silences in the current research on sex education highlight four underexamined questions:

- How should the effects of sex education on students be conceptualized and studied?
- How should sex education be understood as a part of a school system and culture (as opposed to a stand-alone program implemented in a school setting), and how ought the effects of sex education programs within this broader system be analyzed?
- How can the consequences of community-school and teacher-student interactions around sexuality and sex education best be examined?
- How do school systems and cultures interact with, become affected by, and affect the broader social, political, economic, cultural, and policy environments in which students, teachers, parents, communities, and schools operate?

Encouragingly, a small but important literature does examine sex education policies and practices as part of social structures and school cultures, curricula, and practices.[4] Whatley's (Whatley and Trudell 1993; Whatley 1988) content analyses of sex education programs and curricular materials, for example, were pathbreaking in analyzing the sociocultural constructs underlying popular AOUME curricula. Her work laid the foundation for later content analyses that reshaped the sex education policy arena (most famously, the Waxman Report), and widespread state adoption of laws requiring that sex education curricula be "medically accurate."

Other researchers, including di Mauro and Joffe (2009), Irvine (2002), Moran (2000), Patton (1996), Sears (1992), and Trudell (1985), have examined the political histories of adolescence, HIV/AIDS, and sex education policies and programming. Their accounts revealed the social, political, economic, and cultural forces that shaped the sex education debates over the past centuries and into the present across diverse communities. These histories provide important information about the social constructs (such as "adolescence") and forces (such as political movements) that underpin our national discussions about sex education and our schools' sex education practices. The research described in this book drew on these authors to understand factors such as student-teacher positionality in schools, community-school interactions around sex education, and the divergent responses of district, state, and federal actors to research indicating that AOUME programs are generally ineffective at meeting their stated health goals.

Other researchers, including Bay-Cheng (2003), Bettie (2003), Elia (2000), Fine and McClelland (2006), Milner (2004), Pascoe (2007), Sears (1992), and Walkerdine (1990), have examined teen sexuality and gender relations (often in their complex interrelations with race, class, sexual identity, and ethnicity) and how they interact with, shape, and are shaped by school and sex education practices. These studies, often based on qualitative research and drawing on feminist, queer, and critical (race) theories, have revolutionized our understanding of students' differing experiences of sex education and schooling. They have explicated links between sex education research and broader issues of social, health, and economic inequity and justice. Some researchers working from more philosophical traditions, such as Mayo and Pruitt, have examined the implications of current sex-education programs as they relate to constructions of citizenship (e.g., Rhoads and Calderone 2007; Mayo 2006) or health (education) (e.g., Pruitt 2007), and have reached similar conclusions about the need to link studies of sex education to broader analyses of social inequity and justice in the United States. These accounts stand in sharp contrast to studies of sex education that take the institutional space of the school for granted, assume "sex education" is just the official curriculum, and claim that the official outcomes of sex education are the only consequences that should be evaluated.

Lastly, a smaller number of researchers, including Fields (2008), Fine (1988), Trudell (1993), and Weis and Carbonell-Medina (2000), have utilized ethnographic approaches to explore sex education as an embodiment of and in relation to sexuality, gender, race, and class practices in US schools. These studies draw conceptually from the broader field of qualitative research conducted on teen sexuality (Tolman's work on gender, sexuality, and adolescence is paradigmatic here),[5] but provide particular insights into how schools as institutional spaces and sites of state-community interaction shape practices of teen sexuality, sex education, and gender, race, sexual identity, and class. A much smaller number of these studies have utilized comparative ethnographic or qualitative research methodologies to examine contemporary school-based sex education practices across educational settings and across sex education program types. Fields's (2008) research in three North Carolina public and private middle schools that offered a range of sex education program approaches is exemplary here. Taken together, this research has significantly expanded our understanding of how sex education programs in the United States *school* students in (often quite conservative) sexuality and gender norms, pathologize teen (particularly female, queer, and black) sexuality, create sociopolitical panics that schools must navigate in providing sex education, and result in undemocratic school policies and practices that sideline students' and many parents' voices.

The research that is described in this book draws heavily from these approaches, which in turn link methodologically and topically to a growing body of ethnographies and qualitative studies that link classroom and school interactions to macro-level social, economic, and political processes in their analysis of the consequences of US public school practices. Studies such as Pope's (2003) ethnography of "doing school," Demerath's (2009) study of the lessons that high school students learn about success, competition, and social equity in the United States, Varenne and McDermott's (1999) study of schools' production of "successful failure," Lopez's (2003) study of race and gender in the construction of student experiences and educational dreams, and Staiger's (2006) multisite study of diversity-in-practice represent the types of school ethnographies that informed my methodological approach, and from which I modeled the micro-macro-analyses conducted herein.

This Research

Building on these studies, this book argues that we need to more fully understand the similarities and differences in students', teachers', and communities' sex education experiences across the United States in order to better inform efforts to improve sex education for all students. By conducting systematic, comparative ethnographic research to identify and analyze the consequences of diverse sex education programs, we see that CSE and AOUME approaches often result in quite similar consequences despite their hotly contested ideological differences. We see that, as with all arenas of school policy and practices (e.g., Ball 1990), the messages that students receive about sex and sexuality may not always be those that are expected or desired. Only by understanding the daily practices and full consequences of formal and informal policies, curricula, and practices can we improve sex education.

COMPARING POLICY EFFECTS: POLICY AS/IN PRACTICE

This research reflects my longstanding interest in understanding how top-down policies aimed at transforming schools actually affect people's daily lives. In the case of sex education, I wanted to understand if and how federal funding for AOUME interacted with state, district, school, and classroom practices to shape students' experiences with sexuality in schools.[6] AOUME funding is one example of a broader shift in federal rationality concerning school and individual governance, in which official policies grow in importance because they represent the framework through which public and private practices are understood and judged.[7] There has been little discussion of how these changes play out in sex education practices at the school or district level.[8]

For this research, I adopted an anthropological approach to understanding policy that capitalizes on what Peacock (1986, 113) terms anthropology's capacity to "broaden the framework of discussion" by examining lived realities (policies in practice) as rooted in the broader forces (including official policies) that shape them. I drew particularly from the anthropology of policy literature that examines the roles of official policies in promulgating (neoliberal) governmental rationalities.[9]

I paired this approach with a multisite comparative research framework based on Hart's (2002) ethnographic comparisons of constellations of forces operating in locales. Hart describes her approach as moving away from a comparison of geographical sites and toward a comparison of the interrelated forces that make up the environment within which policies play out. This approach shifts the research focus of sex education from a study of a bounded geographic site (ethnographic models of "school culture" studies, for example) to an idea of place as "always formed through relations and connections with dynamics at play in other places, and in wider regional, national, and transnational arenas" (14). This approach provides a better tool for examining phenomena that are, and are affected by, local, state, national, and international phenomena. Thus, for example, English Learners in California classrooms are not simply and only part of a single California school's fabric; their lives, families, movements, ideas about sex and sexuality, and engagement with sex education instructors are formed through their relations with ideas, languages, experiences, places, and processes that are transnational in scope. At the same time, the school is eminently constituted by students' interactions with each other and their teachers, their walks from home to school and back, the television they watch, the after-school jobs they hold, and the day-to-day of life in their communities in California. The particularity of sex education in any classroom thus "arise[s] through *interrelations* between objects, events, places, and identities, and it is through clarifying how these relations are produced and changed in practice that close study of a particular part can illuminate the whole . . ." (Hart 2002, 14). This type of comparative approach challenges policy literatures that assume a unilinear impact model,[10] which begins and ends with official policy makers, places elite policy "experts" at the center of the policy process, and depoliticizes (through the provision of technocratic rationales) policy outcomes. These top-down approaches are often neither able to, nor interested in, grappling with the broader social, political, and economic structures that affect policies in practice.

Comparative, ethnographic, policy-as-practice research approaches are particularly appropriate to studying sex education in the United States because of the remarkably wide range of constellations of forces that influence classroom and school practices in the more than 15,000 school districts that compose the highly decentralized US school system. Neither top-down policy studies nor narrowly geographically bounded ethnographies can begin to truly explore the breadth and diversity of student, teacher, and community experiences in US schools.

Comparative policy-as-practice research does not provide parallel stories of how classrooms in different schools and states function in each setting, nor simply a comparison of official district policies. Instead, it identifies which forces come together in different places to shape daily sex-education practices. In one community, a group of parents and official state policy might be the primary forces determining sex education practices in a school. In another school, a loose set of official policies, an administrator's bias against one group of students, and teachers' overburdened schedules may be the primary forces that shape quite different sex-education experiences across different classrooms in the same school. This type of study helps us understand the uneven movement and effects of policies, resources, structures, and ideas across settings and groups, while illuminating underlying consistencies that hold across quite different constellations of forces.

Research Design: Obstacles as Evidence

This book is informed by two and a half years of ethnographic research conducted between 2004 and 2009 in five states: California, Florida, Wisconsin, Wyoming, and, very briefly until politics closed the door, Maryland.[11] These states represent a breadth of state policy responses to sex education and to federal AOUME funding and policies (appendix 1 includes information on AOUME funding and sex education policies in each state). Recognizing the diversity of school approaches to sex education in most states, I did not aim to conduct research that would be generalizable (in the quantitative sense) to all schools in a state or in the country. Instead, I aimed to compare the constellations of forces affecting sex education experiences in a small number of schools and communities in each state to elucidate some of the different logics and relations among actors and institutions that drive sex education practices in diverse US schools, and to examine analytic themes that emerged across these very different settings. Similarities that arose across these settings would offer evidence of underlying themes that might elucidate broader macrosocial analyses.[12] Individual schools and communities would thus be illustrative, not representative, of how national, state, district, school, and community policies, actors, and institutions interacted to affect sex education practices.

My intention was to spend an extended period of time conducting classroom and school observations in each state, as well as conducting observations, interviews, and focus group discussions with a wide array of actors and institutions involved in sex education. My previous experiences in southern Africa conducting ethnographic research on educational policy practices had been in communities and schools that were interested in the topic I was exploring and willing to allow me to join them for extended periods of time. This was not the case when I conducted sex education research in US schools and communities.

Research on sex education and students' sexuality, while never particularly welcome in public schools, was especially difficult to navigate in the political and legal climate prevalent at the time of my research, most of which was conducted between 2004 and 2006 (I conducted research in Wisconsin through 2009). Schools were increasingly concerned about community backlash to sex education because of legal threats from AOUME advocacy groups and legal rulings that had penalized schools and teachers for providing CSE.[13] Local and state AOUME advocacy groups often received support from national New Christian Right groups, and therefore often had both a local base of support and strong national networks and resource bases.[14] In contrast, the only CSE advocacy groups that I encountered were nationally based and did not have extensive local connections or organizational capacity. Simultaneously, schools were facing new pressures generated by the No Child Left Behind (NCLB) Act, which, among other effects, made subjects such as science (e.g., Marx and Harris 2006), arts (e.g., Chapman 2004), and sex education (e.g., Kendall 2008a) low priorities for many schools and districts.

The combination of federal and state pressures to focus resources on English and mathematics and the potentially inflammatory nature of sex education made many of the districts and schools that I approached wary of participating in the research. This was particularly true for schools and districts implementing AOUME programs or located in more conservative communities. As one Florida superintendent said to me,

Sex education is not a priority for us. Our kids can't read or write, and we're trying to keep our schools [from being reconstituted per NCLB mandates]. So this research is not our priority. Now also, it could really upset our parents— telling them you are going to talk to their kids about sex. And then we have to handle that situation.

My research was also impeded by district, school, and university institutional review boards that balked at my talking to students about their experiences in sex education classrooms.[15] In Maryland, the Citizens for Responsible Curriculum (CRC), a local AOUME advocacy group that was soon to file a court case against the school district in which I was working, threatened to "investigate" me and to find out which officials had approved my research, in order to mount personal attacks against them. Although these responses made the research process more complicated, they also provided important insights into the broader AOUME and CSE movements' understandings and uses of research.[16]

During the time I was conducting research, a number of reports concluded that there was not yet evidence that AOUME programs were effective at achieving their intended outcomes (e.g., Kirby 2007; Santelli et al. 2006). Quite a few people in the AOUME movement felt the scientists involved in these reports were deliberately attacking and discrediting AOUME. For example, when a report authored by Santelli et al. (2006) claimed that there was no evidence of AOUME program effectiveness, the Medical Institutes of Sexual Health (a New Christian Right–affiliated organization, now called the Medical Institute) released a policy brief that attempted to discredit the Santelli et al. report by presenting an entirely different set of studies (largely unpublished in peer-reviewed scientific journals)[17] that found statistically significant changes in reported attitudes and behaviors resulting from AOUME programs (Hendricks et al. 2006).

At the same time, researchers and other scientists were writing about and organizing against what they perceived as systematic attacks by the Bush administration on evidence-based research (e.g., Markowitz and Rosner 2003). For example, the Union of Concerned Scientists collected over 15,000 signatures for its statement on "Restoring Scientific Integrity," which challenged the Bush administration's involvement in peer review, hiring, and research-dissemination practices in key federal scientific and medical research institutions.[18] Battles over evolution and creationism in schools were on the rise as well (e.g., Gross 2006): sex education and evolution—the "science wars" as an aspect of the "culture wars"—were debated publicly in schools throughout the country.

The New Christian Right has long held that Christians and Christian values are under attack in the United States.[19] This sense of being under attack, of the need to "guard the gates," was evident in many of my conversations with AOUME advocacy groups and educators (though not with private AOUME providers). The translation of this sense of attack into efforts to curtail scientific investigation into sex education, and particularly into AOUME, has been evident in a number of arenas. For example, during the 2000s, an increasing number of conservative schools, districts, and states refused to allow the US government's long-standing national Youth Risk Behavior Survey (YRBS) to collect information from adolescents on sexuality. Similarly, most of the AOUME programs that originally agreed to participate in a congressionally funded randomized controlled trial of AOUME programs dropped out before the results of the trial could be collected and analyzed (Trenholm et al. 2007).

Given these realities, I was not surprised that I found a warmer welcome for my research in schools and districts that were implementing CSE programs. Based on state guidelines and politics, I assumed when I designed the research that I would be working in schools with AOUME programs in Florida and Wyoming, abstinence-plus programs in Wisconsin, and CSE programs in California and Maryland. Instead, I found myself working in schools in California, Wisconsin, and Wyoming that were implementing CSE programs, had extremely limited access to AOUME schools in Wisconsin, Wyoming, and Florida, and had research in a CSE district in Maryland terminated by an AOUME advocacy group's litigation.

My experience trying to gain access to different schools, communities, and districts was, in short, a research process all its own, and one that mirrored broader national trends concerning the relationship among AOUME advocates, sex education researchers, and schools. I learned important lessons about how AOUME service providers and advocates understood their roles in advocating for AOUME approaches. I also learned about teachers', principals', school boards', and district officials' concerns about sex education as a potential legal distraction to their central mandate, and about schools' concomitant efforts to regulate discussion and research about sex education in areas with perceived community or state support for AOUME.

Though I was able to access AOUME curricula and speak with private service providers freely, the restrictions on my access to AOUME classrooms, schools, and districts limited what I can say about the classroom-level consequences of federal AOUME funding. In contrast, my access to a range of CSE classrooms, schools, and districts allowed me to learn a great deal more about how CSE was being practiced in light of federal support for AOUME, and how the varied community and school relations that characterized the research settings in each state affected sex education in practice. My limited access to AOUME versus CSE settings thus paralleled Kirby's finding that we can say much more about the effectiveness of CSE programs than we can about AOUME programs, because few AOUME programs have been (I would add, have allowed themselves to be) rigorously evaluated (e.g., Kirby 2001, 2002).

My analysis of CSE programs in California, Wisconsin, and Wyoming is rooted in extended classroom observational research and interviews with teachers, students, parents, school and district education officials, CSE service providers, CSE and AOUME advocates in the district and state, state education officials, and sex education organizations and advocates. I also conducted curriculum and policy document reviews across these institutions.

I observed at least two sex education instructors and/or two formal sex education classes in each CSE school, which helped me compare microsocial interactions and constellations of forces affecting formal sex education practices within and across schools. I also participated in and observed informal events and spaces at each school (school dances, cafeterias, school hallways, sporting events, and so on) and attended school board meetings. I observed students in all of these settings (as I discuss below, my ability to talk directly to students was limited) and listened as they talked to one another about sexuality, school, and relationships.

In all of these states, I easily gained access to the CSE-teaching schools and districts in which I spent time, but in these same states, public schools and districts implementing AOUME would not grant me access. (I was, however, able to speak with private AOUME service providers.) In Florida, where the state received significant federal AOUME funding and was actively involved in creating an AOUME movement, I also had very limited access to schools and classrooms. A research associate was able to observe one AOUME lesson in one classroom, and I conducted interviews with a limited number of principals and teachers from four schools and students and parents from one district. In contrast, I had extensive access to public, state-funded AOUME events and curricula and to the private AOUME service providers funded by the state. This access helped me understand the state's role in shaping the political, social, economic, and legal milieus in which Florida public schools were making decisions about sex education.

Although I saw students in action and heard their voices through extensive observations in each state, my data are dominated by the voices of adult policy makers, classroom teachers, parents, community members, and sex education service providers and advocates. This was an effect of both the research design, which looks across multiple actors, settings, and institutional levels (and therefore never intended to focus only on students), and, more significantly, the constraints placed on the research by school districts and institutional review boards, who were not willing to let me speak directly to students under eighteen years of age about sexuality.[20]

In addition to the research conducted in each state, I conducted interviews with national AOUME policy makers and AOUME and CSE nongovernmental organizations involved in sex education advocacy. I talked with researchers who had recently studied sex education and conducted literature reviews. The analytic heart of the research, however, is the observation of schools and sex education classrooms and trainings that I conducted in the four states. (Additional information about these school, district, and state data collection activities may be found in appendix 2.) I coupled these observations with a review of the content of twenty well-known, popular, or widely disseminated CSE and AOUME formal curricula, including many of the AOUME curricula officially sanctioned by the state of Florida, to provide a general sense of how what I was seeing did or did not reflect discourses and activities common in nationally recognized and widely implemented AOUME and CSE programs.

Over the course of my research, I was able to travel back and forth among school and state settings, which provided an opportunity for me to reflect on how each setting's story related to the others' and to see how processes or practices I was observing in one setting were or were not playing out in others. I also attempted to engage the same actors and institutions across settings, if only briefly, to double-check my findings of which actors, institutions, ideas, and resources mattered to the stories about sex education arising in each school and community. The group with whom I was least able to do this triangulation was students: for the most part, it was luck that dictated whether I heard conversations about sexuality-related topics outside of classroom settings. When I overheard in one school, for example, that students were furious about the dress code, I could not instigate a conversation about this in the other schools. Certainly, then, not only the initial data collected, but also the analytic themes I developed by working across sites over time, were less rich than they would be if I had been able to talk to students freely.[21]

Situating Research Schools and Programs

My findings are contingent on and determined by my access to participants, but this condition is not new in ethnographic research. The openings and closures that I experienced are in fact an important part of the information

I have available for analysis. It is hard to see how comparative, multisited research on daily practices associated with controversial topics such as sex education could achieve uniformity, as the different ideologies, resources, and experiences of actors and institutions involved in these debates fundamentally transform researcher access. In this case, for example, the deeply held conviction on the part of many AOUME supporters that researchers were out to prove AOUME approaches "wrong" resulted in my lack of access to these programs, whereas CSE supporters' fundamental belief in the power of "scientific evidence" to inform their own practices and to prove CSE approaches "right" resulted in fuller access. Both because of this lack of ideological uniformity among research participants and because of my deliberate effort to capture diverse experiences related to sex education practices, this multilevel, multisite, comparative research approach—with a sample contingent on ideological barriers—was the only feasible research design. It was also a more powerful (and realistic) research tool than a top-down case study approach aimed at collecting the same type of information from the same actors across all sites. Not only would this not be possible for the reasons stated above but also what might appear to be a consistent, systematic research plan involving an equal number of AOUME and CSE sites in each state would actually be a highly biased sample, masking the selection bias in replacing twenty or thirty AOUME rejections with CSE programs that would agree to participate.

There is a danger, of course, that the ideological basis of access that shaped the research will result in an inequitable analytic treatment of sex education approaches. CSE programs come under much greater scrutiny than AOUME programs because of my greater access to CSE schools and classrooms. I cannot ignore the differences in the conclusions I can reach with these different data, but I have tried throughout the book to account for the ideological stances that underlie these differences and to clearly explicate their effects on pedagogical practices, curricular materials, official policy-making approaches, and community-school relations.

CLASSIFYING RESEARCH SETTINGS

The sex education programs I observed can be classified in many ways, including by official identification, level and type of privatization, level of school support for sex education, length of program, and so forth. For the purposes of situating the programs in the sex education debates, two classifications are useful: first, how the schools defined their programming; and second, where their official curricula fell on the ideological spectrum described in the introductory chapter. Using the first criterion, the following categorization emerges: Florida, AOUME; California, CSE; Wisconsin, CSE; Wyoming, CSE. Using the second criterion, the following categorization emerges:

AOUME ————— abstinence-based education ————— CSE
Florida   Wyoming   Wisconsin   California

I use this second categorization to order the state chapters in the book, but I distinguish the Wyoming, Wisconsin, and California approaches as "abstinence-based sex education" versus "CSE" only where significant differences existed between the approaches. Otherwise, the term "CSE" refers to Wyoming's, Wisconsin's, and California's programming.

PART ONE

Microanalyses of Sex Education

Florida's "It's Great to Wait" Campaign: The State as Manager, Marketer, and Moral Arbiter

Introduction

In 2004, Florida received the second-largest amount of federal Title V AOUME funding (second only to Texas). These funds require states to partially match them. Both during and after Governor Jeb Bush's administration (during which time I conducted my research), the Florida state legislature actually provided *more* than the required matching funds for AOUME. Additional funds were often taken from other federal programs designed to support families living in poverty (SIECUS 2009). The state thus prioritized AOUME as a key mechanism for educating youth about sex *and* for addressing the needs of marginalized families and children.

This chapter focuses on the state actors and institutions that built Florida's AOUME movement, and the federal and state resources upon which they drew. It examines the state's "It's Great to Wait" campaign, which aimed to reeducate people about sexuality; the private, "grassroots" AOUME movement that the state fostered and managed; and the private AOUME service providers who became the key implementers of the state's new pedagogy. Though the efficacy of AOUME funding in alleviating poverty or improving youth's sexual health is far from clear, I will argue that federal AOUME and Healthy Families funding to Florida was employed in a coordinated, state-led effort to grow, mobilize, and privatize an AOUME movement that will likely survive future funding ups and downs. The state's efforts to establish an AOUME movement had shifted the calculus that the school officials I spoke with used to judge the risks and benefits of providing one type of sex education over another, and thus state and national actors played key roles in determining what students learn and from whom they learn about sex.

This chapter is quite different in tone than the next three state chapters. In Florida, where policies and practices were heavily shaped by federal and state actors and schools were responding to top-down dictates, my analysis begins with the state and works "downward" to districts, schools, and communities. The narrative and flow of this chapter is therefore more directive and analytic, and less about relationships and the daily rhythm of schools, than the other state chapters. Just as I did, the reader may feel removed from the day-to-day of sex education classrooms, though I will argue that the state practices described deeply affected classroom policies and practices. In contrast, in Wyoming, Wisconsin, and California, policies and practices were more decentralized and locally rooted, and so my analysis begins with classroom and school practices and traces outward through school, district, state, and national policies, and flows of resources, ideas, and discourses.

This chapter is also broader in scope than the remaining state chapters because I use this space to accomplish two goals. First, in service to the book as a whole, I lay out the core components of AOUME's directive policy and pedagogical approaches so that readers can compare it to the CSE approaches described and analyzed over the coming three chapters.[1] Second, in service to my research in Florida in particular, I describe how, utilizing directive policy and pedagogical approaches, the state was attempting to transform the social, political, economic, and cultural arenas in which Florida sex education occurred and to create a new "common sense," in which AOUME was the default setting for sex education and sexual morality, and other options were viewed as potentially dangerous by schools, parents, and students.

Research with One Right Answer

Florida was the first state in which I conducted fieldwork for this project, and it was almost the last. I was an assistant professor at Florida State University while conducting the research, and through the university I had connections with researchers, school districts, and teachers in Florida. Nonetheless, I soon discovered that the schools and districts with whom I made contact were actively opposed to having a sex education researcher working in their schools.

At first I thought I was approaching schools inappropriately or explaining the research in a way that was setting off unnecessary alarms. But when I began contacting CSE districts and schools in other states, I did not encounter similar problems. After many months, I finally gained research approval from one school district in Florida, but then could not gain principal approval in any of the high schools that I approached—another issue that I did not face in any other state.

Direct research access to public schools was, in the time and with the resources I had, not possible in Florida. But private AOUME providers went into schools regularly, and I soon learned that through them, I could partially access public schools. Schools were willing to have me conduct research on sex education if I could minimize their risk by limiting my observations to the (privatized) formal sex education curriculum provided by an outside organization. This would have allowed me to operate without sending notifications of my research to parents (something an institutional review board (IRB) would allow if I was observing *only* the private service provider, not the teachers, students, classroom, or school).

The strong negative response to my requests for public access to classrooms and schools was indicative of a culture of silence and fear surrounding teen sexuality in AOUME schools. This culture was promulgated by wary school leaders and fed by state political and legal activism around sex education and high-stakes testing (required by the state and No Child Left Behind (NCLB)). It was also indicative of the central ideological tenets of AOUME: centralized control over messages, secrecy concerning sex and sexuality, and a belief that the movement is under attack and must be protected.

The AOUME and New Christian Right movements embrace the idea that they are under attack and that this attack is at least in part spearheaded by liberal university types, who promulgate scientistic approaches to evaluating (moral) programs like AOUME. For example, one principal participating in a 2004 Florida AOUME conference with me said that, in his district, schools were only accepting researchers who had been approved by known church leaders, so as to ensure that the research would be "fair." This would sound like anathema to researchers concerned about objectivity, but such concerns reflect CSE epistemic approaches to research. From AOUME advocates' perspective, because there is only one story about the effects of AOUME that can be viewed as morally correct, encouraging people to search out alternate stories through research is not only a waste of time, it is dangerous.

I did not choose to follow private AOUME providers into Florida schools. These providers were being trained in and were implementing (as my research associate's observation of a middle-school classroom demonstrated) directive AOUME approaches that they learned in state-sponsored AOUME workshops, and they were receiving hundreds of thousands of public tax dollars to provide AOUME services to public schools. Thus, the most important story about sex education in Florida schools that I felt I could tell was a story about the state's efforts to create and support an AOUME movement, replete with new advocates, educators, and institutions. I therefore focused my research on state-sponsored events for educators, parents, students, and advocates, and on talking to as many public school administrators as I could to understand if they perceived the state to be advocating for AOUME, and if they did, how they were responding to this advocacy.

Private, but state-funded and state-sponsored, actors and institutions were more than happy to be interviewed and have their activities observed— largely, it appeared, because they had no doubts about either political support for their work or the truth and goodness of their message. Public actors and institutions, in contrast, were full of doubts. Many public school actors with whom I spoke were unsure that AOUME programs could meet their students' needs, but they were fearful of AOUME activism, which they felt could significantly weaken their institutions financially and politically. Because both public and private actors and institutions appeared to be heavily influenced by state activities, my research needed to map and analyze the different positionings and roles of these actors, and to trace the lines of power and authority that silenced some actors and institutions and empowered others.

In order to do this, I attended two "It's Great to Wait" regional conferences on abstinence, beginner and advanced abstinence-educator training workshops, a teen rally, and a parent conference. I conducted interviews with personnel from three private sex education service providers that received AOUME funding from the state; public school actors that were served by these AOUME organizations; CSE service providers that did not receive state funds; school and district personnel in rural and urban areas; high school students, teachers, and parents from one urban Florida school in a historically conservative region of the state; and state-level personnel involved in AOUME activities. I collected and analyzed information and images from the "It's Great to Wait" media campaign (billboard messages, pamphlets, screenshots, and so on). And I attended a conference jointly funded by "It's Great to Wait" and President Bush's Strengthening Families Initiative, which provided additional insights into the social changes the state hoped to advance through AOUME.

Directive Teaching: Ideology as Pedagogy

AOUME approaches rest on a number of ideological assumptions about teaching, learning, and teens. These include that there is only one appropriate sexual state for teens—abstinence—and that "traditional" Judeo-Christian social hierarchies should shape church, family, school, and nation. Just as the father should direct the family and parents should direct children, so too the teacher should direct students through loving, but clear and firm, guidance.

TABLE 1. Sex education teaching models

Non-Directive	Directive
• Teacher's principle [sic] role is as Facilitator.	• Teacher is Director giving guidelines, standards, and reasons.
• Knowledge is aimed at awareness.	
• Knowledge is key—more information and awareness given to the student.	• Knowledge is aimed at prevention.
	• Knowledge alone is not enough—clear direction must be given.
• Sex education is taught without moral distinctions.	• A clear message is always given. No "neutral" position.
• Affective—emotions, opinions, feelings predominate.	
	• Effective—truth predominates.
• Public classrooms are not the appropriate place to give directions for expected behavior.	• The classroom may be the only place some teens are ever exposed to expected standards of behavior.
• Decision-making skills encourage young people to consider all options, enable and encourage youth to make "appropriate" decisions.	• Decision-making skills which lead young people to make good healthy decisions are taught.
• Over-emphasis on non-judgmental attitudes.	• Judgments of behavior, not persons.
• Contraceptives discussed with emphasis on use; failure rates downplayed. Little emotional distress discussed.	• Risks, diseases, emotional distress, and failure rates of contraceptives are discussed.
	• Most teens do abstain while many others respond to "Secondary Virginity" and start over again.
• Most teens will be sexually active, and the best that adults can hope for is that they will act "responsibly."	• Abstinence is presented as the goal.
• Abstinence is presented as a choice.	

Source: Table copied from the Teen-Aid website (http://www.teen-aid.org/), which states the following: "Please feel free to copy any of this document. It was produced with funds from Title XX through HHS [the Department of Health and Human Services] and by the gracious permission of Dr. Onalee McGraw at Educational Guidance Institute."

This pedagogical approach is described by Teen-Aid, a leading provider of AOUME programming, in table 1.

The directive pedagogical approach was evident throughout the state's "It's Great to Wait" activities, all of which promulgated one clear, top-down message: AOUME is the only approach to sex education that the state supports, and the AOUME message must be transmitted clearly and consistently by adults to students.

Building a Movement: The Rise of AOUME in Florida

While I was conducting research in Florida (in 2004 and 2005), Governor Jeb Bush was attempting to make the state a leader in a number of social initiatives advocated by President Bush's administration, including the Healthy Families Initiative, AOUME, and NCLB. In addition, a number of conservative social movements and organizations with roots in Florida were mobilizing legal and political support for Bush's "compassionate conservative" agenda. This led to an influx of resources for faith-based, socially conservative, and AOUME organizations in Florida. In contrast, traditionally CSE-oriented organizations, such as Planned Parenthood, struggled with shrinking budgets and increasing legal attacks.

With Governor Bush at the helm, state Department of Health personnel were, in their own words, trying to create an AOUME movement that "can't be stopped," regardless of future federal support or changes in the political climate. Their multifaceted efforts to create this movement were largely organized under their "It's Great to Wait" program.

"IT'S GREAT TO WAIT"

Florida's "It's Great to Wait" campaign (http://www.greattowait.com) was a multimedia effort to mobilize, train, and support a new generation of AOUM advocates, educators, and citizens, and to "brand" abstinence. The campaign's website states:

> Abstinence (Ab-sti-nence) is defined as a positive lifestyle for an adolescent that promotes self-control, character and a solid foundation for friendships and for committed love within the context of marriage. Abstinence is the commitment to not participate in sexual activity, which may include intercourse, genital contact, or other sexually arousing activities.[2]

At the time of this research, the "It's Great to Wait" program included the following:

- Statewide public awareness media campaigns, including teen and parent rallies, billboards, and distribution of "It's Great to Wait" paraphernalia
- Free abstinence-educator training programs, at the end of which each individual or organization was given a voucher for $250 to use toward the purchase of a state-approved AOUME curriculum
- State funding for public, private, and community-based organizations to provide AOUME to children ages nine to eighteen, parents, and community members
- Support for the formation of a network of AOUME advocates and service providers

The state claimed the following results from these efforts in 2007:

- More than 350,000 youth have participated in state-sponsored abstinence-only education classes and activities.
- A total of 22,247 parents have participated in health fairs, educational classes, and workshops since 2000.
- The state has created a mailing list of over 5,000 organizations and individuals to whom information about AOUME funding opportunities is provided.
- The Florida Abstinence Education Association (FAEA) was formed in 2002 to help community- and faith-based organizations and businesses collaborate and build their capacity to "enhance abstinence-only education in Florida." (Florida Department of Health 2007, 11)

The state estimated that by 2008 more than 350,000 young Floridians had received the "It's Great to Wait" message either directly from the state (for example, through a teen rally) or from one of its sponsored AOUME service providers (for example, through school-based sex education) (Florida Department of Health 2007).

Commenting on these efforts, one AOUME service provider involved in FAEA said, "We only need a few more years, and we won't need more [federal] government money. We'll have totally changed the [sex education providers] in Florida, and they'll be our kind of groups."[3] State personnel were increasingly able to rely on a state and national network of trained and funded AOUME speakers, materials, and organizations to support this effort, thus creating a positive feedback loop that sidelined CSE advocates and providers in terms of funding, policy making, and organizational legitimacy, and that placed additional pressure on schools to utilize state-sponsored AOUME materials and service providers.

In the following sections, I examine the different roles that the state played in fostering changes in the sex education arena. I begin by describing the state's efforts to educate and organize a new cadre of AOUM educators and activists.

Creating a State Market for AOUME

State actors with whom I spoke talked about sex education as a market. Instead of passing new laws or directly providing AOUME training or curricula to schools, the state adopted a marketizing managerialist role designed to increase public schools' demand for AOUME and the supply of private AOUM educators.[4] By increasing the supply of and demand for private AOUME providers and advocates, the state could transform schools' and students' behavior without major legislative changes.

On the supply side, the state subsidized the creation and growth of private AOUME service providers, curricula, and other products; trained a new cadre of AOUM educators; and created a network of AOUME advocates who could, as external lobbyists, pressure the state for resources and policies that would strengthen private AOUME organizations and their access to public schools.

The state also attempted to influence demand for AOUME. It adopted the federal A-H guidelines in its state monitoring, endorsed (and subsidized the purchase of) a range of national AOUME curricula for use in Florida schools, and supported political and legal efforts in Florida that would discourage schools from adopting CSE approaches.

Based on my interviews with school and district personnel, the state appeared to be successfully transforming schools' perceptions of the risks associated with not implementing a state-approved AOUME program. For example, an employee of a long-standing CSE service provider reported that she was having increasing trouble securing private funding to provide free CSE programming to schools, and there was, of course, no state funding for CSE programming. She reported that schools in which she had worked previously were now less willing to offer CSE programming:

> You know the state now has this list of approved curricula, and we don't use any of those because they're all abstinence-only. But because of all the litigation here, you know, schools want that safety, to know that the state has certified it [the curriculum]. Because then if parents come [to complain about the programming], they say, "This is state certified." I'm not saying they think these [AOUME] are better programs, I mean I've had teachers tell me they are so worried because they know their students need this [CSE], but it's too much risk.

Her comments point to the transformation of the sex education market across institutional levels. Even well-established CSE providers were being squeezed out of schools by new AOUME providers. In some cases, new AOUME providers were receiving state support to transition from tiny one-person operations into large institutions receiving hundreds of thousands of dollars for AOUME provision.[5] In more than a few cases, these were organizations with no previous experience in public schools and no background or expertise in public health, but they were rapidly gaining access to schools with their offer of free, state-approved sex education programming.

In Florida, the boundary between state and private AOUME funding, actors, and organizations was more blurred than in any other state in which I worked. Also, more than anywhere else, CSE providers reported feeling under attack by a well-funded and well-organized legal and media effort to discredit and legally inhibit their work. School officials commonly described themselves to me as caught in the middle of this battle and struggling to stay on task in addressing their core educational responsibilities—which did not include sex education. The easiest thing to do, in such a situation, was to go with the market flow and accept the free services of a state-endorsed AOUME group.

Transforming the Sex Education Service Provider Arena: The State as Gatekeeper and Funder

The state played an active role in training, equipping, and providing guidance to up-and-coming AOUME groups as part of its effort to expand the "supply side" of AOUME. The most visible of these efforts was the state's AOUME training series, which was free to all who wished to attend. The state offered beginning and advanced abstinence educator workshops; I attended both. At the end of each workshop, participants received a certificate of training and up to $250 toward the purchase of a state-approved AOUME curriculum.

"IT'S GREAT TO WAIT" BASIC ABSTINENCE EDUCATION TRAINING

The training for basic AOUM educators that I attended took place on a warm spring day in a large conference center in central Florida. We participants were a motley group of about thirty, of whom the majority were either church youth ministers or pregnancy crisis center employees; a smaller number were teachers or district school officials. The trainer was a vivacious national speaker who had been involved in AOUME for decades. He began by telling us:[6]

> I attended a [1992] abstinence summit. No one here was at that meeting. But abstinence education is becoming more acceptable; we're fighting harder now. It's a grassroots thing that's growing now, every day. If I ran to New York and tried to tell Jennings or Brokaw about this movement, they'd say, "Ah, it's just a few zealots." We're the underdog in this fight, we're the David. But you have a chance to make a real difference.

The speaker's comments highlight trademark AOUME themes, of supporters as underdogs, biases in the mainstream media, and the power of "grassroots" movements to reshape social morality.[7] The speaker also told us that we would learn the "paths of least resistance" to get into schools, where to look for federal AOUME funding, and how to be good AOUME instructors—in other words, how to help build and maintain a sustained AOUME movement.

We began the workshop by introducing ourselves and our goals in attending the workshop. One participant, an AOUME coordinator for a southern Florida school district, explained to the group, "I felt Jesus was moving me to do this work. It helps people lay up treasure in heaven." Her goal in attending the workshop, she said, was to spread the Word: "We can't say 'Jesus' or 'God,' but we're here to bring this message to all children." A health educator who had in the past conducted abstinence-plus sex education in Florida said that he wanted to collect more information about AOUME approaches. His organization was having an increasingly difficult time getting into schools, but he hoped that with an AOUME makeover and the state's imprimatur it would have more luck. A third attendee was a private AOUME service provider who conducted school-based trainings for about 10,000 children a year. She wanted to upgrade the information she used in her presentations and receive certification for having completed the state's training. I introduced myself as a professor at Florida State University who was trying to understand how and why schools made decisions about what forms of sex education to provide their students.

Our trainer began the session with an overview of the development of CSE ("nondirective") approaches. Such approaches, he said, had been developed based on the work of Alfred Kinsey, who "only studied the gall wasp but had a fetish with sexuality." He explained that "nondirective education presents a lot of ideas and concepts—intercourse, oral sex, anal sex, abstinence," noting that abstinence was one among many choices. He said that if a teacher mentioned abstinence, it had to be qualified with a "but," and "a child's belief is destroyed with that 'but.'" In contrast, the core belief of AOUME, which he referred to as the "directive" approach, is that oral, anal, and vaginal sex are not allowed before marriage. Beyond that, he said,

> Because media is full of sex, the focus [of sex education] has been on the physical aspect of teen sex. This is shallow. Condoms offer little, if any, protection for six of the eight major STDs, and there is no clinical proof of their effectiveness. In the dominant public health [field], the belief that condoms are protective is foundational. But in NIH studies, condoms are 85 percent effective against HIV. Using a condom is like getting on a plane of 100, where 15 seats will pop out. . . . And this is in theory! In actuality, humans make mistakes. Condoms are risk reduction. Abstinence is risk elimination. Condoms do not protect against four-fifths of the consequences of sex; they don't protect against the social, emotional, spiritual, or intellectual consequences at

all. . . . We don't help kids recognize the consequences, which are much worse for girls than for boys. . . . Tolerance and diversity are important, but so are our social norms.

In this speech, the presenter made a series of arguments that were common throughout the AOUME programs I attended and curricula I reviewed: first, that although the general public and the public health fields have been focused on the physical outcomes of teen sex, AOUME is concerned with a much broader array of outcomes. Second, even if only looking at the physical outcomes of sex, contraceptives regularly fail, and fail by official public-health (e.g., CDC) standards.[8] Third, issues of sexuality are issues of moral and social norms, not issues of individual health behaviors. Fourth, "tolerance and diversity" in addressing teen sex is impossible, because there is only one appropriate sexual ideology.

The speaker expanded on this ideology throughout the workshop. He explained how the AOUME definition of gender, family, and sex should be understood as, in his words, "traditional family values." He then emphasized that AOUME supporters needed to learn how to express the values underlying the AOUME approach in terms of "public health language" and the social concerns important to the general public and "the opposition." For example, biological differences between male and female susceptibility to STIs could be used to support AOUME's (moral) claim that women are weaker and need greater protection than men. Differential HIV and suicide rates between self-reporting gay and straight boys could be used to support AOUME's (moral) claim that homosexuality is destructive of individuals and society.

The speaker repeatedly emphasized the centrality of marriage and traditional gender norms in healthy sexual relationships. He described boys as near-animals with barely leashed sexual impulses that only girls could tame. Girls' abstinence saved boys from enslavement to their natures and gave girls what they needed from relationships: long-term commitment and deep emotional connections. Girls who had sex before marriage ceded power to men by "giving pieces of themselves away" through sex. In contrast, once married, when they "fully [gave] themselves" to their husbands, they gained the ultimate freedom of having a man to protect and care for them.[9]

The speaker then spent about an hour reviewing information about STIs—not including HIV because, he said, it is a relatively rare STI in the United States.[10] He emphasized repeatedly how much riskier—physically, emotionally, socially—sex is for women than for men. The handouts on HPV that we were given, for example, included the following information:

Since HPV is spread by skin-to-skin contact, and condoms do not cover the entire genital area, condoms are likely to be less effective in reducing the risk of HPV transmission than with other sexually transmitted infections. A few studies have shown that condoms may partially reduce transmission in men, but their effectiveness has not been demonstrated for women.

This, according to the CDC, is simply incorrect;[11] condom use has been associated with the clearance of HPV infection in women and regression of lesions among men. The reduction of transmission from female to male or male to female has to do with whether the infected area is covered or not, not the sex of the person involved. A consistent declaration of the higher risk for women, however, laid the groundwork for arguments about expectations for women's behavior and social roles that are central to AOUME models of traditional family values.[12]

The speaker closed the conference with two points that refocused the workshop on translating AOUME's central message into pedagogical action. The first was that teens, especially girls, are looking for clarity and guidance, and that abstinence provides a directive, clear, easy message for kids to follow to protect their bodies, hearts, souls, emotions, and reputations. The directive pedagogical approach to addressing teen sexuality is central to achieving the goals of AOUME.[13] It aligns with AOUME's ideological assumptions about appropriate ("traditional") family and social hierarchies (e.g., Bartlowski and Xu 2000; Wilcox 1998), and it protects children from morally incorrect messages and the confusion they cause.

Second, the speaker said that the "other side" is trying to draw AOUME supporters off message by saying that AOUME is only religious education. The speaker emphasized that it was our responsibility to stay on message when talking in public about AOUME: "This is about health. There's no answer that detractors can give when we say abstinence is always 100 percent effective. Nothing else is." The speaker thus cautioned us to be aware that our public explanations of AOUME needed to emphasize its health, not its moral, benefits, despite the fact that most participants were advocates of AOUME because of the moral ideology it embodies.

"IT'S GREAT TO WAIT": ADVANCED ABSTINENCE-EDUCATION TRAINING

The advanced abstinence-education training, also run by a national AOUME speaker, covered many of the same themes as the basic AOUME training. It emphasized the gender-inequitable consequences of premarital sexual activity for girls and the negative influence of the media and corporations that "market sex" to youth. The presentation also included an extensive "medical update" section, which provided new data on STI rates around the country, and led the presenter to comment "how unfair STDs are; women get it [*sic*] much worse than men."

The advanced training also included new themes, for example, that immoral and uncaring adults (single mothers, absent parents) cause negative sexual behavior in and outcomes for teens:

> Teens are not feeling love. They have single-parent homes—or two parents, but the parents are working all the time. They look for intimacy and fall for sex, look for love and fall for lust. But there is no love without respect. All boys are mistreating girls, 'cause there's no love. . . . Teen sex is a correlation, not a causation, of depression. Sex outside of the right and proper context has no foundation, no basis, so then it increases depression. We overlook these symptoms and say they don't exist, but this is real. There are emotional consequences to sex.

He then listed the consequences of sex before marriage—worry, guilt, depression, girls "6X" more likely to attempt suicide, boys "5X" more likely to use alcohol and drugs—and gave three examples of how boys are affected by premarital sex and pregnancy. All three involved the boys physically assaulting others, including, in one case, a boy beating his newborn to death.

The presentation ended with a mentoring session for participants on how to apply for federal and state funding for AOUME programming. The presenter reviewed the A-H guidelines, and then one of the state representatives attending the training said,

> Abstinence as a movement and as a message is about to turn a corner. I will share this database—our names, affiliations, and addresses—with you so that you can all network. Make your message prominent and positive. Develop a relationship with local media people, get to know your legislators, spend time with your community leaders. Stick to the health issue. This is not about religion. That's why the DOH [pointing to the state Department of Health representative] advocates this message. Don't argue ethics, and pay careful attention to medical accuracy so that you are not drawn into an argument.

The message was clear: in order to succeed, AOUME advocates needed to adopt a public health rationale in their pubic discussions about AOUME. Though this rationale captures very little of what AOUME supporters believe or are attempting to achieve through AOUME, the presenter and state representatives argued that it provides the best platform from which to launch AOUME programs in public settings and with public funding.

Fostering "Grassroots" AOUME Advocacy: The State as Convener and Manager

While the state was transforming the supply of and demand for AOUME providers, it was also attempting to transform the networks among AOUME providers and advocates and to foster the growth of an advocacy organization that could draw on private funding and lobbying strengthen state support for AOUME in the future. To achieve these goals, the state played a key role in helping to organize a "grassroots" AOUME advocacy group—the "grassroots" partly belied by its government backers and connections to national AOUME organizations. The Florida Abstinence Education Association (FAEA), named in 2002, is described by the Florida Department of Health (2007) as

> a collaborative group made up of over 100 non-funded and state-funded community-based and faith-based organizations, businesses and other entities supportive of abstinence-only education. The organization, which meets on a quarterly basis, was formed to share information, build capacity, network and to explore other funding opportunities among its membership to enhance abstinence-only education in Florida.

FAEA's leadership, along with many of its members, are involved in local, state, and national abstinence-only movements and organizations. FAEA has advocated for continued state funding for AOUME, shared federally and state-funded AOUME curricula and other resources among members, and created a network to identify AOUME opportunities and advocate for legal changes to sex education.

By providing support for the group during its infancy, the state aimed to create a locally sustained advocacy movement that could lobby the legislature for continued involvement in AOUME. Through the FAEA, private sector partners with strong ties to national organizations could support up-and-coming AOUME service providers and advocacy organizations in the state, socializing them into the AOUME movement. Over time, smaller organizations could converge into a more powerful vehicle that could share resources, present a united lobbying front, and create a pressure group for AOUME in Florida schools and communities. AOUME service providers and advocacy organizations would also benefit from strong ties to the business community, which could provide additional lobbying power and resources to fund AOUME activities.

By most measures, the state succeeded in its goal to transform the advocacy networks around sex education. The FAEA became an active organization with solid ties to national abstinence organizations (for example, a previous president of the FAEA was elected president of the International Abstinence Organization). It had over one hundred members, from small community organizations run entirely on a voluntary basis to large organizations that received federal and state funding and provided sex education in multiple counties in Florida, that were well networked and in contact with one another. A recent SIECUS report (2009) found that AOUME resources are often shared throughout the state and that AOUME organizations often partner to increase their reach throughout the state. At least some of this activity is likely due to the contacts and networks fostered by the FAEA.

Similarly, my own research and the SIECUS report indicate that during the time of state involvement in organizing the FAEA, more schools started drawing on federally and state-sponsored curricula and programs in their sex education programming, and more schools began adopting an AOUME approach. In interviews, school administrators said that they were concerned that AOUME activists, such as some of the members of FAEA, would cause trouble for them if they were not implementing state-approved AOUME programs.

Marketing Virginity: The State as Moral Arbiter and Salesclerk

The state took its AOUME message directly to the public through an "It's Great to Wait" mass media campaign. This campaign offers perhaps the clearest indication of the market-based approach underlying the state's AOUME activities. Its direct marketing campaign to teens and parents conceptualized teens as consumers of ideas, trends, and peer influences, and adopted social marketing techniques to reach its audience.

As opposed to viewing teens as rational consumers and providing them with "complete and correct" information to inform their own decisions (the "nondirective" CSE model), the directive social marketing approach of "It's Great to Wait" focused on norming abstinence as cool, desirable, and an unquestionable good whose alternatives were unthinkably bad for teens. Teens (particularly girls) were conceptualized as emotional consumers in need of firm guidance and clear messaging, which were provided by producing and distributing a dizzying array of branded "G2W" ("Great to Wait") goods at teen and parent rallies; bringing in TV and radio personalities and local musicians to provide personal testimonies of the power of abstinence; putting up billboards and buying radio, TV, and movie advertisements; creating and hosting an interactive website; and hosting statewide teen and parent rallies.

The state worked in partnership with Group 5, an advertising firm, on the campaign. Of its work for "It's Great to Wait," Group 5 said,

> Group 5 developed a two-phase statewide advertising and public relations campaign in English and Spanish. Phase I targeted teenagers via television, radio and cinema ads and directed them to GreatToWait.com to "get the facts" about teen sexual behavior. Phase II targeted parents, educators and influencers via direct mail, community forums and outreach to encourage them to bring their teens to one of a series of motivational rallies across the state.
>
> Creative was developed, tested and redeveloped to ensure it perfectly resonated with the target audiences. The teen-targeted, "I Wish I Would Have Waited," featured teenagers sharing personal stories of their sex consequences. The adult-targeted, "Scary, Baby," shared facts about Florida's teen pregnancy and STD transmission rates . . .
>
> Results: The website received over 1.4 million visits during the campaign window. More than 4000 teens and adults attended the seven statewide abstinence rallies, reaching maximum capacity in each city. The television commercials won an American Advertising Federation ADDY Award and the Florida Public Relations Association Golden Image Award as the year's best public service announcement.[14]

This consumer model constructs teens and parents as target audiences whose responsiveness to messages (Go to this website! Go to this rally!) becomes the central and most appropriate measure of consumer-driven change. The intervention is the message; the outcome is people hearing it. Below, I describe the messages transmitted through one of the "It's Great to Wait" teen rallies.

REACHING YOUTH: RALLYING FOR ABSTINENCE

The "It's Great to Wait" teen rallies, designed to market abstinence to teens and "convince them that virginity's not a dirty word," contained a mix of popular consumer and evangelical messages, including many that were also evident in the AOUM educator conferences. The rallies, however, focused more on personal decision-making and morality and less on social relations (e.g., parent responsibilities, unequal gender roles). They also emphasized redemptive second chances, something seldom mentioned in the educator workshops.

I went to a teen rally in spring 2005, after attending the earlier parent education workshop. When I arrived, hordes of young teens were entering the rally venue. As they entered, they received free G2W items, including plastic wristbands, Frisbees, water bottles, car window shades, and pens, all packaged in G2W tote bags. Inside the rally room, music with abstinence-friendly messages blared as teens mingled and waited for the performance to start. The lineup for the rally included a locally popular rap group, an ex–reality television competitor, and a national beauty pageant winner, as well as a number of interactive games and exercises for participants.

Many of the rally events included individuals telling their personal stories of redemption following premarital sexual intercourse. These narratives drew heavily on Christian evangelical forms of storytelling and included calls to those who had strayed to return to traditional social values (through, for example, secondary virginity), and powerful warnings to those who had not yet lost their virginity about the dangers of premarital sex. The stories pronounced marriage to be the ultimate state of fulfillment for all people and enthusiastically described the joys of sex in marriage. For example, the former reality-TV presenter talked about his descent into drug and alcohol abuse. He vividly detailed the parties he attended, the sex and drugs in which he engaged at the parties, and the health problems he developed as a result. Because the story was personal, he also talked openly about finding Jesus Christ and becoming born-again. He described the personal and professional transformations that had occurred after his rebirth and concluded,

> I'm married now, to the most beautiful woman in the world. But one of the hardest moments in my life [he chokes up] was when I asked her to marry me. I had to look her in the eyes and beg her forgiveness. Because I wasn't strong enough, I didn't love her enough and believe enough to wait for her. I wasn't pure. I begged her forgiveness, and she forgave me. That's the power. And there is nothing better, there is nothing out there that comes even close to sex when you have pledged your life to each other. Everything before that, it didn't mean anything.

Continuing the theme of the redemptive power of abstinence and the benefits of waiting to have sex until marriage, another presenter urged,

> There's a lot of things that you can do [to support yourself in abstaining]. When you go on vacation with your family, you can keep a journal to your future spouse. Tell them how you are feeling and how much you want to meet them. You can buy a present that reminds you of the vacation that you are taking so that you can show it to your spouse, so they know you were thinking about them. You can make a scrapbook that you can go through together. I

bought presents for my future wife when I traveled. By the time we got married, I had twelve presents, one for each month of our first year of marriage, to give to her. She knew that I hadn't met her yet but I was thinking about her.

The personal narrative provided presenters, many of whom were AOUM educators because of their religious beliefs, an otherwise unavailable opportunity to present religious information they felt was critical to students. As one AOUME presenter who regularly spoke in public schools said, "We can't talk about religion in public schools, but if you ask someone to tell their story and their story is about the power of Jesus Christ [as] savior, that's their personal story." The personal narratives appeared to hold a great deal of rhetorical power for students, building as they did on current cultural references and a reality TV–like format.[15]

These narratives offered perhaps the clearest elucidation of the state's marketing of the concept of abstinence as "waiting," and the idea of "waiting" as safe, healthy, spiritually and emotionally powerful, and pleasurable. In the rallies, teens were urged to wait for the "right one," for marriage, for the opportunity to fulfill their social, spiritual, physical, and emotional selves within the context of a traditional family arrangement. The consequences of not waiting were presented as horrific for individual teens, their families, and potentially their future spouses and children. In exchange for shallow and fleeting physical fulfillment, they would live a life of regrets, fear, disease, social derision, depression, and unwanted pregnancy. Sex outside of marriage was presented as devoid of pleasure, passion, or fulfillment in any sense of the word, whereas the presenters discussed the passion with which they dreamed about their future spouses and future lives, the pleasure they took in preparing themselves to meet this person and in planning for the life they would lead together, and the personal and sexual fulfillment (physical, emotional, spiritual) gained through marriage.

A DISCOURSE OF DELAYED DESIRE

There was, to borrow Fine's (1988) phrase, a "discourse of desire" in the "It's Great to Wait" programming that was almost entirely missing from CSE classrooms that I observed. This discourse was certainly not "thick"—as Fine and McClelland (2006) note, it strips responsibility for teen health and sexual outcomes from the state and re-places it on individual teen girls, and it fails to address the socially, economically, and politically inequitable policies that influence individuals' sexual health—but it did provide a narrative about a desired and protected future (in a loving and safe marriage, not in a protective and productive social space), and a future full of (spousal) desire, for those who behaved "morally." There was no parallel discussion about desire or pleasure in the CSE programs I observed. Educators often said that sex was natural and should be pleasurable, but then quickly moved on to discuss the dangers of teen sex.

The "It's Great to Wait" campaign's discourse of future desire was, of course, limited and limiting. The heteronormative focus on marriage in all the teen rally stories promised perfect sex as a reward for abstaining until marriage. LGBTQ students in Florida can never have a sexual future within this framework. It also silences the experiences of teens who do not want to get married or for whom potential partners might be systematically limited by structural inequities (for example, teens living in communities with very high male incarceration rates); the voices of teens for whom sex outside of marriage has been fulfilling and pleasurable; the myriad voices of adults— particularly young adults—for whom marriage has not been a safe or sexually fulfilling experience; and the voices of those whose sexual experiences were marked by coercion or force, and for whom "choice" was not an aspect of their sexual decision-making. Lastly, though many of the narratives called on both boys and girls to abstain, the stories told about the effects of sex before marriage were highly gendered, and they reproduced assumptions of gender inequity that stifle women's sexual subjectivity (Tolman, Hirschman, and Impett 2005).

Repositioning Sex Education: The State as Categorizer and Social Activist

Most states link sex education to adolescent reproductive health services or to educational issues such as school-based bullying. These links maintain sex education's connection to the health and education sectors, and to social services targeting children and teens. In Florida, however, the state linked AOUME to federal discourses about and funding for strengthening the nuclear family. This reflects AOUME supporters' conceptualization of sex education as primarily a moral issue with public health implications: Florida teens' sexuality shifted, in practice, from a current health issue to a future social issue. Indeed, the very name "It's Great to Wait" signals a similar intent.

In Florida, AOUME was coupled with President Bush's "Healthy Marriage" initiative, which, like the AOUME funding, began as part of a welfare reform act.[16] The Healthy Marriage Initiative aimed to provide educational services to support stable, male/female married and parenting couples, and to "increase public awareness about the value of healthy marriages."[17] Of its seven pilot marriage-support projects, three were in Florida. Florida used

Healthy Marriage, AOUME, and Temporary Aid for Needy Families and Ma-
ternal and Child Health Block Grant funds[18] to attempt to normalize abstinence until heterosexual marriage, and parenting only within marriage, as
part of their programming for needy families. Below, I briefly describe one
of the state-organized Healthy Marriages/AOUME conferences I attended to
begin exploring this shift of sex education from a teen public-health issue to
a multigenerational morality issue.

THE HEALTHY FAMILIES, PARENTING,
AND ABSTINENCE CONFERENCE

The Florida Department of Health, in partnership with (among others) the
governor's Faith-Based and Community Initiative, the Department of Children and Families, and the Department of Juvenile Justice, utilized federal
and state AOUME and Strengthening Families funding to hold a series of
large-scale public events, including the Healthy Families, Parenting, and
Abstinence conference. From the opening speaker, the conference framed
teen sexuality and sex education in terms of sexually conservative morality,
implied that responsibility for providing teens with AOUME lay with families and communities, as opposed to schools, and explicated a vision for improving the nation's spiritual and social health founded on abstinent teens
and two-parent married couples raising children. The conference's opening
address, "Sex Has a Price Tag," was presented by a woman whose biography
included the following:

> In 1964, a fifteen-year-old girl was raped, became pregnant, and decided to
> carry her unborn child to term. Five months after the baby girl was born, in
> an act of courage and love the young mother provided her child a better envi-
> ronment by giving her to an adoptive family. That child was Pam. . . . Pam is
> a dynamic, charismatic and educated expert on Sex, Love and Relationships.
> She understands the perils that young people face as they make adult choices,
> and is dedicated to reviving the character and integrity of today's youth.

Pam is a nationally acclaimed AOUME and pro-life speaker. A woman
of seemingly bottomless energy, possessed of a radiant smile and engaging
presentational style, she bounded on stage and was met with hearty applause.
Pam's presentation began with a discussion about what she described as a
general decline in American culture: sexually active single mothers, high divorce rates, and a socially detrimental media culture. She said that, despite
these factors, youth were beginning to rebuild a more positive culture of abstinence, but that they needed adult help to do it. She urged parents to ask

themselves and their children, "What is [sexual] safety? The piece of latex or the partner?" Pam explained that AOUME programs "tell the students the reality . . . the failure rates [of contraceptive methods]," whereas CSE programs confuse students by talking about "safer" sex with contraception and neglecting to discuss the emotional, social, psychological, and spiritual consequences of sex before marriage.

In this speech, Pam utilized a directive lecture approach to present AOUME's message about teen sex: just don't do it. "It's abstinence until marriage, not until you're ready, or until you're in love. . . . No thirteen-year-old girl can make that decision. Abstinence is not complicated. If you're not married, don't do it. If you are married, go for it." Teens need to hear the same simple message from all of the adults in their lives in order to avoid potential confusion, according to Pam: "I want my kids to hear [my values] in school. If I don't talk to my kids, whatever they hear in school is what they get . . . and they need the same message from everyone." In response to the common argument that teens have sex even if they are consistently encouraged to be abstinent, and therefore need information on how to have sex safely, she replied,

> We don't decide policy based on whether or not people will do it, we make the right policy and then work toward compliance. . . . Kids lack character decisions — that's why they have sex. But sex is more than a physical act, it's also emotional. We are accused of being fear-based; that blows my mind. It's personal, it's relational. Our number-one fear is still pregnancy. I'm shocked. [Pregnancy] doesn't kill you, but diseases these days will. And the number-one indicator of poverty is single-parent households and the age of a girl when she becomes pregnant.

Here, Pam clearly explicates the directive approach to *policy making* that drives the state's AOUME approach: "make the right policy and then work toward compliance." She also clearly indicates that AOUME is a policy aimed at a improving teen morality, by giving kids the "strength of character" they need to avoid sex.

Pam's full speech pointed to a number of themes that arose throughout the AOUME events and curricula I reviewed:

- A focus on girls as the primary agents in improving or destroying men, families, and society
- A focus on STIs as the most significant negative physical outcome of teen sex
- AOUME is primarily moral education; it is fundamentally about training children to return to "traditional family values."
- AOUME is risk *elimination*; everything else is only risk *reduction*. As such,

AOUME is not only morally superior to CSE, it is also the only reasonable public-health response to teen sex.

- The outcomes of sex before marriage are not only, or even most importantly, physical. Psychological, emotional, spiritual, and social outcomes are not regularly measured by sex education evaluations but are extremely important.
- The media is a bad influence and misrepresents the AOUME movement.
- AOUME supporters are the underdogs.

Following Pam's talk, which received thunderous applause, I attended a presentation called "Hispanic Parenting," one of a number of the conference's ethnically themed breakout sessions about family relations. The audience for the talk was made up largely of Latina and African-American women. The self-identified Hispanic speaker[19] began by outlining the goal of the talk: "to acquire knowledge on [sic] the Hispanic culture to enhance parent and child communication on traditional family values." The talk aimed to explain how "traditional Hispanic culture" was largely aligned with "traditional" Judeo-Christian gender and family norms, but that Hispanics were "struggling" when and because their cultural practices were not yet fully aligned with these norms.

The speaker began by making sweeping generalizations about genders and ethnicities, many of which were met with nods of agreement by the audience. She said that Hispanics in the United States tend to have smaller family networks, but "high family loyalty. Family is core to our identity. Hispanics place family's needs before their own and stress interdependence versus individualism. Some people say separation between kids and families never happens for Hispanics." For Hispanic women, she said, this means that "motherhood is highly revered," and that "a woman's role as a mother is more important and valued than her role as a spouse." At the same time, Hispanics "are authority-oriented people . . . Males have a higher status." She described the multiple roles that Hispanic women were expected to play in the home and the issues they faced because they received little help from men or extended families.

She contrasted Hispanic families with "Asian" families, which, she said, "come over in family units and are kept together by family businesses," a tendency she approvingly attributed to Asians being "very traditionalistic." She then compared Hispanics and "African Americans." The comparison was chosen, she said, because the two groups usually have the worst family, health, and economic indicators in the United States. She concluded that Hispanics are in a better position than African Americans to overcome these problems because their families (and by extension their values) tend to be "intact." She argued that by maintaining the traditional family unit, which African Americans had not done but Asians had, Hispanics could overcome the economic and social struggles they faced.

This presentation introduced many of the AOUME conceptualizations of family and society that arose throughout the state-sponsored activities I attended:

- The family is the primary unit of society.
- There is only one right way for a family to be constituted: the male head, his wife, and their children.
- Males and females are inherently different, as are their roles in the family and in society.
- When families don't follow this model, children suffer.
- Women are or should be subservient to men.
- Parents need to control and discipline children.
- Individuals, families, and "cultures" are responsible for the situations in which they find themselves. Traditional family and community structures breed success and happiness for all.
- Sex outside of marriage (and thus all sex between people of the same sex) is physically, emotionally, psychologically, spiritually, and socially damaging.

The importance of abstinence outside of heterosexual marriage was emphasized in every conference presentation I attended. It was what parents needed to be teaching their children, children needed to be learning in school, and unmarried teens and adults needed to be practicing. It was a multigenerational approach to modeling appropriate values in an immoral society. But this state-sponsored vision of a moral society allowed for only one model of family and one form of sex education. Other models and practices—from CSE to single-parent families, to families with two parents of the same sex, to divorced women having sex outside of marriage—were cast out as morally corrupt. Through its denouncement of these other models and its consistent norming of conservative sexual values, the state of Florida attempted to serve as the arbiter of sexual morality through its AOUME and Healthy Families activities.

WHO'S IN AND WHO'S OUT? INCLUSION,
REPRESENTATION, AND THE ONE RIGHT WAY

In all of the Florida events I attended and conversations with AOUME personnel that I had, and in most of the state's AOUME materials, there was a concerted effort to include participants of multiple ethnic, linguistic, and racial backgrounds (particularly African Americans and Latin@s); the AOUME movement provided more opportunities for nonwhite youth and adult voices to serve in positions of leadership and public speaking than any of the CSE programs that I observed. The diversity of AOUME representatives did not mean that there were diverse ways of understanding teens, families, or society's problems, however; there was no space to question the official narrative, and the official narrative reflected and reified a particular social order: one in which heterosexual, married, middle-class whites are at the top, and poor, single, African American women are at the bottom, as we saw in the presentation above. There was no opportunity to explore or acknowledge the raced, classed, and gendered assumptions and hierarchies underlying this official narrative and indeed, AOUME approaches are predicated on the belief that the model is universal.

The state of Florida directed resources to support needy families away from social and economic programming and toward AOUME and Healthy Families initiatives. As Fine and McClelland (2006) and Geronimus and Thompson (2004) point out, what may be most important about this shift is the work the AOUME and the Healthy Family programs do to sever the consequential connections between personal desires, individual outcomes, and neoliberal and neoconservative social policies (for example, NCLB, legal changes to the juvenile justice system, restrictions to teens' access to legal abortion, and so forth), so as to recast "needy families" (and particularly single African American and Latina mothers) as problems and moral failures.

School Options Redefined

Just as the state reframed what kinds of families would be celebrated in Florida, it also reframed what schools felt they could present to students. Before the advent of large-scale federal and state AOUME funding in Florida, there were few sex education service providers who could provide free sex education programming to public schools. These providers generally had a long history of reproductive-health services and sex education provision (though sex education was rarely their primary programming focus), presented themselves as abstinence-based or abstinence-plus education service providers, and were clustered in urban areas. Most school officials with whom I spoke said that in the 1990s, they had either had their own teachers provide the 0.5-credit high school sex education programming required at that time by the state, or invited in one of these private abstinence-plus service providers.

With increasingly tight school budgets, growing legal threats to public schools, and new federal funding for AOUME, options for schools were changing. By 2005, thirty-three groups in Florida were receiving Title V and CBAE funds, and many were using the funds to provide free AOUME programming to schools. There was a concomitant explosion in new AOUME organizations and curricular and program materials around the country, many of which were funded with federal dollars. During my research, schools were opening their doors to this wide range of new state-sponsored AOUME curricula and service providers. The rationale offered by the school officials with whom I spoke was multifaceted, but commonly included the perceived importance of having school curricula or sex education providers that were approved by the state. From the school's perspective, this meant that neither irate parents nor the state could blame the school for the content of their sex education programming.

These were not idle concerns. At the same time that new funding and training resources systemized state support for AOUME approaches, AOUME supporters in Florida and around the country successfully won a number of high-profile legal cases brought against schools and teachers who taught CSE. For example, in one widely publicized case, a teacher was dismissed for showing students how to put a condom on a banana.[20] These court cases were part of a wider effort supported by various neoliberal and neoconservative groups and policies to use courts and legislatures to challenge teachers' status as professionals with the right to some measure of academic free speech, and to challenge the institutions (such as unions) that have historically fought for teachers' rights to academic freedom.[21]

Concomitantly, many public schools were facing harsh sanctions under NCLB, along with threats from state privatization efforts (through, for example, vouchers). As more schools faced sanctions because of NCLB's accountability system (which was based in part on Florida's pioneering high-stakes "A+" system, but which labeled many more schools as failing),[22] there was growing pressure on schools to increase resources for reading, writing, and math. This meant that many schools were offering the bare minimum of sex education required by law. Not only was sex education a low priority for many school officials (and has been for many schools for a long time [e.g., Emihovich and Herrington 1997]), and particularly officials in "failing" schools, it was high risk, because it posed the danger of setting off community agitation around the topic. Thus, schools already facing scrutiny because of NCLB were the least able to take on the additional burden of fighting for more or different sex education than what the state was sanctioning. As Fine and McClelland (2006) note, schools serving the students most in need of effective sex education were therefore those least able to access it, because of the broader structures of inequity in which their schools and communities operated.

PRIVATIZING RISK

Most school personnel with whom I spoke during my research indicated that they were, as one principal said, "taking our cues from the state" when it came to sex education programming, both to avoid conflict and liability, and to minimize the costs to the school. By adopting a hands-off managerial role, schools shifted responsibility and accountability onto state-sanctioned service providers and off of teachers and administrators.[23] Of course, many school administrators favored AOUME approaches for their students because they thought they would be most effective; the movement toward AOUME was not simply a bureaucratic calculus. The language used by administrators in interviews to explain their decisions, however, seldom focused on program goals or outcomes; instead, it addressed the political and economic pressures that administrators felt they must balance. For example, I was informed by the district superintendent for a poor, largely black school district with one of the highest teenage pregnancy and adult HIV rates in the state that his school had recently cut all physical education, arts, recess, and after-school activities for children who were not scoring high enough on the FCAT (Florida's high-stakes high school exam). Did he think his students need sex education? Yes. Were they going to get it? Not until their test scores indicated that they were making enough progress on reading and writing. Until then, he did not feel that the school could spend any resources—time, attention, personnel, funding, or political capital—on the topic.

Conclusion

The state of Florida played an active and multifaceted role in seeding, funding, and institutionalizing an AOUME movement throughout the state. The state organized an AOUME network, trained and funded AOUME organizations, and marketed AOUME to teens and adults—all within a broader activist judicial and educational environment. The state's activities appeared to be encouraging districts, schools, and teachers to privatize sex education and adopt state-sponsored AOUME programs in part to protect themselves from AOUME activism.

The state-directed educator workshops and teen and parent rallies highlighted a number of the themes central to the AOUME movement: directive policy and pedagogical approaches, the centrality of traditional gender and family norms to AOUME ideology, the role played by individual redemptive narratives in shifting responsibility for the outcomes and consequences of teen sexuality onto individuals (particularly girls) and off of the state or systems of broader structural inequity, and the need to cloak the religious and moral bases of AOUME in a public health discourse.

The size and strength of the AOUME movement in states like Florida should be understood both in terms of the clarity and comfort of the message itself—if you abide by this set of moral regulations, you will be safe and happy—and in terms of the movement's openness to a diverse range of people who believe in the power of the message. In Florida, actors at the national, state, and community level coordinated themselves and their actions through a deliberately organized and well-aligned social-pedagogical movement, resourced at various levels and supported by an expanding AOUME product market. There was no parallel CSE movement in the states that I observed.

In the next chapter, we travel inside classrooms in Wyoming and examine how community-school relations and curricular decisions made in a decentralized policy environment affected the sex education approach adopted by a school and its teachers. While the school board adopted a scripted curriculum to try to control the content of the sex education class, the three teachers that I observed created entirely different educational experiences for their students. One adopted a directive approach and presented an informal AOUME curriculum; the other two used the official CSE curriculum, but in different ways silenced their own and students' voices to avoid potential confrontation with community members. The story of locally negotiated sex education in Wyoming thus stands in sharp contrast to the top-down story of sex education in Florida.

4

"It's a Local Thing": Sex Education as Compromise and Choice in Wyoming

Live and Let Live

Granite, Wyoming, is a small town that serves as a gateway to many of Wyoming's natural treasures.[1] With a mix of socially conservative, liberal, and libertarian community members, the town prides itself on letting everyone live as they want, as long as they don't step on others' toes. Granite's residents told me repeatedly that because the town is small and rural, its residents were more interconnected than people in larger towns. As one resident described it, "You can't wall yourself out because you depend on each other. There are issues you can't talk about [with everyone], but that's fine. People try to convert each other [to different political and social positions], but we eventually reach compromise."

I found in my interviews and observations that people with opposing political and social views were often good friends. This differed from the cities where I conducted research, in which people tended to mostly know and socialize with others who held similar political views. The desire to remain on good terms with one's neighbors was central to understanding Granite's and its high school's approach to sex education.[2]

TETON HIGH

I spent part of the 2005–06 school year at Teton High, one of Granite's two high schools. Of all the schools in which I worked, Teton High was the smallest, most rural, most integrated into the community, and best resourced. The school provided its seven hundred students with a wide array of resources, including well-stocked workshops and classes on auto mechanics, woodworking, pottery, glass blowing, visual arts, family-life education, and sports, as well as a school nurse and guidance counselors.

The school served two populations: about 80 percent of the school was white, and about 20 percent was Native American; many of the Native American students traveled to the school from a nearby reservation. Though there were friendships and social relationships among whites and Native Americans, in important ways, students often had very different in- and out-of-school experiences. For example, the school's graduation rate was almost 74 percent in 2003, but when broken down by group, it was 78 percent for whites and 53 percent for Native Americans. Overall, about 70 percent of the school population scored at or above state-determined proficiency levels in English, reading, and math, and about 20 percent of students received free or reduced-cost lunches.

While at Teton High, I conducted classroom and school observations; took part in various school activities; conducted interviews with students, teachers, school administrators, parents, and district officials; and participated in daily life in Granite. Through these activities, I soon learned that a battle over sex education had occurred in Granite well before I arrived and before national debates about sex education took center stage. The battle had been resolved in an eminently Granite-ite way: through a compromise that emphasized individual parental choice and each individual's right to not be constrained by others' beliefs. Unless this compromise was broken, most adults felt there was not much more to say about sex education.

Sex Education in Granite

Sex education became a hot-button issue in Granite in the 1980s. As in schools around the country, Teton's school board was troubled by national and local pregnancy and sexually transmitted infection trends, and decided to incorporate a sex education class into the high school. The school's Physical Education (PE) department was tasked with developing and teaching the class. The school's senior PE instructor, Mr. Lauder, asked Ms. Jeffries, a recently hired PE teacher, to develop and pilot the class. Ms. Jeffries said the program she developed was aligned with the school board's broadly comprehensive mandate and was based on a critical-thinking and decision-making model for students. She designed the course to be largely driven by students' own questions, which would be solicited through their active participation in class. She used various curricular materials from around the country to inform her work, most of it mailed to her by national organizations like the Centers for Disease Control (CDC) and Planned Parenthood. Mr. Lauder described the resulting curriculum as "not just about facts, it was about self-esteem." He approved its use, and Ms. Jeffries piloted it the next semester.

As part of the curriculum, Ms. Jeffries looked to the community for experts to address questions she felt she could not fully answer. She had a lawyer come in to discuss paternity issues (mostly as a scare tactic for boys, she said), asked the school nurse to discuss date rape, and invited in a health professional to provide information about HIV/AIDS. The health professional, as part of her presentation, put a condom on a banana.

The day after the condom demonstration, Ms. Jeffries and Mr. Lauder were called before the school board and threatened with dismissal. A group of parents, quickly organized and led by one of the town's pastors and his wife, had filed complaints overnight about the sex education curriculum, in particular the condom demonstration, and accused the teachers of attempting to corrupt students.

The group, led by the pastor, called for AOUME to be adopted as the only acceptable approach to sex education. Not long afterward, a group of other parents and community members organized a counterattack to resist the imposition of AOUME. Many of those involved in the second group held a libertarian view of the issue. They did not necessarily support CSE, but they viewed the efforts of the social conservatives led by the pastor as being at odds with Wyoming's political and cultural ethos of "live and let live." As one parent described it,

> You find ways to work things out, find an understanding that balances people's rights . . . Especially on this topic, you know, the [politically conservative] ranching community sees sex so differently; it's just natural, what's the big deal? So they were not on board [with the abstinence-only group].

Because the school board controlled decisions about sex education in Granite, it was evident that the sex education battle would be determined by the outcome of school board elections that were soon to take place. Both sides engaged various media, including church bulletins, newspaper editorials, and conversations with neighbors to try to sway people's votes. Both sides also used information from outside sources to claim their stance was "scientific" and externally validated. Those supporting an alternative to AOUME collected information from organizations such as the CDC; those supporting AOUME collected information from New Christian Right organizations like James Dobson's Focus on the Family and Phyllis Schlafly's Concerned Women of America.

In the end, the group organizing against the AOUME proponents won control of the school board. They demanded that the sex education curriculum be examined by the community and recommendations be made for a compromise position. They eventually approved a national abstinence-based sex education (hereafter ABSE) curriculum that did not include condom demonstrations, restricted information about contraception, homosexuality, and abortion to one "pull-out" section of the curriculum, and provided extensive teacher scripting. They then created a menu of sex education choices from which parents could choose. The new school board asked the minister who had led the fight against the teachers to offer an in-school AOUME program to any child whose parents preferred that option. Parents could also opt their children out of the "pull-out" (comprehensive) section of the curriculum but keep them in the rest of the mainstream ABSE class. If parents did nothing, their child was included in all classroom activities. Ms. Jeffries and Mr. Lauder remained tasked with teaching the revised class. For some years, they were instructed to tape-record all class sessions so that any further parental complaints could be reviewed in light of the exact teacher utterances and classroom discussions that led to the complaints.

School board members and teachers active at that time reported that 90 to 95 percent of the students remained in the ABSE classroom for all activities. The other 5 to 10 percent either met with the pastor or were pulled from the school entirely to attend a newly created Christian private school. The PE teachers were not dismissed, but they did have disciplinary warnings placed in their folders and suffered brutal personal attacks on their characters throughout the process.

Church leaders taught an AOUME program at the school for a number of years, but when the minister who led the original charge moved away, no one stepped forward to take his place. The three-track choice system for parents remained in place, but now parents had to individually prepare an alternate curriculum for their child if they did not want the child to attend any of the ABSE class (as before, parents could also opt their child out of the "comprehensive" section of the ABSE curriculum). At the time of my research, the teachers reported that no parent had chosen the option of creating an alternate curriculum. The number of parents opting their child out of the "pull-out" part of the curriculum had increased significantly, however, from 5 to 10 percent in the 1990s to 20 to 25 percent during my observations in 2005–06.

In the interviews I conducted with school officials, teachers, parents, and local leaders about Teton High's historic sex education battles, three themes kept recurring. First, the key issues for the AOUME parent group had been condoms (and, to a lesser extent, other contraceptive methods) and any discussion of sexual orientation. The school board responded to these concerns by walling off these subjects so that they were only discussed at a particular controlled and monitored moment in the formal curriculum.

Second, the attacks made against the teachers and those who supported

ABSE were described by onlookers and participants as "vicious," "brutal," and "highly personal." This type of ad hominem attack was not leveled against those supporting AOUME.

Third, the diverse cross section of community and school board members that organized to fight against the push for AOUME did not strongly support CSE or the PE teachers. Rather, they organized against the perceived imposition of one set of values over others. As one parent described it, "For a lot of us, it wasn't sexuality, it was about control and personal rights. We have the same arguments over grizzlies."

These three themes—"hot topics" related to nonprocreative sex, a much more coordinated and moralistic attack made by AOUME supporters than by CSE supporters, and the particular vulnerability of teachers in such battles—are common to many places in which battles over sex education have been waged. Granite's response to these issues was also not uncommon: adopting a sex education policy and an ABSE curriculum that, at least in theory, structured classroom activities, controlled teacher talk, and increased external oversight of and threat of disciplinary action against teachers' sex education practices. As we will see below, this response had a significant effect on students' and teachers' sex education experiences at Teton High, even decades after the initial battle.

THE COMPROMISE CURRICULUM

Like a growing number of nationally distributed health-education curricula in which sex education is one module, Wyoming's sex education curriculum was designed to allow schools to purchase and use one set of materials to teach both AOUME- and ABSE-based modules. All material viewed as potentially inflammatory from an AOUME perspective is organized into the "pull-out" section of the larger sex education curriculum and offered, in Teton High's case, on two days of the two-week module. This kind of curriculum represents a mainstream abstinence-based or abstinence-plus model: the "based" or "plus" is literally an additional section that can be added or subtracted from what is otherwise an abstinence-only curriculum. The topics, language, values, and activities presented in the balance of the curriculum are therefore considered appropriate for an abstinence-only classroom.

When I asked the district curriculum official to describe the current sex education curriculum and the process by which it had been selected, he cited the process described above. When I then asked him whether he thought there would be a change to the curriculum anytime soon, he responded,

The system is pretty stable now, given the current school board. No one would push to shove the curriculum off this balance point and no one in the community could amass enough direct political pressure to do this. . . . The classic triggers [that might force a battle over sex education] would be putting a condom on a banana, talking about LGBTQ behavior or that implied endorsement [of LGBTQ identities]. . . . abstinence-only [issues] would not draw too much fire—those people [who support CSE] don't get too emotionally cranked up.

His response reflects the perception expressed by most people I interviewed that the only potential threats to the status quo would arise from the curriculum being perceived as "too comprehensive." *Can curriculum be too comprehensive?*

The principal of Teton High, who had come to the school after the sex education battle, believed that the current curriculum kept conflict to a minimum because "70 percent of the sexuality education class is determined by the shared curriculum, while teachers are able to choose the other 30 percent."

The sense shared by the principal and the district coordinator that the current sex education curriculum maintained the status quo and that the status quo was good was widely shared by the administrators and parents with whom I spoke. As we will see below, the teachers reported that they felt this message from the community and the administration clearly. They silenced their own concerns about addressing their students' needs, their students' questions, and their own voices in order to assure that the type of confrontation that had occurred previously did not occur again. Their main task in the sex education classroom, in other words, was to meet the expectations of the adults in the school community by not causing new controversy or conflict.

TEACHER RESPONSES TO SEX EDUCATION AT TETON HIGH

During my observations, three PE teachers, including Ms. Jeffries and Mr. Lauder, were responsible for providing health and sex education at Teton. The third teacher, Mr. Dean, was new to the school. When I conducted research at Teton High, sex education was a part of health education, a required class for all 10th grade students.

Ms. Jeffries and Mr. Lauder spoke openly and at length to me about how much their experience during the battles continued to shape their sex education teaching practices at Teton High. Unlike parents and administrators, who generally expressed satisfaction with the compromise curriculum, Ms. Jeffries and Mr. Lauder were much more conflicted about its effects on students' sex education experiences. Ms. Jeffries said,

deprofessionalized
teachers
panoptic
system

> After the uproar, the original comprehensive curriculum was changed; [the new curriculum] spelled out day by day what could be said. . . . It's interesting teaching sex education at [the high school], but it's like walking on eggshells. We had to tape-record the classes for a while. If something came up, we would refer students to the school nurse or guidance counselor. . . . Generally, we like to pass the buck [she smiles]. They don't pay me enough for these decisions. . . .

In this quote, Ms. Jeffries reflects on the general culture of fear concerning open discussion about sex and sexuality created by the sex education battles and the policing of teachers that occurred after it. She also mentions a trend I will describe in greater detail below: an effort to move discussion of sex and sexuality out of the classroom and into private spaces (for example, a meeting with the school nurse or guidance counselor). She later spoke of how these consequences affected her sense of herself as a teacher:

> I had a feeling that, as a professional, I should do facts-based work. But this changes whenever people don't believe in what they are teaching, because they avoid issues to make life easier. This includes closing off questions. I wanted uncanned stuff . . . some guidelines for kids with license to choose. For instance, there is a very high incidence here of drug and alcohol use. To me, the tie-in with teen pregnancy is so evident. How can you talk about addiction in health and not talk about sexuality? You have to be able to tie these things in, let them talk about it in their lives. We can't.

For Ms. Jeffries, the sex education battles continued to structure the social relations governing policy decisions, curricular selection, and classroom practices. She said that though the time immediately following the battles had been personally painful and professionally difficult, the incident had also created new, very positive, spaces for community participation in the school. She longed for an equally participatory space in her classroom, but felt that the democratic process that had occurred at the school-board level had actually closed off such opportunity for her and her students. Open student participation and discussion had become dangerous, and adult efforts to control it were stifling her ability to teach to her students' actual needs.

Mr. Lauder added another dimension to Ms. Jeffries's concerns about limiting student participation in sex education classes when he reflected on pressures arising from national and state reforms to increase time spent on individualized assessment at the expense of students learning from each other:

> It's much easier to get a canned curriculum by the school board and parents. They know that teachers can inject their own biases, not just in the discussions about sex, but also about drugs and alcohol, and all of these are really touchy

subjects for parents. Before, when we used to have more discussion and there were no health standards, we used to have things more stretched out. We spent three to four days on communication skills, for example, and we had every kid do a personal interview where kids asked each other questions. This meant that they got to know each other. We talked a lot about their goals and plans for the future. . . . Now, there is no time for this at all. The [health] classes are much more impersonal. . . . We have all of the time in the world for assessments, but no time for discussions, role-playing, questions, all of that.

The teachers' remarks reflected their belief that opportunities for open discussion and interpretation of sex education material, such as those built in to the original curriculum, provided the richest learning moments for students. These learning experiences had to be given up, however, because of the potential dangers to them and the school in veering away from a "canned" approach. Moreover, state and national movement toward standards-based education meant teachers were under increased pressure to restrict the time spent on health education at all, and to stick closely to formal curricular materials aligned with state standards in all of their classes. These pressures further limited opportunities to hear from students and to engage them in critical analyses. Though disappointed by these changes, both teachers made it clear that their current approach was an effort to be responsive to parental and community demands—something they both deeply valued. And it was in response to these demands that they stopped trying to create a classroom environment in which students could speak with one another about their questions and needs—the kind of environment they both felt was essential to honest communication about sex and sexuality. They did not curtail these activities because they felt they were adopting a better curricular or pedagogical approach for their students; they curtailed them to be responsive to the community and to state standards.

Mr. Dean, unlike Ms. Jeffries and Mr. Lauder, was not at Teton during the sex education battles and had never received pre-service or in-service training on sex education. He expressed profound discomfort with teaching sex education. According to Mr. Dean, high school students needed to hear one clear message: just say no to sex. He was not comfortable, he said, answering students' questions about sex in or out of class—however, unlike Ms. Jeffries and Mr. Lauder, he felt no pressure to do so. He expressed no concern about community or student response to his teaching style, no concerns with teaching what he felt was important instead of following the curriculum (on which his students were tested), and appeared much less familiar with the official curriculum than the other two teachers.

Despite the imposition of a curriculum designed to control teacher talk

and pedagogical approach, the three teachers' ideological stances toward sex
education, coupled with their previous experiences teaching sex education
at Teton High, significantly impacted how they applied the official curriculum and made sense of their responsibilities to parents, students, and the
school. As a result, an "official" sex education policy and curriculum meant
to be implemented similarly across all classrooms was in practice reshaped
by teacher ideologies and experiences and teacher-student interactions.
The CSE-supportive teachers were silenced, while the AOUME-supportive
teacher was not. Student voices were constrained or silenced across all of the
classrooms, but were more silenced the more aligned teachers' ideologies
were with AOUME approaches.

Official Sex Education Practices at Teton High

In order to better understand the roles that various factors such as individual
teachers, social norms, school policies, and perceived community demands
played in shaping students' sex education experiences, I attended one of the
sex education modules offered by each of the three PE teachers during the
2005–06 school year. I also attended another course offered at the school,
because it provided an alternate model of sexuality education: the Family and
Child Health (FCH) course, an elective taken by a smaller group of students,
mostly girls.

Teton High's official health curriculum calls for twelve hours of class time
to be spent on sex education. In Ms. Jeffries's and Mr. Lauder's classes, all
twelve hours of instruction were delivered. In Mr. Dean's class, this amount
was cut to less than half. This disparity offers some initial sense of how attempts at standardization (in this case, by the school board and the textbook
publisher) are always and everywhere transformed by the "street-level bureaucrats" (Lipsky 1980) who use them. The significant differences in teacher-
student interactions in each classroom, caused in part by the teachers' quite
different pedagogical ideologies, also contributed to the differentiation in sex
education practices evident in the vignettes below.

MS. JEFFRIES'S CLASS: NAVIGATING
DANGEROUS TERRITORIES

Ms. Jeffries was the sole female health-education teacher at Teton High. I
observed her first-period health-education class, which had seven students
in it. It was, she said, the smallest health-education class she had ever taught

and had a "really different feel because of the size. We have conversations that I would never allow in larger classes, because we are small enough that we can listen to each other and respect each other's opinions." This comment points again to her sense (shared by Mr. Lauder) that conversation among students is central to good sex education, but also potentially dangerous without time and teacher involvement to assure the classroom is a safe space for such conversation.

[handwritten margin note: what makes it a safe space? For who? Decided by who?]

The students were a diverse and lively group of four boys and three girls. From a local minister's son to a recent transplant from the West Coast, the students and their political, social, and economic backgrounds appeared to span the range of Granite residents. The students did not appear to be friends outside of class, but within the classroom, they developed relationships marked by humor, gentleness, and a sense of camaraderie that I did not see in any other sex education class that I observed. All seven students participated actively in the class, teased one another gently, and were comfortable enough with each other to talk about their own lives. Ms. Jeffries seldom engaged directly in their conversations about their social relations, but she did sometimes use these conversations as a springboard from which to pose questions to the group.

Over the course of the module, Ms. Jeffries's class viewed and discussed all the curricular materials approved by the school board, including the videos (which contained material not presented in the textbook). Most of each class period was structured around the formal curricular materials, which deliberately limited class time for in-depth discussion. Unlike in the other classes, however, students regularly talked about sex and sexuality, including "hot topics" such as abortion and homosexuality, while engaging with the formal materials. Ms. Jeffries neither persuaded nor dissuaded students from having these conversations, but when they began to debate a topic, she often tried to open up a larger class discussion about it:

MS. JEFFRIES (J): OK, question 7: What is a miscarriage?
MEGAN: (reading from the book) It's when the uterus contracts and expels the lining when a woman is pregnant.
J: Yes, that is called a spontaneous abortion. What other kind is there?
FEMALE STUDENT (I can't see who says it): An induced abortion is the intentional killing of a child in a medical setting.
JEAN: I would say unborn child.
MEGAN: It's still a child, but I think it's a personal decision.
JEAN: Why aren't we allowed to talk about this in school?
JOSH: Because it's so controversial.

MEGAN: Isn't it controversial right now because of that judge [referring to a local court case]?

A lively conversation begins among the class members about responsibility and abortion (for example, if different moral issues are at play if the girl was raped), illegal-abortion deaths, and girls committing suicide because they're pregnant.

JEAN: I don't think people understand it's none of their business; no one knows why a decision is made.

J: And the big question is, when does an embryo become a human? I can't give you an answer—I know what I believe, but it's up to each person to decide what they believe.

In conversations on "hot topics," Ms. Jeffries generally took on the role of moderator, restating what students said and asking additional students for their opinions. She never expressed her opinion on any of these topics, often pointedly telling students that her personal views were unimportant. Although she asked students to be respectful of one another's views, she almost never commented directly on students' opinions. She explained to me that she adopted this approach out of concern that direct comments about her opinion could cause trouble with administrators or parents. The result of her silence, however, was that students regularly expressed views that would usually be considered anathema to CSE approaches. For example, in a class in which two of the seven students had been sent to the library because their guardians had opted them out of the section on contraception, Ms. Jeffries asked the students to review the correct steps to using a condom.

Josh laughs and says he likes this kind of question; Frank replies that boys are just hornier than girls and "that's why 90 percent of rape is male on female." Ms. Jeffries enters the conversation by asking, "Do you think that changes how it feels?" Frank shrugs, but the boys continue talking about rape and how it would take a female bodybuilder to pin them and rape them. Ms. Jeffries asks, "What if it were a man?" The two boys erupt in protest, and Josh yells out, "Man, it's not prison!" Frank laughs and says, "I like to get bit, I like it rough. But from a lady!" Ms. Jeffries looks at me, then turns back to the students and steers the conversation back toward condom usage.

Ms. Jeffries succeeded in creating a space for students to speak openly and comfortably with each other in class, but because of concerns about community response and about making students feel safe and comfortable speaking, Ms. Jeffries did not patrol this space. In practice, this allowed students to make almost any statement imaginable, no matter how xenophobic,

homophobic, sexist, or racist, without challenge from the person in a position of authority over class discussion. The unexamined consequences—the
hidden curriculum—of this approach to monitoring classroom discussion
and engaging students was to validate students' right to verbalize questions,
comments, and concerns related to sex and sexuality, including misconceptions and biases, without fear of negative teacher response. By removing her
own voice and refusing to "pass judgment" on the students, Ms. Jeffries created a space for student participation that was missing entirely in the other
two classrooms at Teton, but this space did not engage students in a critical
analysis of classroom discussion or their own perspectives.[3]

In the paragraph below, I describe Ms. Jeffries's January 2 sex education
class. She was absent that day, so the description provides a good sense of
the students' comfort with each other and engagement with the curricular
material, but not a good sense of Ms. Jeffries's usual skillful management.[4]
Descriptions of the other two teachers' January 2 classes are included below
for a comparison of the classroom environments and progress through the
curriculum on the same date.

> January 2, 2006. First period: Class starts with the national anthem. Josh and
> Luke refuse to sing it, saying they have the right not to do so. Janet (the substi-
> tute teacher) passes out the AIDS study guide. The students begin discussing
> vaccines and whether any medications have worked against the virus. By 8:22,
> Josh is asking Pete what AIDS is; Pete's answer is generally correct. Then con-
> versations begin diverting from the class topic. At one point Lexie says loudly,
> "Yeah, 'cause I have AIDS!" "Ew, that's gross," says Megan. The boys are talk-
> ing about hitting deer while driving. The girls start discussing braces. Tom and
> Luke are trying to answer the question "What do you call a person with HIV?";
> both get it wrong. Tom then asks the class, all of whom are talking about
> Christmas break and the gifts they received: "What is latency? Somebody?"
> Josh answers, "It's when you ejaculate after you pre-ejaculate." Tom: "What?"
> Josh: "I'm just making stuff up." Lexie finds "latency" in the book and reads
> aloud: "Stage where the virus is present but not active." The students write it
> down and return to their conversation about Christmas presents . . . The boys
> start talking about a local man, about forty, who works at McDonald's. They
> are denigrating his work, saying he is "nothing." Lexie exclaims, "Why are you
> so mean?" Josh responds, "I don't know, I need therapy." They all begin to dis-
> cuss therapy, which leads to a discussion about *The Passion of the Christ.* Lexie
> says she does not believe in God; Megan is shocked, and they begin discussing
> the existence of God with Tom (a minister's son) . . .
>
> Megan tells Lexie that her boyfriend bought her a Quarter Pounder with-
> out onions the other day without her even asking. Lexie asks if they are getting

along well; Megan says yes, repeating again and again, "I can't believe I'm dating him!" Some of the boys listen in on this conversation, while Josh and Luke talk about McDonald's. Josh: "Have you been over to the house of the new people in McDonald's?" Luke: "No." Josh: "You should; they're cool." Luke: "I don't like 'em." Josh: "Why?" Luke: "'Cause they're foreign!" Tom: "'Cause they're foreign!" Luke: "Yeah!" The boys begin talking about the guys who work at McDonald's (one is Peruvian, another Brazilian) and denigrating how they "always speak in foreign languages." They make a joke about Mexicans driving badly because they are trying to play "Grand Theft Auto." Josh, who is a Latino newly transplanted from the South, leads this conversation. They then talk about a friend of Lexie's who spent the week tweaking (cocaine) and how dumb they think it is. Lexie then looks down at her study guide and asks the class, "What's the best way to avoid HIV/AIDS?" There is a chorus of "Abstinence" . . .

Ms. Jeffries's classroom evidently fostered an environment in which students were comfortable talking with each other about their relationships and their peers' behaviors. It was also a site in which students used homophobic, xenophobic, and sexist language. Such statements were consistently treated by adults in the school as "joking," neither to be taken seriously in terms of the school climate nor to be incorporated into the formal curriculum. Students were not challenged to examine their own views on these topics, nor to systematically consider the social, cultural, economic, and political inequities that shaped and were reproduced by their statements. In the classroom, this meant that student voice was simply that—students could give voice to their ideas, but were seldom asked to critically analyze either their own comments or the curricular materials. When they were asked to do so—as when Ms. Jeffries asked the boys, "What if it were a man?"—conversations were usually short and consisted of students restating their own opinions. The broader consequences of almost all sex education instructors I observed not critically engaging students' comments or beliefs are addressed in the book's concluding chapter.

The next day, Luke, who had been sent by his parents to live with his aunt in Granite, learned that his aunt had opted him out of the "pull-out" section of the curriculum:

January 3, first period: Ms. Jeffries begins the class with a quiz. Luke is sent out of the class to work on the AOUM section of the curriculum. Luke is very upset, saying that his aunt is retarded, he has already covered these materials in his previous school, and his mother always lets him hear this kind of information. Ms. Jeffries replies, "Yeah, I know, but this is what we have to do." Josh is riling up Luke, telling him that he can't learn about "sexual intercourse." Ms. Jeffries tells Josh that he is being inappropriate, and he quiets down. Josh then turns to Luke and says, kindly, "Don't worry, I'll give you the lowdown after class." They smile at each other, and Luke walks out.

In this encounter, Ms. Jeffries restated the power of parents and community members to determine student involvement in the sex education classroom, and, by having the opted-out students leave the classroom, she maximized opportunities for the rest of the students to engage in conversation about the "pull-out" comprehensive materials. She was the only teacher who had the opted-out students leave the room so such engagement with the curricular materials could occur. Luke and Josh's conversation also points to the centrality of student-student interactions around sex and sexuality; the formal sex education classroom is only one of many settings, and certainly not the most important or readily available one, in which students talk to each other about these issues.

MR. LAUDER'S CLASS: AN UNSPOKEN AGREEMENT

The two other classes I observed were larger than Ms. Jeffries's class (more than twenty-five students each). These classes included Native American students (Ms. Jeffries's did not) and provided almost no opportunities for content-related student participation or questions. Whereas Ms. Jeffries' class sometimes felt like a barely contained but often quite invigorating free-for-all, in Mr. Lauder's class, it felt like a silent agreement had been struck: he would not embarrass the students by making them talk about sex, and they would not embarrass him by asking questions about it.

Mr. Lauder was a very popular PE coach who enjoyed good rapport with many of the students, particularly those involved in sports. He made it clear throughout the sex education module that he didn't want to be teaching this any more than (he assumed) the students wanted to be hearing it from him. Though Mr. Lauder completed the entire sex education unit, class discussions were often about other topics (particularly sports), and a number of students wore earphones throughout the class. In most of the class periods I observed, more time was spent on administrative details than talking about sex or reviewing the curricular materials. When on-topic, students were usually working individually on worksheets or taking quizzes. January 2 was a typical mix of individual work and limited conversation about administrative details:

Second period. (17 students present at the start of class.)

MR. LAUDER (L): Get your books out, give me one minute, and we'll take
care of everything that we need to know for the rest of the semester.
Wednesday we will meet in the auditorium from 8:10 to 9:40 to deal
with STDs and contraception. Then on the 5th, [the school nurse] will
be in here going over the AIDS presentation. She goes around to post-
ers that she puts up all over the room. You probably won't have any
questions when she's done.

JOE [in a falsely bright tone]: Sounds like fun.

L: Then the test is on Friday. On the 9th, you can work on assessment 9.
The tenth is a review. Then we have our exam days. Assessments 1
through 9 must be in for you to get credit for this class. [Assessments]
19, 20, 21, 22, 29, and 30 are the chapters that will be tested on Friday.
All of your assessments must be in on Friday. And if anyone misses the
assessment on Friday, you don't get the easy test, you get the hard test
that Ms. Jeffries made.

He then asks who has the papers that he passed out on Friday. Most
students do not have them, so he begins passing them out again. One girl
says loudly, "I hate school." There is no response. Mr. Lauder goes to get the
AOUM materials for the students who were opted out of the general curriculum and tells everyone to stay in the room and work alone on section 19 of
their workbooks. There is almost no interaction among the students during
this time.

Frank asks Mr. Lauder why he has a different book than others. Mr. Lauder
shows him the form that his parents signed saying he should have the AOUM
curriculum. Frank looks confused, then tells Mr. Lauder, "It's really OK, I
can do the regular book, it doesn't make a difference to me." Mr. Lauder tells
him it is his parents' choice, not his. Frank starts to protest. Mr. Lauder cuts
him off:

L: Look, the six of you [who were opted out], your parents said you can't
cover the same things that the rest are covering today. What is not being discussed, but only covered in the reading for the rest of the class,
is birth control, definitions for sexual orientation, definitions of some
stereotypes, abortion, sexual abuse, date rape, and rape. OK?

As long as they can opt out of the relevant bits

[Unlike Ms. Jeffries, Mr. Lauder does not have the opted-out students
leave the classroom. This means the rest of the class cannot openly discuss
these topics even if they want to. Mr. Lauder does not discuss either set of
materials out loud.]

Students begin working silently on their study sheets; it's 9:40. Three of
them have iPods in and on. By 9:55, two girls are done, and a third (who never
received a handout from Mr. Lauder and did not ask for one) is playing soli-
taire on her iPod. By 10:00, about 80 percent of the students appear off task;
some are chatting quietly with their neighbors, some are resting their heads

on their desks, some are doing homework for other classes. With the exception of Joe's and Frank's comments, there has been no student discussion in the class.

Mr. Lauder was a dedicated and well-respected teacher at the school, and in the interviews I conducted with him, he expressed support for sex education. Nonetheless, and although he talked about the influence of his pre-service CSE training on his approach to sex education, he said he was not comfortable answering students' questions because of the battle that had occurred in Granite. Like Ms. Jeffries, Mr. Lauder felt the changes to sex education that had occurred over the years had made it harder to connect with students. In Mr. Lauder's case, he no longer appeared to try to foster the kind of classroom he said he felt students needed, because he felt the restrictions the curriculum placed on them made it impossible to do so. It did not let teachers hear students' voices or needs or address misconceptions. He said that he felt confident that most students were able to access the information that they needed about sex and sexuality anyway, from family, friends, media sources, and individual staff like the school nurse. Thus, he did not feel that that the limits placed on sex education at Teton High had tremendous negative effects for students; they simply rendered the sex education module useless. Still, he covered all of the official curricular materials, including the videos, in class before the final exam.

His concerns, as well as his discomfort with the class, were evident. When students asked questions or made comments that could lead to conversations about sex, Mr. Lauder largely ignored them. For example, during one class, as Mr. Lauder was passing out worksheets on contraception (or abstinence for the opt-out students), one of the students, Julia, said to him, "Abstinence is the only kind of birth control, Mr. L." Another student, Annie, responded, "No, it's just the only kind they teach in school." Mr. Lauder responded to neither comment, and continued to pass out the worksheets. In another session, Mr. Lauder asked a student to drop a question she was raising about the morality of premarital sex, saying to the class that he did not feel comfortable discussing the issue with them.

[handwritten margin note: silencing student and teacher voice]

While Ms. Jeffries addressed her concerns about community response by fostering student conversation but rarely inserting her own voice into the classroom,[5] Mr. Lauder controlled class discussion and discouraged students from talking about sex. Students' voices, when heard, generally probed administrative details, such as the timing of tests. During the entire sex education module, I never once heard a Native American student, and only a small percentage of the white students, speak. In this sense, Mr. Lauder's classroom most closely mirrored the school board's goal of regulating the materials presented and the conversations held through the official curriculum: students came in (silent) contact with all official curricula materials and did not hear Mr. Lauder's or each others' opinions about any of it. Mr. Lauder's students were learning important "hidden curricular" messages, however, concerning the apparent danger of speaking openly about sex and sexuality at school, and teachers' discomfort engaging with them on the subject. These were lessons that the students with whom I spoke felt permeated their experiences at Teton High.

MR. DEAN'S CLASS: UP CLOSE AND PERSONAL WITH AOUME

Mr. Dean, the oldest in years but the most recently hired PE teacher, was the only one of the three teachers with no formal sex education training. Hired to coach some of the boys' sports teams back to state prominence, he had not taught sex education as part of any of his previous coaching assignments. Mr. Dean was the most visibly uncomfortable of the three when teaching the sex education materials, and he spoke openly about this discomfort in interviews. He began the sex education module almost a week later than his colleagues; his class (which usually consisted of about twenty-four students) did not cover most of the curricular material and did not watch any of the videos; and in those classes where he did cover sex education topics, he provided no opportunity for students to ask questions or make comments.

Unlike the other two teachers, who very deliberately removed their opinions from the classroom space, Mr. Dean often told stories from his personal life, made normative comments about sexuality and family, and openly expressed his opinions on matters related to sexuality; it was evident throughout his speeches that he was strongly supportive of an AOUME approach to sex education. Although all three teachers were mandated to teach the same ABSE curriculum and although all students took the same test based on this curriculum, Mr. Dean presented only part of the official curriculum to his students. He expressed no discomfort with doing so and no concerns about community responses to his teaching, which included the open use of religious terms and language, avoidance of official curricular materials, traditional gender norming, and an obfuscation of facts related to sex and sexuality. These are all hallmarks of a more conservative sexual ideology than that formally approved by Teton High's school board, and they were all on clear display during Mr. Dean's January 2 lesson. This was the start of the second week of the sex education module, at which point his class was about five days behind in the curriculum:

Third period.

> MR. DEAN (D): OK, we have five chapters to cover this week on sexual education. On Wednesday, you have [a local health care provider] presenting on STDs and contraception. All of the assessments are due by Friday. If you have to go past that, it's OK, but I'm giving you a due date. Remember, Coach Dean is nicer than the other teachers—I didn't make you turn them in, but let them pile up. OK, how many people don't have assessments? [He passes them out.] OK, turn to page 435. We're going to go through this a little faster. . . . Hopefully, you've all taken a shower and know if you're male or female. I don't know if it's the good Lord that created these bodies or who, and we're not getting into that here, but these bodies . . . we laugh, love, hug, play basketball, go on vacation, and so forth as a family unit. We all reproduce. We go through stages in life and get to the point where we're old and mature enough to reproduce, to make babies . . .
>
> Chapter 19 talks about the reproductive system. The male's reproduction system is the simplest. The male produces the sperm from testicles from the chemistry of the body. We can get so complicated about how this happens. But we're not getting into that. Then the sperm is injected into the vagina, and it all meshes. The male system is very simple, as it should be. Males are not very smart, and we only have one goal. If the timing is right, you get the start of the greatest thing in the world: the fetus, the baby. The male has the easiest time of reproductive life. We inject semen into the female and we're done. Kind of like salmon, where the males die after injecting semen. We're lucky we don't die, too! [Giggles from the class.] Page 437 shows a picture of the penis, testicles, and all of the stuff that leads to erection and depositing semen in the female. [I am embarrassed, as are most of the kids, by their looks, as is Mr. Dean.] Then things are back to normal and we go on with our lives . . .

In this monologue, Mr. Dean presents traditional gender norms, obfuscates biological facts related to reproduction, and mentions God in his discussion of human sexuality. Later, he again clearly expresses core AOUME values, including the sexual danger of almost any male-female contact, even conversation; the failure of contraceptive devices to lessen sexual risk; and abstinence as the only appropriate adolescent sexual behavior:

> D [talking about the senses and sex]: If you see a gal dressed in tight clothes and we have our value system and have control of ourselves, but what

if we varied a bit on our ability to refuse that sense [sight]? Eventually, the consequences can be drastic, even of conversation. It's like a ladder, climbed one rung at a time, it's a progression. That's the way life and sexuality is. If we allow our senses to progress in the wrong direction, we would never get ourselves back on track . . .

If you know there's a bad situation, don't put yourself in there. Avoidance, refusal skills, we can't say it enough. When we talk about sex, abstinence is such an important word—just don't do it! . . . On Thursday [the nurse] will be in here talking about STDs. You will find out about contraceptives and the worries we have with having sex. It could be a death experience.

Mr. Dean also often talked about his own life in class, a trademark of AOUME approaches also on clear display during the student rally in Florida. This led to some unusual conversations for a high school sex education class, which as a rule try to convince students how easy it is to get pregnant, sick, or in trouble. Instead, in the following story, Mr. Dean talks about infertility and difficulties getting pregnant—subjects that are almost never discussed with teens but impact over 10 percent of adult couples' lives:

My wife and I, we got married when we were twenty-two. We decided we didn't want kids right away—we wanted to live a little bit and enjoy ourselves and save up. Laura was on birth control but I don't know what kind. We waited eight years before deciding to start a family. We'd purchased a house and we could provide for a family. All that time we'd guarded against pregnancy. We decided to go! [He shoots his fist up in the air and holds it aloft for a few seconds.] But nothing happened. Look at page 444—a woman's reproductive cycle is twenty-eight days. Day fourteen to sixteen or twelve to sixteen, ovulation is starting to happen, the egg is presented and a woman can become pregnant. As you go through life, your wife, hopefully it's your wife, won't necessarily become fertile then. That's when it's supposed to be, but you can't count on that calendar. OK, so we're counting, today we have to have intercourse because it's the magical time. But after two years, nothing. So we went to doctors. We did everything checking this out. It was kind of embarrassing. We even had one doctor say we might be allergic to each other. Well, we come to find out, when Laura was in high school, she had an appendicitis attack. Then on page 443, there are two little tubes called fallopian tubes floating around in there. When the sperm is injected, they come down and attach to the ovary. Laura's tubes were hung up on scar tissue and couldn't attach. So they did a laparoscopy. Bam! As soon as they got those released, magic happened. She was able to conceive, and our daughter was born. So it's not automatic that everything will be OK. More couples have problems getting pregnant than we realize. Everything has gotta be just right for it to happen.

One could imagine this narrative being used in a sex-positive CSE classroom to critically examine why teen sex education is so closely tied to discourses of fear and why conversations addressing common sexual experiences (such as infertility) are so seldom allowed. I never heard a single mention of infertility, however, in any of the CSE classrooms I observed, nor did I hear any effort in any classroom to destabilize assumptions about the inherent dangers of teen sexuality (this story refers to marital sexuality, which is viewed as inherently safe).

Mr. Dean's insertion of his own views and avoidance of the official ABSE curricular materials had a number of effects. For many students in his class, the periods during which Mr. Dean did talk about sex (and his own sex life) were intensely uncomfortable: students looked away from him, put their heads down on their desks, and otherwise disengaged. He made comments that visibly annoyed some students, including ones that supported gender inequitable stereotypes. Because he talked throughout every sex education class, students were left no time to discuss the materials or ask questions. Students, usually girls, did occasionally try to challenge him when he made factually incorrect statements or when his comments directly contradicted material in the book, but Mr. Dean silenced their questions, allowing students to speak only when he posed a direct question to them. I did not hear a single Native American student's voice. Like Mr. Lauder, Mr. Dean did not ask students who were opted out of the CSE components of the curriculum to leave the room; but in Mr. Dean's case, it wouldn't have made a difference because he did not have students interact with the official ABSE materials during class time. Not only did Mr. Dean's students have few opportunities to interact with the formal curricular materials, because they started the sex education unit so late, they covered only about a third of the materials covered by the other two classes. Nevertheless, they still had to take the same final exam. Students expressed fury at this course of events to Mr. Dean and to each other during class, but to no avail.

Mr. Dean's directive approach to teaching is a central component of AOUME approaches, which emphasize the transmission of one clear message from teacher to students and provide few opportunities for student challenges. AOUME emphasizes the dangers of teen sexuality and of open discussion about the "details" of sexuality (such as reproductive biology or definitions of sex acts), and it consistently and deliberately presents a set of norms and values concerning sexuality that are predicated on the male-headed nuclear family model. These values were evident throughout Mr. Dean's class.

"CANNING" THE CURRICULUM

Though from the principal's and the district coordinator's perspectives the curriculum was "70 percent canned," in practice the sex education class-rooms differed radically in tone, patterns of student and teacher talk, and students' opportunities to engage with the official curriculum. Mr. Dean's directive teaching approach stifled students' questions and comments, Mr. Lauder's approach limited them largely to administrative questions, and Ms. Jeffries's approach provided the only opportunity for students to actively discuss curricular materials and topics. Mr. Lauder and Ms. Jeffries silenced their own opinions about sex, sexuality, and teaching sex education in order to avoid potentially negative community reactions, while Mr. Dean's AOUME opinions were front and center during his monologues. These pat-terns of student and teacher silences reflect the district curriculum specialist's sense that AOUME proponents could "cause trouble" if CSE messages were "overdone," while supporters of the current curriculum would not mobilize against AOUME messages.

All three teachers constrained what students learned and how they were allowed to interact (or not) with each other, with their teachers, and with the official curricular materials in order to avoid CSE programming and commu-nity mobilization. Students' needs and questions were consistently silenced in two of the three classrooms, as were their voices in deciding what materials they wished to access.

TETON HIGH'S OTHER SEX EDUCATION CURRICULUM:
MRS. CURRY'S FAMILY AND CHILD HEALTH CLASS

While all students at Teton High were required to take the health educa-tion class that included the sex education module, Mrs. Curry's Family and Child Health (FCH) class was offered on an elective basis. The class provided insights into a potentially different model of sex education programming. Most of the students who took FCH were girls and a fair number were Native American. The class environment was very different from the required sex education classes; here, the class size was smaller, students cooked together and talked about topics related to family life, and often spoke to Mrs. Curry before or after class about their relationships, their families, and their plans for the future. During the weeks I attended the class, there were open discus-sions among students and between students and Mrs. Curry about pregnancy, marriage, domestic abuse, and family financial planning. I saw Mrs. Curry talk with students about relationship issues, and I observed students coming in to ask her how to handle stresses they were facing in their daily lives. These one-on-one and group conversations were significantly different than those I observed between students and the health teachers.

At the time of my research, Mrs. Curry was new to the school but well aware of the politics surrounding sex education; as with Ms. Jeffries and Mr. Lauder, this played a key role in her curricular choices and interactions with students. Mr. Dean described himself as a coach who was uncomfortable with and had little interest in sex education. Ms. Jeffries and Mr. Lauder talked about themselves as health and PE teachers who cared about students' health needs but had been tasked with teaching a scripted sex education curriculum that did not let them address those needs. Mrs. Curry talked about herself as a student ally who was trying to get students to think carefully and critically about their future families and communities. She fostered personal relationships with students who were open to it or whom she felt were in need, and she generally viewed her FCH mandate as expansive within the area of current and future relationships—with some exceptions, including most sex education "hot topic" triggers: ongoing sexual or child abuse, students' personal sexuality or sexual experiences, sexual identity, and contraception.

To me, Mrs. Curry emphasized that she was careful not to discuss issues related to sex and sexuality that fell outside the FCH purview, but that she felt the FCH's focus on "physical, social, and emotional wellness" evidently had many connections to sexuality. Mrs. Curry reported that she received a lot of questions about pregnancy and abortion from students: "Can you get pregnant at twelve?" "Can you get pregnant when you have your period?" Of such questions, she said,

> Those are the cases I answer in relation to what we are studying, so it's almost a biological explanation of what is possible. I try not to answer in terms of birth control, because that falls outside of what I teach, and I don't want myself or the district to get in trouble. I will tell kids that I know the answers, but that my classroom is not the appropriate place to get the answers.

[handwritten margin note: If not the school then where do they go for answers?]

When student questions fell outside the FCH purview, Mrs. Curry directed students to talk to other school personnel or adults in the community. An important component of her class was fostering these linkages with supportive adults: "The personal relationship between a student and the resource people—a nurse, a counselor—is absolutely central to what they can do. I have the nurse come to class so that the students know who she is, and each student has to ask her three questions." This effort to foster familiarity with adults in a position to answer students' questions differed significantly from the sex education classes in which resource experts conducted presentations, answered topical questions, and then left.

Mrs. Curry named two reasons for fostering relationships between students and other adults. First, she felt it was impossible to know which students would feel comfortable discussing issues with which adults, so introducing students to a range of potential mentors was important:

> There is real variability in which students feel comfortable going to which adults. Some are viewed as judgmental, others as helpful, and that differs for kids. The Native American population as a whole tends to be very reticent and hesitant to share personal things. They may not have as many people with whom they have close connections. But [the Native American counselor] has a very close relationship with a lot of students and is also very involved in outside activities.

Second, because of the politics related to sex education at the school, Mrs. Curry was adamant about not talking publicly with students about issues such as sexual abuse or contraception. She noted that these issues were often the most pressing ones to students but constituted areas of silence at the school. She said she could not "violate" these silences, because topics like pregnancy and abortion were "private" issues. Most of these hot topics were not covered in the FCH curriculum; those that were, such as child abuse, were covered in an in-depth but theoretical manner deliberately disconnected from students' lives. For example, in the classes I observed on child abuse, the students were cast in the hypothetical role of future parents and asked to think about what might lead parents to become abusive and how they might respond to such behavior in themselves or a spouse.

With the important exception of these structured silences, Mrs. Curry's classroom provided opportunities for students to interact with her and each other on many of the issues related to sexuality that were sidelined in the official sex education classrooms. These included the personal experiences of teen mothers, in-depth discussions about the prevention of child abuse, and conversations about stressors on family relationships (particularly teen parents), such as finances. Mrs. Curry's class did not include information about reproductive health, STIs, and so forth, but students were given opportunities to talk about and reflect on the reality of multiple models of sexual and familial relationships, in all of their complexity. Because of this, students in Mrs. Curry's class were interacting with, and appeared to be reflecting on, issues related to sexuality and relationships more regularly and profoundly than in the official sex education classes I observed.

In the official classes, the prescribed curriculum kept most class periods focused on the biology of sex and sexuality, with little space built in for students to talk about their own lives and relationships. In Mrs. Curry's class, the course material revolved around relationships, and the "biology" of sex and sexuality was addressed only as it related to specific relationship situations. The kind of comprehensive relationship education that Mrs. Curry provided at Teton High is supposed to be an integral component of CSE approaches to sexuality, but as we see in Wyoming and throughout this book, constituted a very limited part of CSE curricula in practice. Similarly, the close relationship that Mrs. Curry formed with some students, which allowed them to more safely discuss personal questions and concerns, provided a different model of teacher-student relationships than that observed in the official sex education classrooms. We can thus understand Mrs. Curry's class as a different relationship (and sexuality) education model, with both official and hidden curricula and pedagogical practices quite distinct from official sex education classes.

Privatizing Hot Topics

In all four observed classes at Teton High, students were not permitted to openly discuss certain topics, their own experiences with abuse, sexual activity, and sexual identity foremost among them. Mr. Lauder and Mr. Dean told me they were seldom approached by students with questions about these topics; Ms. Jeffries said that on the occasions she was approached, she directed students to the guidance counselor. Mrs. Curry also dealt with these issues by "privatizing" student concerns and experiences: whenever the subject was personal or directly related to sexuality, she would talk with students only outside of class and one-on-one. For example, child abuse prevention could be discussed in class, but personal concerns or experiences had to be brought to her privately after class, or more likely referred to other adults at the school, such as guidance counselors or the nurse.

Students received strong messages through this privatization process that many topics related to sex, sexuality, and violence were taboo in public school spaces. The silencing of students' experiences and needs was not felt equally. Students who were viewed as violating gender or sexuality norms, students who were sexually active or being bullied by peers about their sexual identities, and students who were or had been sexually abused received strong messages that their experiences and concerns were not valid issues for public discussion within the school setting, and that their experiences of inequity or abuse—even when occurring at school—were not appropriate topics for discussion or potential change.

Outside the Classroom: Unofficial Sex Education Practices at Teton High

The majority of students' experiences with sex and sexuality at school occurred outside formal sex education classroom settings—in their interactions with each other and with teachers, through educational materials in all subject areas, and in structured and unstructured in- and after-school activities. These "unofficial" sex education experiences are central to understanding how students perceive the place(s) that their experiences, concerns, and questions about sexuality have within the school context; their understanding of how school authority figures feel about teen sexuality; and the messages they receive and give concerning gender and sexuality norms.

In interviews, teachers and staff at Teton High expressed a wide variety of opinions about teen sexuality and its appropriate place in the school. Some felt that any action overtly related to sex or sexuality (from holding hands to wearing tight jeans) should not be allowed at the school, while others said they thought the school had a responsibility to engage students in open discussions about issues such as drugs and sex, teen pregnancy, sexual identity, and abortion. *All* of the teachers, however, expressed the view that "the school" did not foster open discussions about student sexuality.

Most of the students with whom I spoke felt they had no real opportunities to ask questions or express concerns about sexuality in the school and believed that violating unspoken adult social and sexual norms would result in harsh consequences from teachers and peers. Although the sex education curriculum was officially "comprehensive," most of the students with whom I spoke felt that the textbook was extremely limited and that neither during health education class nor in other school settings did they have a chance to discuss their questions and concerns with teachers or other adults. The official sex education classes were roundly dismissed as "boring" and out-of-date. When asked whether they thought the sex education curriculum should be changed, however, a number of student interviewees said they were not sure that changing the official curriculum would have much of an impact on students' opportunities to engage in conversation, particularly given the widespread sense that school staff and teachers wished to avoid discussion about students' sexuality. As one recent female graduate said,

> There's no really helpful sexual education stuff because it's been the same talk since fifth grade, including the condom stuff. "Don't have sex or you will get AIDS and die," like in *Mean Girls*. Kids think it's stupid or don't care. Sexual education could be important if they taught us stuff we didn't already know. Or maybe stuff just isn't said enough, like rephrase it from our point of view. It's useful to show putting on a condom, and refusal skills are also good, [but]

there's lots of problems with the school's response to us being sexual. Like last year, my friend wore an off-shoulder shirt, it wasn't too sexual, but she almost got a Tuesday/Saturday [detention] because they said it didn't help boys concentrate on their schoolwork. This tiny patch of skin influences the boys? Those boys [who would be distracted] don't do their work anyway! And boys wear shirts with women on them and nothing is ever said . . . and then last year, I got a short haircut and everyone thought I was a lesbian with my best friend and that we did drugs. No one bothered to check the truth, and it was just wrong.

Students were well aware that the formal curriculum was operating within an institutional environment in which those in positions of authority—teachers and administrators—were wary of talking to students about policy and practical concerns related to sexuality (such as the dress code). Students were also well aware of the effects of this environment on their personal expressions of gender and sexual identity, and on the school community's ability to address well-known issues related to sexuality at the school (such as homophobia and Native American girls' high pregnancy rates). Some of the students felt misunderstood by teachers and peers, but, due to the prevailing silence concerning teen sexuality, felt unable to address these misunderstandings or fight against perceived prejudices.

While peer norms concerning personal expression and sexual behavior differed among student groups at the school, students perceived the adults as propounding homogeneous, restrictive, and "fear-based" norms related to student sexuality. Though a number of students identified individual teachers or guidance counselors whom they felt were exceptions, they noted that their interactions with these adults always took place in private. In other words, in public adults were a homogeneous group tasked with suppressing student sexuality, and only in private could some adults be approached about these topics.

Of course, not all students' experiences or concerns at Teton High were patrolled or silenced in the same way. Below, I briefly describe the stories I was told about Native American girls' experiences related to pregnancy; in chapter 9, I discuss patrolling and silencing that students experienced related to sexual and gender identity.

NATIVE AMERICAN GIRLS AND PREGNANCY

Teton had high teen pregnancy rates throughout the 1980s and early 1990s; as in the rest of the United States, these rates fell during the late 1990s. When I visited Teton in 2005, I was told that the school no longer had a "problem" with student pregnancy, and that therefore pregnancy rates were no longer officially addressed—yet at that time, five Native American girls were or had recently been pregnant.

Data on pregnancy rates in Wyoming and the county indicate that teen pregnancy rates declined between 1988 and 2007, but they declined much less than throughout the United States because they rose between 2000 and 2008, unlike in most of the United States, where rates continued to decline. Moreover, pregnancy rates declined less for Native American girls than for white girls. When I asked school staff why they thought Native American girls' pregnancy rates had not declined as rapidly as white girls', they generally agreed on one reason: culture. Specifically, they said that Native American families saw nothing wrong with letting boyfriends stay overnight with girlfriends, or with their teen daughters becoming mothers. As one teacher explained: "On the reservation, there are a lot of grandparents and extended families raising kids. Having a baby is very accepted. The girls usually stay at home after birth, and the mom helps them raise the baby. It's nothing for the boyfriend to be living in the house with her—it's not called 'living,' it's called 'staying,' no matter how long they've been there. We can talk about contraception, but pregnancy is just not considered that big a deal."

Because most school personnel considered the roots of Native American teen pregnancy to be "cultural," they talked about it as difficult to change and almost inevitable; school efforts to support Native American girls before or after pregnancy were viewed, therefore, as inherently ineffective.

In fact, Native American girls' experiences with sex, family, and school were virtually absent from official school policy and practices. Most teachers appeared to have little understanding of the lives of students on the reservation, few networks with Native American students, and no contact with the parallel health-care and welfare systems on the reservation. Even formal attempts on the part of teachers to address teen pregnancy and high school dropout, which disproportionately affected Native American students, seldom actually included Native Americans. For example, a series of presentations on child development in the FCH class, in which mothering teens came to talk to the class about their experiences, was composed entirely of white girls.

A number of school support staff members worked directly with Native American students; the Native American liaison, who was the only Native American staff member, worked most closely with them. These staff members' explanations of Native American pregnancy rates challenged other teachers' and administrators' naturalization of a deficit cultural model as the primary cause of higher pregnancy rates. For example, the Native American liaison explained:

> Girls used to disappear when they got pregnant. Title IX brought girls back in school. I've not heard of any giving the baby up, so whether the baby disrupts the school process a lot depends on the family support. A lot of the girls say that they care about school, but it's very hard—even getting to this high school from the res is hard. There's lots of violence and fighting in a lot of the homes, and the houses are often very small and dirty. It's a hard environment and it's easy to slip into poverty.

Here the liaison points to a set of structural constraints, including poverty and its effects on home environments and transportation on the one hand, and a set of shrinking support systems for parenting students, such as Title IX, on the other hand, to explain why Native American girls might stay in or drop out of school following a pregnancy. She went on to identify changes in local and national school policies that were once supportive but now constrained the school's capacity to address Native American girls' educational futures:

> What school does is give her a chance to come and be a kid—there are no responsibilities here. She gets to be a kid going to school. But it becomes such a hassle—the baby is sick, there's too much homework—and a lot of the flexibility we used to have has been cut out by NCLB and the need to meet so many standards and requirements. We just have less flexibility to be as creative as we need to be.

She also pointed to the need for open and honest discussion about how a primarily white staff could better serve Native American students, and how staff could gain a better understanding of students' lives:

> I would love to do diversity training for the teachers and school staff . . . As a district, we are really working to try to open people's eyes to what kids' lives are like. For Native American kids, if we want sex education to be useful, we need to involve elders in this, bring them in, bring in people from Indian Health, let the kids know what's available at the clinic, because kids here won't go into town to use that clinic, they don't have transportation to it. We also need to tell them what to do if they're pregnant—for example, prenatal care.

The liaison also highlighted a different set of cultural concerns than those mentioned by the white teachers and administrators. While the white teachers focused on "cultural differences" that, from their perspective, encouraged girls to become pregnant, the liaison highlighted the interactions among sociocultural, geographical, and political-economic structures that shaped girls' and their families' understanding of and response to pregnancy. In the liaison's view, pregnancy was not itself a purely negative issue. Neither was the derided (by white faculty) practice of teens of opposite sexes staying over at each other's homes. From the perspective of some white teachers, this was an example of Native American parents encouraging immorality. From the perspective of the liaison, the practice was complexly related to conceptions of caring for other community members; the interaction of poverty, transportation, and geography; and different cultural norms for parenting and its social roles.[6]

Perhaps most importantly, some white teachers' assumptions about Native American culture wrote off pregnant girls as students and as full members of the school community. The school's sex education curriculum did not provide girls with the information or opportunities for discussion that could, according to the liaison and sex education teachers, potentially affect their sexual decision-making. It also did not provide opportunities for teachers to learn about students' questions or experiences, or to question their own assumptions about pregnancy and schooling. For example, the liaison emphasized that girls often wanted to stay in school after giving birth, but the school no longer supported their return, and family dynamics and poverty made it hard for girls to return without such support.

The experience of Native American students at Teton High serves as a parable for the entire sex education enterprise. Because the sex education classes at Teton High lacked a connection to most students' actual experiences of sex, relationships, and family, they appeared unlikely to effect change in student behaviors. Furthermore, they were based on a particular model of sex and sexuality that privileged white, middle-class, straight, adult conceptualizations of "good" and "bad" sexual decision-making, behaviors, and outcomes. Therefore, they failed to address the experiences of many students at the school, but they particularly failed students whose lives did not fit this model. Teen mothers' experiences highlight the extent to which students who were viewed as violating these norms were dismissed and, at the extreme, literally cast out of the school. Most teen mothers, Native American and white, were either no longer attending high school at all, or they were attending the alternative high school in the area, which had remarkably fewer resources (including, even, meals) to meet the needs of their students.

Conclusion

This chapter described how community mobilization around sex education created and maintained an official ABSE regime in Granite, and in turn, how the implementation of this regime by three different teachers affected students' official sex education experiences at the school.

Decades after the battle that occurred at Teton High, the compromise reached by adults in Granite over the sex education curriculum appeared to be holding up. The curriculum is essentially the same scripted, nationally produced program that was agreed on after the battle, and students' voices and needs remain largely ignored or actively silenced. For many of the students with whom I spoke, though, their primary concern was not the formal sex education curriculum but how the school's adults chose (or failed) to interact with students about issues of sexuality in everyday school events and practices.

Adult responses to teen sexuality at Teton High often appeared to be motivated by fear: either of teen sexuality itself, or of the potential for negative community responses. The result was an effort to silence discussion about potentially dangerous topics. Two of the three PE teachers, for example, mentioned their concern that something said in a sex education class would rekindle the sex education battles, and a number of teachers made comments in individual interviews about the danger of students' sexuality and the need for careful adult patrolling of, for example, student dress. The adults who *were* able to connect with students around issues of sexuality (the guidance counselor, the Native American liaison, the FCH teacher) did so in settings that were deliberately privatized. This fear of publicly addressing teen sexuality and teen desire has been noted in other adult-managed settings (e.g., Schalet 2004; Tolman 2002), and permeated the school's sexuality policies and practices.

Students reported that there were significant issues related to gender and sexuality at the school that adults refused to address. Although all the students with whom I spoke felt that the imposed norm of silence around issues of student sexuality was sometimes difficult and unfair to them, students who were breaking gender or sexuality norms, who were not white, who were experiencing sexual abuse, or who were poor were particularly affected by these silences. These students' experiences were officially invisible, resulting in an environment that was markedly less able to meet their needs.

Teachers echoed students that public discussions of sexuality or of issues such as abuse, social and cultural norms, and family dynamics were considered close to taboo, and this taboo appeared to apply as much to the sex education classes as to other spaces. Few formal settings allowed students to talk openly about issues they were facing in their own lives, even when they were affecting their educational performance; teachers seldom used students' interests to shape lessons about sexuality; and the broader social or economic inequities that impacted students' sexuality were not discussed.

Just as some students' experiences were silenced more than others, so too the voices and concerns of CSE-supportive teachers were silenced more than those of AOUME-supportive teachers. The official curriculum attempted to structure and script teacher-student interactions. But, as we saw, only teachers who were concerned about being seen as too supportive of open discussion about sex and sexuality felt constrained by these materials. While Mr. Dean's AOUME beliefs were expressed without concern, Ms. Jeffries' and Mr. Lauder's more sexually liberal beliefs and their concerns about the unmet educational needs of their students were silenced.

The current state of sex education at Teton raises a number of questions that face many schools implementing ABSE programs: What are the values that underlie these programs? What are the school's goals in implementing the program? What information and experiences do school leaders think will actually change student sexual behaviors and outcomes? How are these beliefs related to students' perceptions of the sex education programming? What models of participation and democratic decision-making underlie sex education policy-making practices?

For the most part, teachers and pupils disagreed on the answers to these core questions. Granite community members and school leaders felt that the current sex education program represented a democratically negotiated middle ground among (adult) stakeholders in the sex education battles. The curriculum was viewed as flexible and able to accommodate various parental demands, and was structured to silence teachers' (value-laden) opinions. For most students, on the other hand, the sex education classes represented at best a waste of time, at worst a denial of their experiences and educational needs. Their concerns about sexuality were silenced in the sex education classes and in the wider school environment.

In practice, the sex education programming at Teton High did appear to meet the expectations of a broad range of parents and other adult community members, and this meant that sex education materials remained in the official curriculum and were accessible to all students. However, the price of this democratically reached consensus was that inside sex education classrooms, there was little space for democratic functioning: teachers' and students' voices were silenced in the decision-making process and in the classroom itself. The school environment fostered the privatization of discussion about teen sexuality, which meant that the hidden curriculum of the school embodied a central AOUME message: sex is private and secret and should not be discussed openly. As discussed in chapters 8 and 11, this status quo raises important questions about school models of democratic participation, and about the messages that students receive concerning their potential rights, responsibilities, and roles as members of a democratic institution, be it the school or the state.

No Idea Is Bad, No Opinion Is Wrong, but Knowledge Is Power: Sex Education in Wisconsin

COAUTHORED WITH KATHLEEN ELLIOTT[1]

Wisconsin Sex Education Policy

In the previous chapter, we went inside three classrooms in Wyoming, each taught by a different teacher using the same district-mandated curriculum. In this chapter, Kathleen Elliott and I examine one classroom that was, at the time of our joint observations, being co-taught by two teachers at Fontaine High School in Wisconsin.[2] During the 2009–10 academic year, the classroom teacher, Mrs. Shane, was hosting Mr. Kelly, who was completing his student teaching. This situation allowed for a fruitful comparison of two teachers' curricular and pedagogical approaches and classroom-management styles as directed toward the same group of students, and a comparison of the same students' responses to two different teachers.

At the start of our research, Wisconsin schools and teachers had broad leeway in determining the shape and scope of their sex education programming. Schools were not required to provide sex or HIV/AIDS education, and if they did offer it, they could give it any emphasis and offer it at any grade level they chose. Though the state guidelines tightened and shifted over the years during which I conducted research in Wisconsin (2004–2009), this history of decentralized control over sex education had shaped a diverse set of sex education practices in schools and classrooms. The only unifying theme across district and school personnel with whom I spoke was, in fact, the lack of resources offered by the state to support sex education, which meant that schools and districts struggled to update curricula and provide professional development. As I surveyed districts to determine where I might conduct research, I found some that offered no sex education programming at all (often citing lack of funds as the reason), some that provided no guidance and left it up to the school or to individual teachers to decide what to do, and some that provided policy guidelines and other sex education resources (professional development on health education, curricular materials, and so on) to schools. I found teachers within the same school presenting entirely different programming (for example, one all-AOUME and one all-CSE curriculum), and teachers, particularly in urban areas with more private sex education service providers, who were bringing in as many different perspectives and resources as possible. As one AOUME service provider explained, "It's really frustrating, because we go into classes where the day before they had Planned Parenthood in, and the day after us they have some gay rights group coming in. We tell them [the teachers] that it hurts kids to get these mixed messages, but they say that they don't want to be biased." Variation within school and classroom sex education approaches appeared to be based on several factors: district guidelines and resources, teachers' beliefs about what constituted a good curriculum, teachers' expectations of community responses, and the resources teachers could access at no or low cost.

Fontaine High's sex education programming reflected many of these trends. Mrs. Shane and Mr. Kelly were not required to work within any particular curricular or pedagogical framework, and while the district offered limited sex education guidelines and materials that they could use in their classroom, they were free to choose other materials. Though both teachers were teaching the same class, each selected the materials they would use for a given lesson.

Sex Education at Fontaine High

Within a patchwork of state, district, and school sex education approaches, Fontaine High had maintained the same official CSE approach for many years. The approach enjoyed community support and benefited from Mrs. Shane's extensive experience. The lead sex educator for Fontaine High, she had been teaching sex education for almost twenty years. She and other high school and district personnel said they took pride in their program because they felt it addressed the health implications of students' sexuality but went beyond that to ensure that students had opportunities to reflect on sex and sexuality, to think about and practice relationship skills (such as "saying no" and recognizing abusive relationships), and to master a body of knowledge and a way of learning about sexuality that would serve them well for the rest of their lives.

This approach to sex education was based on the behavior-change theory common to CSE programs: that learning *how* to master, and mastering, a continuously changing body of scientific information about sex and sexuality would give teens power over their sexual decision-making and lead to positive health outcomes.[3] Mrs. Shane described her approach as follows:

My main priority . . . is to let them know that they can find the information from reputable sources and not depend on their friends for sources. Especially if I'm talking about drugs and sex. Because all of them listen to their peers more than to anyone else at this age, and I want them to learn that—and they hear it all the time—"Knowledge is power, knowledge is power," and they all know that. But I want them to know that they have to find the information and, you know, where to find the information and make sure it's correct information because it will affect their health for the rest of their lives if they make the wrong decision. Because I know, if you talk about other subjects, you just get the information, this is how it is, that's how it was, that's it. And health changes all the time, so, I tell them, "What I teach you today might not be the same in a couple years. There might be another STI." There used to only be two or three STIs. Now there are forty-five-plus STIs. It's changed that much. There never was HIV, now there's HIV that can kill you. So I said you have to be able to research and find the information and keep up with it. So my goal is just to make sure they understand that health changes all the time and they need to find the information.

The five-week sex education program that we observed in a ninth-grade classroom in 2009 was officially taught by Mr. Kelly, but Mrs. Shane played an active role in all of the classes and taught portions of most of them. Mr. Kelly and Mrs. Shane appeared to have a comfortable relationship. Mrs. Shane regularly interjected during his lessons to follow up on student comments, present her opinion, or correct Mr. Kelly. Mr. Kelly regularly asked for her help but also pulled the class back to a subject he wished to pursue if her comments led the conversation in a different direction. The two teachers had very different styles; this was partly based on their vastly different levels of experience, which were reflected in their mastery of the content and their interactions with students. It was also due to their very different sexual and teaching ideologies. Exploring the similarities and differences between Mrs. Shane's and Mr. Kelly's teaching approaches and interactions with students elucidates how the dynamics of student-teacher interactions affect students' sex education experiences, and provides particular insight into how teacher-student relationships can transform students' engagement and sense of safety in the class.

CLASSROOM DYNAMICS WITH MRS. SHANE AND MR. KELLY

When Mr. Kelly was "in charge" of the class, students were much less likely to speak up or to talk with one another than they were when Mrs. Shane was controlling the conversation. Not only was the total amount of student conversational time significantly reduced when Mr. Kelly was in charge, but the students who participated and the types of student comments were quite different than when Mrs. Shane led the class. Students were much less likely to challenge Mr. Kelly's statements (often simply remaining silent) than Mrs. Shane's. Female students of color, when they did speak, were repeatedly and actively silenced by Mr. Kelly but not by Mrs. Shane.

Mr. Kelly had just received his undergraduate degree and planned to become a PE teacher. As a teacher trainee, he had much less pedagogical practice than Mrs. Shane. He was visibly focused on completing his lesson plans, which consisted of leading students through various handouts and worksheets he had selected from the district's sex education resources library and materials he had found online. In conversations, he was clear that he viewed himself as a PE teacher, not a health teacher. Nonetheless, he did not refrain from offering his opinions on topics related to sexuality in class, sometimes drawing on stories from his own experiences to illustrate his opinions. His personal views were quite sexually conservative and aligned more closely with an AOUME approach than a CSE approach. Though his pedagogical approach was more directive than Mrs. Shane's, it was not clear how much this was due to an ideological alignment with the approach, and how much it was due to his inexperience. He seemed comfortable allowing students to share their opinions, for example, as long as the time spent on student conversation did not disrupt his lesson plan. He was not directive in his teaching in the same way as was Mr. Dean in Wyoming, but he was certainly less interested than Mrs. Shane in fostering discussion or debate.

Mrs. Shane was a health teacher with almost thirty years of experience, twenty-five of which had been spent at Fontaine. She was one of only two full-time teachers that I met during my research who said that she had wanted to teach health and had been trained to do so. She expressed many of the same concerns that sex educators from other states reported, such as wide differences in students' developmental levels ("In ninth grade I think they're too immature to catch on. They're still goofy. Even though, you know, we have pregnant ninth graders."), the negative influence of the media and peers on students' perceptions of sex and sexuality, the sense that students' morals and values regarding sex differed significantly from hers, and the negative effects of drinking and pregnancy on students' lives. She spoke reflectively in interviews about how sociocultural, economic, and religious norms affected students' lives and sexual decision-making, but focused her teaching on driving home the negative physical repercussions of sex and how they could be avoided through improved rational decision-making—a method she perceived to be universally applicable and useful. For example, she said,

And I don't think they [students] see the consequences [of teen pregnancy], or they think, in some—I don't know if it's a culture thing or if it's just kids— but I think they think, when they see that, I know I've seen girls dote on girls who are pregnant. "Oh, you're pregnant. That's so cool." And, "Can I touch your belly?" And they think of it as a symbol instead of, oh my gosh, you're going to be stuck with that thing for eighteen years. And you're only fourteen? And I don't know where their thinking is or what they're thinking. I don't know if it's a gender thing or a generational thing or it's a, a, cultural . . . it's hard to figure out because it's all different kinds of races and ages.

In Mrs. Shane's view, sex education should lead students to question assumptions and dispel myths, resulting in expanded knowledge. For this reason, and because of her conviction that every person has an equal right to voice their ideas, Mrs. Shane was also a strong proponent that no idea was bad—or at least that airing ideas was never bad—and that encouraging students to explore their ideas in and out of class was central to their growth. She described her teaching philosophy as follows:

That's what I think I'm trying to teach—that they have the brains and the minds. Use them. Find information. Go search it out for yourself, you know. I have the information and I'll give you information about it but, you know, these guys need to develop into adults and at this stage is when they should develop. . . . If you walked in [to the classroom] sometimes you'd go, "What the heck is going on? They're all talking." It's, like, OK . . . I could be mean and strict and come in with a gavel and sit there and go, "Sit down and be quiet!" But I think that cuts them off. And then they don't participate.

As a result of this philosophy, Mrs. Shane's classroom was dominated by student conversation. Mrs. Shane often picked up themes from students' conversations to explore further and tried to get students to discuss traditionally "hot topic" issues such as gender stereotypes and homophobia; however, these conversations seldom took off. Classroom interactions seemed to be marked by a push-pull between her and the students. Consider the example of the class activity and interactions below:

Mr. Kelly separates the girls and the boys and asks them to come up with lists of "what they are looking for in a boyfriend [the girls] or a girlfriend [the boys]." The groups then share their lists with the class. While the boys' list includes more items related to sexual behaviors than the girls', both lists include physical attributes, sexual characteristics, and personality characteristics. After both groups share, Mr. Kelly summarizes by saying, "As you can see, there's a difference between how a lot of guys think and how girls think. Guys think sexually and think about sex more often. Girls should be careful and cautious. You'll think everything's OK, but all he wants is sex." Mrs. Shane interjects,

"Be aware of what's going on. I hear it from girls all the time. Guys are more interested in the physical part of a relationship than girls are. Guys don't think with this head [she points to her head], they think with the other head. Generally girls' lists will be more emotional and boys' lists will be more physical." Theo jumps in, "We're just made that way," he says, eliciting laughs from the class. Shurita disagrees. "Not all boys are made that way," she says. No one responds to her assertion, and the class moves on to a handout activity.

Here, Mrs. Shane attempts to connect with students about sex and relationships in a way that draws on her experience and connects to students' experiences. However, she does this by presenting stereotypes about boys' and girls' different sexual "natures." When Shurita challenges the assumed gender stereotypes, she is ignored and the conversation dies. The space that Shurita's comment could have opened for discussion or debate about the realities of teens' sexual feelings and gendered expectations in relationships remains closed.

Mrs. Shane prided herself on connecting with her students and creating an environment in which they felt could talk freely in class. Students generally did seem to feel comfortable in her classroom and with her, and, as described above, regularly challenged Mrs. Shane's assumptions about teen social relations. While she consistently allowed these challenges, she was seldom responsive to them. Mrs. Shane said that she never wanted to make students feel they could not express their opinions, and therefore never cut them off. At the same time, she wanted students to "know the facts" about sex: a set of facts that she viewed as correct and appropriate for teens. These two impulses were sometimes at odds.

ENGAGING STUDENT VOICES

As in Ms. Jeffries's class in Wyoming, students in Mrs. Shane's class spoke freely and frequently about their lives, families, friends, and school experiences. Unlike Ms. Jeffries, Mrs. Shane actively engaged with students during many of these conversations, pushing back if she felt students were being disrespectful to each other or if she felt they ought to clarify (or change) their positions. This offered the most opportunities that I observed in any classroom for students to engage with each other and with their teacher around issues of sex and sexuality. It was also the most emotionally safe space I observed; for example, the following conversation about families took place during one class:

After an activity that asked students to rate their relationships with their family members on a scale of 1 to 5 [1 for a bad and 5 for a good relationship], the class discusses their answers. Andy shares that his mom is an alcoholic and not around, but that he lives with his dad and his dad is good. Another boy says that his dad had recently left and gotten a new girlfriend before he divorced his mom. He says his dad yells a lot, but that his mom is a 4. A girl shares that her dad is an alcoholic. A couple of students say that their parents get angry at each other and take it out on them. Mr. Kelly asks, "Have you tried talking to them?" Mrs. Shane adds, "Try to open up and talk to them and be honest. Sometimes it's hard, parents start yelling, I know. But it's good to try."

Mr. Kelly then asks the class, "How many of you feel loved and respected?" Almost all raise their hands. He calls on a boy who didn't and asks why not. The student explains that he doesn't feel he can trust his parents, and that they don't trust him. The boy whose father had recently left raises his hand to share. He says, "I don't respect my father or trust him because he's lied about a lot of things. He lied about quitting smoking, he lied about . . ." He gets quiet and starts to cry, though he is visibly trying not to. Mrs. Shane gets up and walks over to him. She squeezes his shoulders in a half hug and asks if he wants to step out of the room. They leave for a bit. The students are quiet as this is happening. There is no joking or making fun of him. They remain quiet after he leaves the class as well. Mrs. Shane returns to the room after a few minutes, and the boy comes back a little while later. Mrs. Shane later tells Kathleen that she hugged him and asked if he wanted to talk and then told him to take however much time he needed.

Many of the classroom interactions embodied what we came to think of as a contradiction between Mrs. Shane's efforts to foster an environment in which each student felt safe to share his or her ideas and where different opinions were valued, and her (and the broader CSE movement's) understanding of students as rational individuals who could only be empowered through the provision of "complete and correct" information. On the one hand, Mrs. Shane was supportive of an ideal of free thought and speech, but she also believed strongly that certain opinions were more valid than others, that there were Facts and Truths and a body of information that, if incorporated into her students' decision-making processes, would transform their sexual health. It was the dissemination of untruths or misunderstandings (through, for example, the media and peers) and a lack of correct knowledge that resulted in poor student sexual decision-making and health. In order to dispel these misunderstandings, students' misconceptions had to be heard publicly so that they could be corrected.

No Idea Is Bad, No Opinion Is Wrong, but Knowledge Is Power

The complexities of student and teacher conversation in CSE classrooms I observed arose from three ideological dilemmas that CSE—but not

AOUME—educators faced. First, teachers' perspectives on what constituted "complete and correct" information were shaped by the norms and values underlying CSE programs and their own experiences and beliefs. In practice this usually meant that CSE approaches embodied white, middle-class, straight, middle-aged, politically middle-of-the-road sexuality norms. While CS educators and programs recognized diversity and claimed to value it, the assumptions underlying their instruction remained largely unexamined and excluded many students' experiences.

Second, CS educators supported students' right to (at least ideally) freely and fully express themselves, even when such expression conflicted with teachers' beliefs or the values that underpin sexually and socially liberal ideologies. This is a classic liberal dilemma that underlies discourses and relations of race, class, and gender in the United States, and is complicated in sex education by arguments among CSE and AOUME supporters concerning the goodness, naturalness, and social acceptability of a broad range of sexuality and gender roles, norms, activities, and topics (e.g., Gutmann 1995).

The CSE teachers I observed practiced a version of Amy Gutmann's argument (1987) that, in a democracy, in order to allow each student to fully explore his or her identity, students' right to express opinions that limited other students' opportunities should in turn be restricted. However, CSE educators' understanding of what might limit other students' opportunities was, in our view, quite narrow: teachers disrupted some conversations that challenged group rights (discussed further in chapter 7) and stopped physical assaults among students, but otherwise did not intercede in students' "private" interactions. This resulted in classroom environments in which stereotypical, biased, or phobic comments were viewed as normal, and often joking, interactions among peers. This meant that teacher judgments about whether to respond to such statements rested largely on their understanding of the relationship between the person making the statement and its addressee. If two students were friends, or the interaction did not seem to be confrontational, then the statements were usually described by teachers as "joking among peers." In the name of valuing all voices, CSE classrooms and schools were ironically full of sexist, heteronormative, homophobic, and racist student talk that undermined the CSE ideology of valuing all people as equals.

Third, CS educators faced tensions with the information they were tasked to impart: their valuing of "complete and correct," scientifically validated information; their need to winnow information and topics to fit within the limited hours of the sex education schedule; their understanding that the science behind many of the topics covered was actually quite complex and seldom as straightforward as it was presented; and their desire to balance the ideal of scientific rationalism with ideals of human rights and tolerance for diversity. Mrs. Shane gestured to this last tension as follows:

> [The] teen years is kind of experimenting and finding out what do you like and what do you not like, and the argument about homosexuals—if it's genetic or if it's not. I still don't know. Research shows different things. So, OK. The idea is you have to find the information and find out. Because you saw how many different kids had different opinions. One of them said in the womb, the testosterone [determined sexual identity]. One of them said well, it's the hypothalamus. Another one said it's in our DNA sequencing. They're very smart and they're looking up this information. But it's just that we want to get them to be accepting of everybody's differences. I mean, a favorite saying of mine is, "People are different. Expect it. Respect it." But some kids . . . you'll always have kids that don't. But talking about that more openly is, it's getting easier.

As in this example, CSE teachers often resolved the dilemmas that resulted from having two strongly held ideals that were in tension with one another by saying that they focused on teaching students how to find new information for themselves within a framework that both valued "scientific truth" and was respectful of people's differences, regardless of the "science" behind the differences.

AOUM educators did not face these tensions because biblical truth, well established through exegesis, constituted the sole moral framework and set of ethical and topical guidelines of these approaches, and directive teaching approaches framed student participation and voice as dangerous and potentially harmful to students and society.

FACT, MYTH, AND OPINION

For CS educators, the tension between human-rights ideals and scientific rationality made it much harder to navigate questions of fact, fiction, myth, and opinion than for AOUM educators. Any five-week class, like the one offered at Fontaine (not to mention shorter programs), designed to cover human development and sexuality is by necessity limited in scope. Teachers must decide which subjects they will address and which they will not, which facts to present and which not. This process is particularly complex in environments like Fontaine High, where Mrs. Shane and Mr. Kelly were able to draw on an almost unlimited range of curricular materials.

There are few simple facts and even fewer eternal truths in the scientific fields from which sex education draws. While there is always a process of selecting information in teaching, the process of taking complex bodies of scientific knowledge and winnowing them down is even more difficult in sex education classes, because the process is informed by the history of activism and legal challenges to teachers' and schools' sex education programming.[4]

Engaging in the process of distilling knowledge while balancing CSE tensions between human-rights ideals and rational individual models was a daily challenge for CS educators like Mrs. Shane, especially when discussing topics—such as the basis of sexual identity—about which students had differing opinions and an array of "scientific facts" could be presented to support these opinions.

The CS educators I observed often attempted to resolve these tensions by emphasizing (1) a basic, simplified, introduction of a topic, including defining terms, categorizing types, and presenting "facts" associated with the topic, and (2) methods through which students could learn more about these topics on their own (such as through visiting health clinics, speaking to their parents, and conducting their own research). For example, Mrs. Shane gave students worksheets that asked them to define terms, such as the following, based on definitions in their textbooks:

- Sex
- Sexuality
- Contraception
- Effectiveness
- Laboratory effectiveness
- User effectiveness
- Abstinence
- Virgin
- Monogamous
- Heterosexual
- Homosexual
- Gay
- Lesbian
- Homophobia
- Bisexual
- Asexual

The definitions in the textbooks were written in medicalized language and drew from scientific, public health, and legal frameworks. Such worksheet activities do not allow students to generate their own definitions, challenge the book's definitions, question how they were developed, or explain how they might disagree with a particular definition. The emphasis on apparently hard-and-fast textbook-based definitions and categorizations limits the possibilities for discussion of topics that are, in practice, disputed and difficult to categorize or distill. To give a simple example, the common public-health definition of "sex" is in direct conflict with the understanding held by many teens (as well as former President Clinton) of sex as including only penile/ vaginal penetration. Nonetheless, the definition of sex appears in the above exercise to be predetermined and unquestionable. Other complex issues were often presented in a similar style that allowed for only one right answer and thus constrained opportunities for debate. For example, Mr. Kelly regularly used "Mythbusters" worksheets, which aimed to correct inaccurate information that students were presumed to have. One worksheet told students to label statements, such as the following, as either true or false:

- Once you stop being a virgin, abstinence is no longer an option.
- It is unhealthy to become sexually aroused and not have an orgasm.
- A monogamous, committed relationship is key to satisfying sexual relations.
- It is self-esteem, not physical makeup, that determines sexuality.
- Many products can be purchased to increase sexual ability.
- Homosexuals are all artists and dancers.
- Medical experts believe masturbation can be helpful in many situations.
- Pregnancy can only occur with ejaculation

In the attempt to distill myths, complex debates, and scientific knowledge into simple true/false statements, the material was sometimes rendered incomprehensible (what, for example, does "It is self-esteem, not physical makeup, that determines sexuality" mean?). In other cases, honest differences of opinion about whether a statement was true, false, both, or dependent on the situation were likely to be shaped by people's sexual ideologies. The exercise, however, leaves no room for discussion of how the questions are presented, what myths they are trying to dispel, or how students might read them critically or differently from how the formulators intended them to be read.

Simply introducing and defining some terms (such as *homosexuality* and *transgender*) has been cause for court cases throughout the country, so we do not mean to dismiss the power of introducing and defining terms. However, the effort in all of the observed CSE programs to "scientize" topics— including sexual identity, family types, STI types, types of penetrative sex, contraceptives, relationships, and abortions—in order to categorize and contain them, and thus to make them politically and discursively manageable, often did not reflect the range of scientific knowledge about a topic or the realities of students' experiences with the topic.[5]

In Mrs. Shane's class, the scientization of complex topics compromised her goal of teaching students how to find and assess accurate information. For example, Mr. Kelly passed out an STI handout titled "Just Thought You Oughta Know: STI Facts" that was produced by the Medical Institutes of Sexual Health (MISH), a conservative think tank. The handout presented information that was technically true, but that implied a number of falsehoods. For example, it included the statistic that "250,000 women each year die of cervical cancer due to HVP [sic]." There were an estimated 274,000 cervical cancer deaths globally in 2002 (Parkin, Bray, Ferlay, and Pisani 2005), so the fact as presented was technically (close to) correct, but it misrepresented the data in two ways. First, it was surrounded by statements referring to the US population, such as "about 50 percent of all Americans between the ages of 15 and 19 are virgins" and "1 in 5 of every Americans [sic] over the age of 12 has genital herpes. 90 percent do not know it," which would lead students to assume that the data refer to the US population only. However, in the United States only about 4,500 women die each year of cervical cancer.

Second, the fact sheet mentions that HPV is incurable and cites the number of deaths it causes per year, but it does not say that the majority of HPV infections are asymptomatic and resolve without negative health effects (CDC 2004). Moreover, domestic and international studies have shown that (1) cervical cancer rates can be reduced dramatically through regular HPV screenings and treatment for precancerous abnormalities (cervical cancer deaths are low in the United States thanks to such screenings; most deaths occur in women who have not received a Pap test in at least five years), and (2) the new HPV vaccine, which MISH strongly opposes, can render negligible girls' risk of developing cervical cancer as a result of HPV.

Despite the fact that many CSE supporters have grown increasingly concerned about the negative effects of misusing scientific evidence for ideological ends (e.g., McClelland and Fine 2008), none of the CSE classes I observed included a critical analysis of presented materials or data, or discussed this issue with students. The worksheet provided an opportunity to discuss how to interpret data, how data might be (mis)represented to serve particular ideological positions, and how various data sources on the same topic may conflict; instead it was offered without critical comment.

To further complicate the issue, in Mrs. Shane's classroom there was a clear pattern of teachers and students adopting scientific language to argue for some points, and "opinion language" to argue for others (even when the "truth" of all points was equally open to debate). Students were less likely to be questioned by the teachers when they adopted opinion language, but because the teachers treated similar comments made by different students differently, there was confusion about what was being presented as fact and what as opinion, and how facts or opinions could be challenged. For example, Mrs. Shane consistently questioned student comments that she judged to include factually incorrect information, but when she judged a student to be expressing an opinion instead of stating a fact, no questions were asked. Take, for example, the following conversation, which occurred during a lesson about abortion, in which Shurita tells a story and Mrs. Shane responds to it by questioning the "facts":

> Shurita tells a story about a girl who drank diluted bleach to try to "kill her baby." Mrs. Shane questions her, saying that that sounds very dangerous for the girl and ineffective as a method—"How would drinking bleach kill her baby? They're two different systems." Shurita says she doesn't know, but insists it was just a small amount of bleach diluted in water. Mrs. Shane remains skeptical but responds, "Oh, in a lot of water."

Mrs. Shane could have used the story in any number of ways: for example, as an opening to discuss the (ineffective) things that girls may do when they are pregnant and scared. Or it could have been used to interrogate assumptions about how girls react to finding out they are pregnant, or as a cautionary tale about what *not* to do if you find yourself pregnant. It might also have been used to celebrate the importance of legal abortion. Instead, Mrs. Shane turned a story about a girl involved in a deeply emotional act into a scientific question for Shurita—"How would drinking bleach kill her baby? They're two different systems." When Shurita could not answer this "factual" question, the story was left hanging—it was unclear to everyone present whether the story was judged to be fact or myth, important or unimportant.

FACT, OPINION, AND INEQUITY

Like all teachers, Mrs. Shane and Mr. Kelly had individualized relationships with, and views of, their students. These relationships and biases played a key role in how they made sense of which of the comments made in class were "facts" and which "opinions." Certain students could make any comment without being questioned, while others could not. That is, certain students were either consistently judged to be expressing opinions, and/or to be providing "correct" information, while others were not. These differences were more visible in Mrs. Shane's classroom than in other CSE classrooms I observed because she was so effective at creating an environment in which students felt free to speak up. However, these differences reflect tensions inherent in many CSE approaches, and indeed, in many classrooms throughout the United States.

Mrs. Shane's class was composed of thirty students, about equally divided between girls and boys. The class was diverse in terms of race, ethnicity, class, and students' physical development. With the exception of the English Learner (EL) classes in California, all of the classes that I observed in California, Florida, and Wyoming were primarily composed of white students, and student voices, when heard, were predominantly white. Not so at Fontaine, where the class was controlled by Theo, a high-status African American athlete who had a snappy comeback to every teacher comment; Cornell, an African American senior who was re-taking the class and who, between extensive under-the-table text-messaging activities, delivered spot-on commentary; and Shurita, a lower-status African American girl and her white friend, Julia, who lived together in a nearby housing complex and who both spoke up frequently, often sharing personal stories and commentaries. The classroom functioned largely as a series of exchanges among these four students and the teachers, with regular comments fairly evenly distributed among other students.

Though all four students were highly active in the class, the teachers' responses to their comments differed substantially. Mrs. Shane did not actively silence any student, but while she never challenged anything that Cornell said, and challenged Theo only once (when he made a comment she considered gang-related), she regularly challenged Shurita (for example, her challenge to the bleach story). As with the bleach story, her challenges to Shurita consistently questioned the veracity of Shurita's stories, even though the stories were often about Shurita's own family and neighborhood. Although these challenges did not appear to lessen Shurita's comfort with speaking to Mrs. Shane, and indeed Shurita and Mrs. Shane appeared to have a caring relationship, they did consistently position Shurita's comments as questioned by authority, while Theo's and Cornell's comments were not.

Similarly to Mrs. Shane, Mr. Kelly never challenged Cornell or Theo, and he actively defended Theo when he felt Theo was being questioned by other students. Mr. Kelly supported most other students who spoke in class, but he actively silenced and marginalized Shurita, as in the following example:

> The kids have been asked to rate their parents. Jihye says that her father lives in Korea and her mom doesn't have time for her and "just gets mad at me every day, but she's always there for my brother. She yells at me for not doing things, but she never yells at him." . . . Shurita nods her head during Jihye's story, and then says that her mom is always angry with her, too, and is always asking her to look after her younger siblings. Mr. Kelly jumps in, "Now, your relationship with your parents, it can be good or bad because of how you behave and the things that you are doing, too, so it's not always just their fault. I would say that in Jihye's case it's probably not her fault."

Mr. Kelly also made comments directed at other students that positioned Shurita as a second-class student, daughter, or woman. Over time, Shurita's behavior changed as a result of this response: when Mr. Kelly was leading the class, Shurita directed fewer comments toward the whole class, sometimes spoke directly to Mrs. Shane even when Mr. Kelly was leading the class, and sometimes began speaking to seatmates but not the whole class. We never saw these speaking patterns when Mrs. Shane was leading the class.

Teachers' gendered, raced, and classed responses to students and their differential judgments of the veracity and quality of student comments are certainly not unique to this class. There is an extensive literature on how student identities and teachers' perceptions of students' experiences and knowledge interact to shape students' school experiences,[6] and on the processes of othering that produce and reproduce inequalities in sexual scripts and classrooms (e.g., Schwalbe et al. 2000). Although the literature on teacher-student interactional inequities has seldom examined sex education as a class subject, there is also an extensive literature on teen sexuality, and particularly about the raced, classed, and gendered assumptions that shape public discussions of and responses to teens, and teens' responses to these sexual scripts (e.g., Stephens and Phillips 2003; hooks 1992). Assumptions about African American girls, such as that they are disruptive and commonly engaged in dysfunctional relationships, were evident in Mr. Kelly's responses to Shurita, just as were assumptions about Asian American girls' sexual and social naivete in his responses to Jihye.

The presence of both Mrs. Shane and Mr. Kelly in the same class provided important comparative insights into how teacher-student interactions can transform students' experiences and create or close opportunities for diverse students to speak comfortably in sex education classes. The fact that I did not observe enough teacher-student interaction in other sex education classes to examine and compare these dynamics across teachers and programs highlights the general silencing of students that I observed across ABSE and AOUME classrooms and programs and the work Mrs. Shane was doing to create opportunities for students to speak in her classroom.

EXPERTS IN THE CLASSROOM

Sex education classrooms are regularly permeated with outsiders brought in to provide their expertise about a particular topic. An examination of the effects of these outside presenters on students' engagement in class and on students' understanding of what constitutes expertise, opinion, and knowledge is important to understanding students' sex education experiences and to more carefully examining the effects of different instructor approaches on students' experiences.

In Wyoming, the teachers brought in "medical experts" (a doctor and a nurse) to talk about contraceptives and HIV/AIDS. Mrs. Shane also invited a number of outside speakers, but most of Mrs. Shane's experts were "identity experts": people who were HIV-positive, identified as queer, or had experienced sexual assault. Their expertise was based not on a claim of greater scientific knowledge, but of greater personal experience. This approach to expertise had the benefit of allowing students to ask speakers about their embodied experiences of HIV/AIDS, LGBTQ issues, and sexual violence. It also, in situations where the speakers displayed a lack of respect for equal human rights (e.g., sexism, homophobia) or a lack of scientific knowledge, further muddied the waters concerning fact, myth, fiction, and opinion.

Whereas in the Wyoming classrooms the presence of outside speakers did not particularly change classroom dynamics—students were already silent, and stayed silent during these presentations—in Wisconsin there was a marked difference in students' engagement with the outside speakers versus their regular teachers. The easy and open rapport students had with Mrs. Shane disappeared, and students seemed to adopt the role of critical, but largely silent, consumers. Their interactive style more closely resembled their engagement with videos than it did their engagement with Mrs. Shane or Mr. Kelly. With the exception of a presentation on rape (discussed in chapter 9), the classroom shifted from about 70 percent student voice to about 20 percent student voice, and the kinds of open questions that students regularly posed to Mrs. Shane were withheld (and often directed to Mrs. Shane later). For example, during the class session with an HIV/AIDS speaker, the following interaction occurred:

> The speaker says that there are three categories of ways that HIV/AIDS can be spread. He talks about mother-to-child transmission and blood-to-blood transmission. The students are quiet throughout this portion of the presentation. Then the speaker gets quiet and doesn't seem to know how to continue. He asks, "And the third?" The class responds, "Sexually." He then says, "Now, this could be awkward . . ." He says it haltingly and does, indeed, sound awkward. Theo speaks up: "We talk about sex enough in this class it's not awkward anymore." The speaker responds, "OK, yes, it's transmitted sexually . . ." Theo interjects: "Oral sex, anal sex, vaginal sex." The presenter seems shocked. "I've never heard anyone just say these three right out loud," he says. He then continues on, restating that he thinks the conversation about types of sex will be awkward. Theo and the rest of the class become entirely quiet, observing him.

The outside presentations threw into relief some of the contradictions in classroom practices concerning CSE approaches to scientific knowledge and CSE ideology concerning human rights and respecting diversity. Although the outside speakers at times said things to which Mrs. Shane was visibly opposed, and/or that were factually incorrect, Mrs. Shane never challenged them directly. This differed from her usual interactions in class, when she challenged Mr. Kelly and students if she felt they were giving incorrect information about which she was confident of her knowledge. For example, during Mr. Kelly's presentation on abortion, the following exchange took place:

> Julia says, "I heard that when you have an abortion you can hear it [the fetus] scream. Is that true?" Mr. Kelly turns to her and says, "I don't know about that . . ." Mrs. Shane interrupts him: "No," she says bluntly.

However, when Mr. Kelly was presenting his opinions, either in class discussions or in his selection of materials for the lessons, Mrs. Shane did not challenge him, allowing him the same opportunity to air his opinions that students and all outside speakers were granted. In the same abortion lesson, the following exchange occurred as the class discussed an extremely graphic handout on partial-birth abortion:

> Theo asks, "What's the difference between killing it [the fetus] with its head inside [the woman's body] or not?" Mr. Kelly answers, "My opinion is it's killing a baby either way." Mrs. Shane asks: "When is it a person?"

As she often did when students aired opinions with which she disagreed, Mrs. Shane did not challenge Mr. Kelly's stated opinion, but diverted the conversation toward a discussion of definitions and categories. In response to her interjected question, "When is it a person?" various students offered opinions about when life began, and all of these opinions were aired without comment.

In allowing everything said by all outside experts to pass without comment, Mrs. Shane's behavior could be understood by students to indicate that the presentations represented opinion, that Mrs. Shane felt the presentations were factually correct, or that Mrs. Shane wanted to be polite to guests (as she referred to them), which meant not questioning them. For students, Mrs. Shane's and Mr. Kelly's responses followed a different pattern: students and teachers had the right to air any opinion they wanted; claims to facts, however, could and should be challenged by the teacher if they were incorrect. As described above, student identity and positionality in the class played a key role in determining whether their responses were understood to be fact or opinion, and therefore whether they could be challenged. Thus, in practice, judgments about fact versus opinion, truth versus falsehood, were infused with the relations of power and authority that structured the classroom. Though diversity and self-discovery are ideological cornerstones of CSE approaches and were highly encouraged by Mrs. Shane, in practice, students learned that some people's opinions and knowledge were consistently more validated, or at least less disrupted, than others.

Conclusion

We have argued that the interactions and conversational patterns in Mrs. Shane and Mr. Kelly's classroom were shaped by a tension between CSE ideals of human rights and equality on the one hand and of scientific truth and rationality on the other. The process of translating these ideals into classroom interactions was influenced by relations of power and authority among teachers, students, and visitors, each of whom was marked by their age, gender, race, class, sexual identity, and life experiences. Similarly, the teachers' judgments of their students' capacity to make healthy decisions, to contribute usefully to the class's construction of knowledge, and to treat others fairly were based on the ideal of human equality, but in practice were always differentiated by the (raced, classed, gendered) social norms for "appropriate" behavior and sexual scripts that shaped their daily interactions with students (e.g., Ladson-Billings 1999; Zeichner 1998).

CSE teachers like Mrs. Shane face tensions between two ideals, and between each ideal and its practical ramifications, in their classrooms. While students in Mrs. Shane's classroom were afforded opportunities to emote that no other students I observed had, they were given few opportunities to critically examine issues or to debate what constituted "fact" versus "myth." Students received the message that, although opinions about sex and sexuality should always be valued, in the end there *was* one right way to understand a situation or question. For Mrs. Shane, this "right way" represented her particular reading of a body of scientific literature and of the sexuality norms promulgated by CSE; in Mr. Kelly's case, it represented his particular reading of a body of data largely considered unscientific and more aligned with an AOUME position than Mrs. Shane's. Mrs. Shane challenged students when she felt they were making "fact" claims that were incorrect, but when they were expressing opinions, she did not intervene because she wanted to keep them engaged and feeling empowered to express themselves. Because Mrs. Shane fostered open dialogue—a pedagogical approach aligned with CSE's ideological stance that students should be empowered with complete and correct information, and the tools to find this information—students in her class could and did question their own and their teachers' statements about "scientific" and social facts, but their challenges were neither addressed nor debated.

That our observation of Mrs. Shane's classroom could yield such rich information about some of the tensions in teacher-student interactions in CSE classrooms was itself due to Mrs. Shane deliberately fostering student questions, debate, and discussion. This environment was a much richer pedagogical, interactive, and democratic learning space than those created in Florida or Wyoming. It also, by providing space for student voices, revealed how teachers' own beliefs, ideals, and biases concerning teen sex and sexuality, as well as race, gender, class, and religion, transform the learning environment for students, creating opportunities for conversation and peer and teacher validation for some but not for others. These patterns raise questions about the facile assumptions common in the CSE literature that curricula, conversations, and interactions in CSE classrooms are empowering to all students. At the same time, they throw into sharp relief the deep student silencing created by AOUME's directive teaching approach.

Engaging Diversity: Sex Education for All in California

Sex Education at Jefferson High

Jefferson High is an old, well-established, and well-respected high school that, like many schools in California, serves an increasingly diverse student body. It is located in a politically liberal, ethnically, racially, and economically diverse neighborhood. The school had won numerous state and national awards for teaching excellence, parental involvement, and student performance. It had, at the time of my observations, a lower student-to-teacher ratio than the state average, numerous in- and after-school arts and sports programs, and an active parent organization.

Jefferson, and the school district in which it is located, had embraced the state's mandate to provide "medically accurate" sex education and to address issues of bullying and gender identity in schools. Conducting research at Jefferson therefore allowed me to better understand how sex education functions in practice when there is general policy alignment at the state, district, and community levels in support of CSE, and a perception of diverse community sociocultural beliefs and practices related to sexuality. Did alignment around CSE policies create an environment in which the school and teachers felt comfortable expressing CSE views without worrying about negative responses from officials or parents? Did instructors feel that the CSE programming approach (providing rational individuals with the same "complete and correct" information and teaching tolerance for diversity) was responsive to the needs of a diverse student body?

At Jefferson High, sex education was offered as part of the science curriculum. Although the classroom teachers were required to provide students with an introduction to reproductive biology before the sex education unit began, the sex education programming itself was provided by Come On In!, a private, nonprofit service organization. Come On In! offered a two-week CSE program to all of Jefferson's ninth-grade science classes. The program was free for the school thanks to funding that Come On In! received from private foundations and donors.

Come On In! is a self-described CSE "learning organization" whose central goal is to provide "science-based, comprehensive sex education" to adolescents, teachers, and parents in the region. It has won local and national awards for its work, and at the time of my observations provided CSE to hundreds of schools in the area annually. They had worked in Jefferson High for years.

While Come On In!'s instructors certainly aimed to maintain a good relationship with teachers and school administrators (if they did not do so, they would likely lose access to the school), their relationship with the school and the community it served was less direct than that of the school's teachers. This meant that they might be less constrained by concerns about negative responses to their programming than teachers might be, that they might more consistently and deliberately foster student discussion and debate in the sex education classroom, and that they might more directly engage with and address students' diverse beliefs about and experiences with sex and sexuality. I observed the two-week Come On In! program in four different science classes in order to explore these questions. To situate the classroom data, I conducted interviews with district education and public health officials, CSE and AOUME advocacy groups and service providers in multiple school districts around Jefferson High, and a number of other private CSE service providers in the same metropolitan area as Jefferson High.

Come On In! the Classroom

My observations of Come On In! classes at Jefferson provided an opportunity to examine the intersection of two important educational policy issues. First, Come On In! met the criteria of a "best practice" school-based sex education program (as defined by Kirby's [1997] meta-analyses) and identified itself as an "evidence-based" program. Second, Jefferson's student population embodied some of the most significant demographic trends occurring in US public schools in this decade: the typical US student is increasingly nonwhite, an English Learner (EL), and qualifies for free or reduced lunch. As in many of the schools with more diverse student bodies in the United States, Jefferson's internal academic-tracking system resulted in significant racial, linguistic, and class segregation among students throughout much of the school day.

Given that the Come On In! program was offered to all science class tracks, each composed of a demographically different student body, I was able to examine how student-instructor relations interacted with an "evidence-based" CSE program designed to be relatively uniform across classrooms. For example, did students in different science tracks have significantly different sex education experiences? If so, were these differences efforts to respond to different students' needs? Did these differences appear to render the program more or less effective? How did instructors balance the tension between addressing different students' needs and meeting the criteria that evidence suggested made Come On In! effective in changing students' behavior, on average?

One Come On In! instructor, Emily, taught three of the four classes that I observed: the mainstream higher-track science class, the 75 percent Spanish/25 percent English language class, and the 75 percent English/25 percent Spanish language class. A second instructor, Ginnie, taught the mainstream lower-track class, which I will not discuss here.

Jefferson's English language–education services primarily addressed the needs of its first-generation Latin@ population. Students with limited literacy skills worked one-on-one in the school's library with tutors to gain basic literacy and numeracy in their mother tongue. Students who arrived at the school already literate and numerate in a language other than English (most often Spanish) were tracked into a series of bilingual classes conducted in Spanish and English, which moved students from a 75/25 to a 25/75 Spanish/English class and then to a mainstream, 100 percent English instruction class. The EL classes, which covered material in all subjects, ran parallel to the mainstream courses. All of the mainstream and EL science classes participated in the Come On In! program.

School staff indicated that they invited Come on In! to provide sex education at the school because teachers had limited or no professional development opportunities in sex education, and they felt this was a topic better left to experts. The school had an attached health clinic and often invited in health professionals from the clinic to talk to students about health issues. Sex education was viewed as a health topic for which there was external expertise and that science teachers (many of whom did not have training in sex education) could easily farm out to a respected organization. Science teachers, who except for the EL teacher were not actively engaging with students during the Come On In! class sessions, appeared to use this time primarily to prepare future lessons and catch up on administrative duties. Unlike in Florida, school staff at Jefferson did not mention concerns about community responses as a reason for privatizing sex education; instead, they talked about levels of instructor expertise and interest and the availability of free, high-quality private providers.

The Come On In! program consisted of a collection of curricular materials and activities that instructors could use to tailor topics to their individual classrooms. The instructors made use of a variety of pedagogical approaches in the classrooms I observed: mini-lectures, small and large group discussions, and individual work; an anonymous question box; distribution of information pamphlets; and quizzes on local reproductive-health and human-sexuality resources. Many of these pedagogical tools were standardized across the classes and designed to provide students with opportunities to ask questions, talk with each other, and participate in student-led classroom activities. All four classes jointly attended a teen-mothers' panel (held in English). Other materials were developed by educators in response to particular groups' perceived needs. For example, Emily identified and used audiovisual and online resources in Spanish for the two EL classes; these resources were not used in the mainstream classes.

Instructor-Student Interactions across Classrooms

In California, I observed Emily interacting with three different groups of students. Building on the analyses conducted in the previous state chapters, these observations bring into sharper focus the central role that teacher-student interactions play in determining the official content, hidden curriculum, and classroom experiences of students. Because of these tensions, and as in Wisconsin, the observations revealed the tension in CSE programs among the ideals of respect for diversity, provision of "complete and correct" information, and rational individualism. As in Wyoming and Wisconsin, the Come On In! instructors did not create classrooms in which students' diverse experiences and needs were fully heard or incorporated into the programming, and they did not provide opportunities for students to construct or question the "facts" about sex and sexuality that were presented to them. This was more evident in California than in the other states because I could observe the same teacher try to address the needs of three different groups of students. In order to focus fully on these issues, in this chapter I will only discuss the three classrooms in which Emily was the instructor: the higher-track and the two EL science classes.

In the following sections, vignettes of Emily's three classes reveal the similarities and differences in the formal curriculum, pedagogical practices, and educator-student interactions that occurred across classes. Each class had about twenty-five students in it. The higher-track science class was composed primarily of students of Asian and Caucasian descent; the two EL classes were composed almost entirely of Latin@ students, although each class also had a few Pacific Islander students.

Emily's Spanish-language skills dated to rudimentary classes in high school; at the time of my observations, Come On In! lacked instructors fluent in Spanish.[1] Not having a Spanish-fluent educator may seem strange, considering the district and schools in which Come On In! worked, yet the program's resource constraints and lack of previous engagement with EL students mirrored the school's own constraints. Jefferson had only one bilingual education teacher. She reported not feeling confident in her mastery of all content areas, and she left at the end of the year because she felt "overworked and underappreciated." The year that I observed was the first one in which Come On In! was asked to work in the EL classrooms, and the organization was aware of the constraints Emily faced in communicating freely with students. Since my observations took place, Come On In! has hired Latin@ educators who are fluent in Spanish.

Above and beyond the language barrier, as the following vignettes show, there were significant differences in student experiences, questions, and ways of engaging with adults, fellow students, and course materials between the higher-track and the EL classes. These differences were central to shaping Emily's responses to students, and to students' opportunities to address their own questions and share their opinions about teen sex and sexuality.

THE HIGH-TRACK SCIENCE CLASS

Emily was a gifted instructor who built good rapport with all of her classes. Her teaching approach reflected the Come On In! program's goal of empowering students by providing them with "complete and correct" information, creating a classroom environment in which students would reflect on this information and its potential effect on their behavioral choices, and training students to search out additional knowledge and resources themselves. For example, Emily spent a significant amount of time ensuring that students were aware of local resources (school and community health clinics, websites, and so forth) they could access on their own. This, she told me, ensured that students were not dependent on any one adult for additional information about sex and sexuality. This was particularly important because the school's sex education services were privatized. The Come On In! instructors were only on campus for two weeks a year, and the students did not have structured conversations about sex and sexuality with any of their regular teachers.

Emily's emphasis on getting students to understand the scientific facts (that is, the "correct" information) about a subject, and on encouraging them to seek out additional information, was evident in nearly every activity undertaken in the classroom. For example, Emily ended each day by answering questions from the anonymous question box. One day, the questions included the following:

- How long does sperm live outside the body?
- Does sex hurt?
- Does childbirth hurt?
- Is there a certain time when it's best to get pregnant?
- Do diaphragms work against pregnancy?
- Can a father infect a baby with HIV without infecting the mom?
- Is putting a Nuva ring in and out painful?
- Why might you have delayed start of period?
- What is contraceptive foam?

All of Emily's answers reflected her emphasis on providing students with complete, scientifically validated, and "empowering" information so they could reach their own conclusions about these questions. For example, when answering the Nuva ring question, Emily said the following:

> No, it shouldn't be painful, and it's pretty easy to do. [She describes what people usually say about the ease of use.] Clinics will often let you practice while you are still there so that you can ask questions if you need to. So make sure you get help from them if you need it.

Her answers implicitly propounded the benefits of information-seeking behavior and of individuals making informed decisions based on their own analysis of information. This approach to understanding student empowerment is fundamentally different than that adopted by AOUME supporters, who conceptualize empowerment as arising from a moral transformation that provides students with absolute certainty concerning appropriate sexual behaviors and beliefs, and which, therefore, renders dangerous any conversation about sex and sexuality or search for additional opinions or information.[2]

Emily held many of the traditionally progressive views that AOUME advocates associate with CSE: she was supportive of equal rights for LGBTQ people and of girls' and boys' rights to choose (be it abortion, contraceptive use, or expression of sexual identity), and she did not view teen sex as only negative (though she viewed its outcomes as largely negative). These views also aligned (or at least were not in conflict) with California state legislation on sex education. They also appeared to generally align with the high-track students' views on these issues. In the high-track science class, then, perceptions of teen sex and sexuality were well-aligned from the state through the district, school, classroom, instructor, and, apparently, student levels. This resulted in a classroom environment in which neither instructor nor students appeared to feel constrained by concerns about external actors' responses to the Come On In! programming.

This lack of concern in expressing the values underlying Come On In!'s programming, and the sharp divergence in these values from those underlying AOUME programming, were evident in Emily's vocal support for equal group rights. For example, when answering the question about when it is best to get pregnant, Emily had the following interaction with students:

> EMILY: Life-wise, when do you think it's a good time to get pregnant?
> GIRL: When you're married or mature enough.
> EMILY: The last part of what you said is the best.
> BOY: You should probably be married.
> EMILY: What about gay or lesbian couples?
> GIRL: When you're in a committed relationship.
> GIRL: When you're financially set up.
> EMILY: Great. Now, if the question meant "when during the month," yes, there are times when you are more likely to get pregnant. [She reviews the ovulation cycle.]

In contrast to the teachers in Wyoming, when Emily felt that a student remark infringed on equal group rights claims, she challenged students in the higher-track science class to reconsider their answers, and students consistently reframed their responses to address her critique. Similarly, when students responded to a question in a way that, as she explained, "doesn't get at the decisions and situations they face," she pushed back, usually by providing students with facts that she felt should inform their views and then asking them to consider these facts in making their decisions. For example, in one class she asked students to comment on a scenario in which their best friend, a fifteen-year-old girl, is dating a twenty-one-year-old man who is pushing her to have sex. The students were told to assume they "have a bad feeling" about the guy and were asked if they would say anything to their friend. The students had strong and diverse opinions about how to respond.

> One girl said, "It says you have a bad feeling, and I trust my bad feelings. If she is really my friend, I need to talk to her." Emily replied, "I really like what you said. You trust your intuition—listen to that, it's good self-protection." Another girl said, "I wouldn't do anything, because my parents have a seven-year difference." Emily responded, "But remember, developmentally, what happens over time matters. Fifteen versus twenty-one is a big age difference at that stage of development." A boy jumped in: "Also, he may be kind of buying

her. It says he has a car, is buying her things. She's kind of powerless without a car." The second girl said again, "I don't think ages should matter." Emily responded: "OK, well, what is illegal between a fifteen-year-old and a twenty-one-year-old is having sex. If he really likes her and is not planning on having sex, is planning on waiting until she is eighteen,[3] OK. But most teen pregnancies happen between guys who are older and younger girls. So, it is really important to be educated about this and to think about why that's the case."

Emily's focus on providing students with information on the basis of which they would be better able to make their own decisions is itself an ethical stance, but not one that necessarily indicates equal comfort with all decisions. As McKay (1998) discusses, the liberal sexual ideology underlying this approach assumes, in fact, a relatively narrow range of acceptable decisions concerning sex and sexuality. So, for example, "scientific information" is constructed in such a way that choosing to become pregnant as a teenager, or choosing to have unprotected sex in anything other than a monogamous, committed, long-term relationship in which the couple is financially and emotionally stable is never presented as a good decision. In the above case, the scenario is designed to convince students of the dangers of teen sexual relationships in which one person is much older than the other. When a student pushes back against this message, Emily provides information that, she feels, should influence their understanding of the dangers of these relationships (i.e., that they result in higher pregnancy rates). She seems to expect that each student will be convinced of these dangers once they examine this information, but she does not ask students to conduct this analysis jointly, nor does she use students' own comments about power dynamics in relationships (such as that the man may be "buying" the girl in the scenario) to investigate why pregnancy rates might be higher in these relationships.

Emily's teaching style focused on engaging students in discussions about the issues that Come On In! (and most evidence-based CSE programs) feel are important for students' sexual health. These include decision making in relationships; the effects of pregnancy on future plans; the "plain facts" about STIs; basic knowledge about a range of contraceptive devices and their effectiveness in preventing pregnancy and/or STIs; information about post-pregnancy options (keeping the baby, adoption, abortion); and general information about sexual identity.

Come On In! and Emily made assumptions about what constituted these issues, their importance in teens' lives, and teens' common misconceptions about them. The assumptions were shaped by mainstream scientific studies and their conceptualizations of the problems and solutions these studies identified. They also reflect what Cahn and Carbone (2007, 2010) describe as a growing politically liberal paradigm for thinking about and forming families:

> With this new set of family values, emotional maturity and financial independence are the sine qua non of responsible family formation. In order to facilitate the investment in workforce potential of both men and women, it is critical to postpone family formation until education is complete and careers are established. Women's greater financial contributions to family income, in turn, require greater male socialization into more egalitarian and companionate relationships. Because marriage and childbearing are postponed until individuals are in their late twenties and early thirties, fertility control is critical: abstinence is unrealistic because of the long gap between puberty and marriage, contraception is not only permissible, but morally compelled, and abortion is the responsible fallback. (Cahn and Carbone 2010, 366–67)

In the higher-track science class, these assumptions, such as that getting pregnant as a teenager was always an undesirable outcome, or that teenagers would, with the right information, always choose to use effective contraceptive approaches, appeared to fit comfortably with students' own life experiences and expectations.[4]

Similarly, Emily's expectations for how students would interact with each other during classes appeared to be shared by the students in the higher-track science class; interactions took place largely during structured group activities and consisted of direct engagement with the materials and activities at hand. Students did not comment on each others' comments, did not speak without raising their hands, and seldom directed comments of any sort at each other unless prompted to do so by Emily or arranged into small discussion groups.

This alignment of cultural assumptions between instructor, curricular materials, and students was much less in evidence in the other three classes, and particularly in the EL classes, which raises important questions about how curriculum-teacher-student norms differentially shape sex education classroom practices, the formal and hidden lessons that students learn in these classes, and the utility of these lessons for students' daily lives.

THE ENGLISH LEARNER (EL) CLASSES[5]

As in the high-track science class, Emily appeared to have a good and comfortable relationship with the students in the two EL classes. Students would often approach her desk after class to ask questions, even though interactions were limited by her lack of Spanish fluency. Emily was well aware of this limitation and did everything she could to provide students with written and visual materials and additional resources in Spanish. She developed a system of writing down questions she did not understand, looking up words overnight, and providing students with answers the next morning. The Latin@ students appeared comfortable with this arrangement. The Pacific Islander students, who spoke neither Spanish nor English, did not participate in these conversations. They were similarly silent in classroom activities for all subjects.

In her EL classes, Emily covered many of the same topics and used some of the same curricular materials and activities as in the English-only classes. Other times, she substituted activities and materials that she felt would address students' experiences more directly (for example, introducing them to Planned Parenthood's Spanish-language website and showing an award-winning video produced by a Latina student about teenage pregnancy in high school). When Emily used the same activities as in the English-only classes, sometimes students in the EL classes responded to them in very different ways.

Many of the students in the EL classrooms were new to the United States, had different educational backgrounds than their peers in the English-only classrooms, lived in different housing and family settings, and were involved in relationships and communities marked by different sexuality, gender, and age norms than were assumed by the Come On In! curricular materials and instructors. One brief example of these differences provides a window into the assumptions underlying Come On In!'s program and most CSE programs. Come On In!'s founder told me that the year before my observations, Pacific Islander students in the mainstream science classrooms were insisting to instructors that if they followed the homework instructions and went home to ask their parents about sex, they would be beaten. Initially, the Come On In! instructors responded to their concerns as they did to white students who expressed concerns about talking to their parents: they told them that their parents might at first resist talking about a taboo subject, but they would in time be pleased that they could talk to their children about sex. Later in the year, because the organization felt that its programming was not successfully reaching Pacific Islander students, Come On In! organized a meeting with Pacific Islander leaders to learn more about the sex and sexuality issues facing teens in the community. They were told that the students had been correct in their assertion that bringing up sex with their elders could lead to harsh disciplinary measures. Come On In! attempted to address this by working with community leaders to create a parent sex-education program that addressed cultural taboos to discussing sex with children. They did not significantly change the programming offered to the students.

Come On In! was aware of and actively tried to engage in discussions with parents about the range of values, traditions, and beliefs they held concerning sex and sexuality. However, these interactions were designed to introduce the project's model of behavior change and convince diverse parents and communities of its benefits. Interactions did not aim to adopt a fundamentally different approach to sex education predicated on different values and beliefs. Take the example above: the ideological stance underlying Come On In! and most CSE programming is that open access to information and discussion about sex and sexuality is fundamental to improved sexual health. When students responded to materials and activities in a manner that indicated that they (or their families) did not hold these values, instructors tried to convince them of the importance of this approach. At the classroom level, when students expressed opinions that Emily assumed were influenced by a different sociocultural model of sexuality, individualism, knowledge, or scientific rationalism than those that undergird Come On In!, she seemed unsure of how to proceed. At times, these interactions threatened to destabilize Emily's control of the class—and her equanimity—and they significantly impacted the lessons that students learned about topics such as sexual identity and gender relations.

There were marked differences between many of the EL students' educational backgrounds and life experiences and the assumptions underlying Come On In!'s approach to sex education. This disjunction meant that, in the EL classes, students asked more questions, offered a wider range of opinions, and were in greater need of certain types of academic information in order to engage with the program's materials than were students in the higher-track science class. For example, students in the EL classes were much less familiar with school representations of human anatomy and biology than were students in the mainstream classes. A number of potential structural causes for these differences can be identified; for example, that Mexican schools many of the students had attended previously had not covered the material, that the school's one EL teacher was not a science expert, or that the EL classes covered course material differently and at a different speed than their mainstream counterparts.

Regardless of the cause, this lack of information led to very different classroom dynamics in the higher-track and EL science classrooms. For example, when Emily presented the causes of STIs in the higher-track class, she asked the students whether viruses have cures, and they answered "no." She asked them if bacterial infections have cures, and they answered "yes." From there, they worked together to categorize various STIs as caused by either bacteria or viruses, thereby identifying which had cures and which did not, and moved on to talk about STI prevention.

In the EL class, these same initial questions received a range of answers. Emily responded by giving a mini-lecture on bacteria versus viruses, followed by an explanation of what this meant for the treatability of infections. A number of students questioned why the distinction mattered; Emily responded by explaining the importance of categorizing the causes of infection in order to determine their proper prevention and treatment. The class session ended before Emily could talk about STI prevention.

Similarly, in the EL classes Emily's presentation on contraceptive use generated many more questions about human anatomy, and students had a harder time categorizing contraceptive methods in the manner that Emily and the curriculum desired. As in the high-track classroom, Emily had the EL students go around to different contraceptive stations and physically manipulate various contraceptive devices. While doing so, they were supposed to talk to each other and fill out a worksheet that indicated whether or not the device was a barrier method. As in the high-track classroom, Emily's presentation on the devices focused on the difference between barrier and non-barrier contraceptive mechanisms, and on the differences among barrier methods.

This is an important distinction from the perspective of getting students to understand the difference between prevention of pregnancy and prevention of STIs. There are studies indicating that teenagers are often confused about the efficacy of condoms versus other barrier and nonbarrier methods in preventing STIs such as HIV (e.g., ASHA 2005). Students in the EL classes, however, responded to the barrier/nonbarrier categorization differently than did students in the higher-track class. They talked about the contraceptive devices not as reproductive technologies to be categorized by mechanism, but as tools whose meanings and uses were always negotiated within relationships. Condoms were viewed as different than pills, for example, because of their social implications in relationships, not the mechanism through which they functioned. Following the class on contraceptive devices and their use, a group of girls from the 75 percent English/25 percent Spanish EL class approached Emily and told her that, once in a relationship that was considered serious and committed, they were no longer able to negotiate condom use, because asking their partner to use a condom indicated a lack of trust. Emily asked the girls a number of questions about why this was the case; the girls replied that, because they could use birth control pills, which were known to prevent pregnancy effectively, the only reason that a girl would be asking to use a condom was because she didn't trust her partner not to have an STI. (This trade-off between oral contraceptive use and condom use in long-term relationships is well documented around the world [e.g., Ott et al. 2002; Holland et al. 1998].) Emily tried to brainstorm with the girls about ways to encourage their partners to consider using a condom, but seemed unsure how to proceed when one of the girls said,

> Our culture is very *machista*. If we ask our boyfriends to use condoms, it's like we attacked them and questioned their honesty. So if we ask them, then they say, "So now you don't trust me?" and there are so many problems. They won't say yes.

The girls were pointing to the complex systems of power, authority, and trust that always shape relationships, and that render condom use in the age of birth-control pills a particularly difficult negotiation in many relationships. This issue is not unique to Latina girls at Jefferson High; women throughout the United States and the world have reported similar issues with condom negotiation. Condom use is linked to relations of power and gender inequity through discourses of distrust, disease, and pleasure, and specifically loss of pleasure for men. A growing recognition of the hurdles women face in negotiating condom use has led to global efforts to develop female-controlled contraceptive methods to protect women from STIs. It has also produced a growing body of evidence about the negative effects of gender inequity on women's sexual subjectivity and reproductive health.[6] The concerns of the girls in Emily's class about condom negotiation are therefore just as (or more) evident in the literature on contraceptive knowledge and use as the finding that adolescents are confused about the comparative efficacy of various contraceptive methods for preventing pregnancy versus STIs. The "scientific problems" taken up in Come On In! and many "evidence-based" CSE programs were not simply the most evident problems. They were the ones that were most easily addressed by an individual making an "informed" decision from a position of power and control over sexual engagement.[7]

What is included and what is excluded from "scientific inquiry" represents the assumptions, or hidden curriculum, of the program. In all of the CSE classrooms I observed, the problems most readily taken up by educators were those for which there appeared to be a simple solution: scientific categorization and "straightforward" information provision. The ones most often ignored were those caused by structural inequities (such as inequitable access to reproductive health information or services) and differences in power and authority within relationships.

This construction of the "problems" teens face with sex and sexuality points toward a set of difficult questions for CS educators: how to translate scientific facts (such as "condoms are protective against STIs and pregnancy, while pills are only protective against pregnancy") and categorizations (such as barrier/nonbarrier) into usable information for students; how to engage in difficult discussions about how scientific information can and should be translated in sexual relations and negotiations; and how to address the implications of factors such as power and emotion in CSE's assumed model of the rational, individual sexual decision-maker.

The girls' conversation with Emily also indicated that the scientific rationality and individual decision-making models propounded by CSE programs are unlikely to lead as readily as expected to changes in student behavior, perhaps particularly for students who share fewer of the assumptions underlying these programs or who actively reject them. Knowing that condoms reduce the risk of STI transmission may indeed help some students negotiate safer sex practices—perhaps particularly students who are involved in shorter-term relationships in which they feel they can actively advocate for their desires, demand use, and easily and without fear of reprisal walk away from the relationship—but this same information may not be as much help to students in relationships in which asking for condom use is viewed as an indication of a lack of trust.

The uses to which students can put information are always related to the personal relationships and social, political, economic, and cultural systems in which they live. These complexities were evident in Jefferson's EL classes because students' experiences of sex and sexuality differed from instructors' *and* because, unlike in AOUME programs, students had the opportunity to challenge instructors' assumptions about the utility of "school knowledge" about sexuality. Students' challenges were not taken up in the CSE programming, regardless of CSE's ideological support for recognizing and addressing diverse perspectives and needs, and regardless of whether social scientific studies supported students' experiences and concerns.[8] The lack of engagement with alternate scientific studies, findings, and framings that might better relate to the lives of more marginalized students (be they marginalized by language, ethnicity, race, class, sexual identity, experiences of sexual violence, or sexual desires) was consistent in all of the sex education programs I observed. This marginalization and lack of engagement occurred by ideological design in AOUME programs, but represented a fundamental tension among CSE's ideological tenets.

The emphasis in all of the CSE classes on categorization and on a scientific rationalization of teen sexuality was clearly revealed, in the EL classrooms, to draw upon a host of assumptions about students' previous educational experiences, ways of categorizing the world, and ways of thinking about individual agency. In the EL classrooms, students were vocal about the fact that the program's categorization of sex education issues was neither particularly familiar, nor always viewed as relevant. Not surprisingly, Emily regularly faced questions and student responses in the EL classes with which she was less familiar and comfortable than in the mainstream class. For example, Pedro, a soft-spoken boy newly arrived from Mexico to the United States, came up to Emily after one class, thanked her for a lesson in which Emily had discussed California's definition of rape, and told her his story about becoming sexually active at age eleven, when he had sex with a much older friend of the family. He wanted to know whether those early sexual encounters, which he described as pleasurable, were considered sexual assault, when "we were just playing around together."[9] For Emily, this was a difficult question, both because she was not aware of the laws governing rape and sexual assault in Mexico, and, she said later, because she did not want to label what might be acceptable "cultural practices" of which she was unaware with the cultural concepts that she and Come On In! took for granted in their programming (for example, that childhood sexuality is a taboo topic [e.g., Angelides 2004; Bullough and Bullough 1994], and that sex between a much older and younger person is always predatory). As with Come On In!'s response to the Pacific Islander leaders, Emily engaged Pedro fully, provided an opportunity for him to talk about his experience, and listened to it carefully, but did not address the issues to which it spoke in class.

Emily was also taken aback by some Latino students' extremely vocal responses to any mention of homosexuality in the class. For example, one of the videos that Emily also used in the high-track science classroom featured a self-identified gay character who talked about his experiences in high school. In the high-track class, the video was screened without a single comment; a number of students appeared to nod off or do other work during the showing. In contrast, in the 75 percent English/25 percent Spanish class, when it became clear that the character was gay, a number of the Latino students began to loudly declare, "Aw, man, no way!" and shout sexual epithets in Spanish. They were disruptive enough that Emily stopped the video, asked them to quiet down, and told them they needed to be respectful of all the people in the video and their classmates' desire to watch it. The boys protested, claiming that being gay was disgusting and that they didn't agree with it. Emily again told them that they needed to be respectful of everyone. This time, she added, "You know, some of your classmates may be gay, some of your family members are gay; you need to be respectful of everyone." The boys responded even more loudly to this assertion, saying that they knew that none of them were gay, and restating their disgust. During this exchange, most other members of the class remained silent. Emily paused for a moment, then repeated that the boys had to be respectful of everyone and that they had to let their classmates watch the video. The boys quieted down a bit, but continued to comment every time the gay character appeared on the screen. They created disruptions whenever sexual identity was discussed in the class, and over time, Emily introduced the topic less frequently.

This stood in sharp contrast to Emily's response to students in the higher-track classroom. When they made comments she found heterosexist or homophobic, she challenged them directly and with the apparent expectation that her challenge would make them reflect on and adopt the universal human rights norms that underlay Emily's and Come On In!'s approach to group rights and equality. Indeed, this was how the students in the higher-track science class responded. Whether they agreed with Emily's statements or not, they understood the response that she expected of them, and they adapted their comments to Emily's expectations.

As the growing body of research on sexual norms indicates, people's conceptualizations of sexuality are raced, classed, and gendered. Take, for example, Talbot's description (2008) of new research on sexual values and class, religious, and political differences among adolescents:

> Regnerus and Carbone and Cahn all see a new and distinct "middle-class morality" taking shape among economically and socially advantaged families who are not social conservatives. In Regnerus's survey, the teenagers who espouse this new morality are tolerant of premarital sex (and of contraception and abortion) but are themselves cautious about pursuing it. Regnerus writes, "They are interested in remaining free from the burden of teenage pregnancy and the sorrows and embarrassments of sexually transmitted diseases. They perceive a bright future for themselves, one with college, advanced degrees, a career, and a family. Simply put, too much seems at stake. Sexual intercourse is not worth the risks." These are the kids who tend to score high on measures of "strategic orientation"—how analytical, methodical, and fact-seeking they are when making decisions. Because these teenagers see abstinence as unrealistic, they are not opposed in principle to sex before marriage—just careful about it. . . . For this group, Regnerus says, unprotected sex has become "a moral issue like smoking or driving a car without a seatbelt. It's not just unwise anymore; it's wrong."[10]

This description of teen values associated with pregnancy, unprotected sex, and abstinence mirrored Come On In!'s materials and the discussions held in the high-track (and to some extent the lower-track) science classes concerning students' future plans. These same "universal" ideals were chal-

lenged by students in the EL classes, who argued that alternate norms or practices were "cultural" and therefore not intelligible within or accountable to
this value system. Emily appeared uncomfortable challenging students who
argued for an understanding of sexual practices and beliefs informed by what
appeared to be other cultural logics, but at the same time, she did not engage
with these logics as tools to reconsider Come On In!'s body of "complete and
correct information" and idealized sexual practices.

Engaging Students

DIVERSITY AND EQUAL TREATMENT

Come On In! instructors talked thoughtfully about the racial and ethnic divisions that existed in many of the schools in which they worked, and the
program deliberately tried to meet the needs of diverse students by learning
about and speaking to perceived sociocultural differences. Nonetheless, in
practice the program was largely predicated on middle-class, white, liberal
assumptions about healthy and unhealthy teen sexuality, and Come On In!
did not address the tensions that arose among the program's norms and values concerning scientific knowledge, universal equality and rights, and respect for diversity.

The Come On In! educators were particularly challenged when students'
life experiences or beliefs differed sharply from their own; all of the Come On
In! instructors I met, including Emily, were white and came from middle-
class backgrounds. They were open about their own backgrounds and encouraged students to view each person's experiences as unique and equally
valid. But, in practice, the CSE ideal of valuing diverse views and opinions
conflicted with instructors' beliefs about scientific rationality and correct
sexual decision-making. The California observations revealed some of the
ways that instructors' and students' interactions were affected when students
who adopted different norms of "doing school" (Pope 2003) and whose experiences of sex and sexuality had been shaped by different sociocultural and
political economic contexts than those assumed in Come On In!, most mainstream CSE programs, and all AOUME programs.[11]

Emily appeared uncomfortable challenging student claims that a particular belief or practice was "cultural," and let student statements about "their
own" practices stand without challenge, even when they violated program
principles concerning universal human rights. We saw similar opportunities
for students in the Wyoming and Wisconsin classrooms. Only in the case of

LGBTQ group rights did Emily seem to feel comfortable questioning students, and even then, her challenges to students varied. While the higher-track science class students were asked whether they supported specific legal inequities for groups (such as denial of the right to marry) and were pushed to consider the legal ramifications of not including one group of people in a supposedly universal right, in the EL classes Emily merely asked students to be respectful of all people and of their classmates' educational experiences by keeping quiet about their feelings. She did not attempt to change their views once they were framed by the students as "cultural," nor did she strongly sanction their behaviors as she did in the higher-track class.

LINKING INDIVIDUAL DIVERSITY TO STRUCTURAL INEQUITIES

Just as the Come On In! instructors appeared unsure of how to address the role that differences should play in moderating universal human rights claims, they and the program materials were also unable to link students' experiences and future aspirations to structured inequities. The instructors argued for each individual's right to information and each individual's responsibility to use that information to improve their sexual decision-making. But these assumptions did not reflect all students' experiences equally well. For example, instructors did not talk about the systematically inferior access non-English speakers and low-income teens in the United States have to quality reproductive health care, though they did say that teens could find out if they qualified for special programs that help teenagers pay for confidential medical services. They talked about the importance of using condoms and each person's right and responsibility to engage in safer sex, but they did not talk about how to negotiate condom use in relationships, assuming instead a model of two equally empowered and rational actors discussing and agreeing upon contraceptive use. They did not talk about sexual violence. They did not talk about sexual scripts, or engage students in discussions about how such scripts and stereotypes affected their own sense of self or their relationships with others. They talked about the deleterious effects of teen pregnancy on girls' and boys' lives, but did not talk about how race, gender, class, and extended family networks interact to shape teens' decisions about and experiences of pregnancy and parenting.[12]

This lack of engagement with structural inequities and relational dynamics affected the sex education that all students received, and at times resulted in the CSE instructors sounding remarkably like AOUME instructors. For example, at one point Emily had the following conversation with her class:

EMILY: Which is the most risky type of sex?

GIRL: Vaginal.

EMILY: No, anal is actually the riskiest. Why do you think this is the case? [No response.] The vagina is a very elastic part of the body and has natural lubricants, so it's not as likely to tear. The anus has erogenous tissue, so it's normal to have sexual feelings when it's touched, but it's not designed for penetration. It's more likely to rip and tear, so it's really important that you use lube and protection. The tears aren't even visible, but they are there. A person receiving a penis has a 1 in 50 chance of becoming infected [with HIV] in a single encounter. With vaginal penetration, it's more like 1 in 1,000 or 1 in 10,000. It's not about who we are, it's about which behaviors we choose. How can we make each type of sex safer?

This discourse about the dangers of sex not being "about who we are" but about "which behaviors we choose" is almost word for word the argument used by AOUME groups as evidence that they oppose LGBTQ identities on health-related, not moral, grounds. Emily made almost the same statement to counter student assumptions that (1) being gay is "risky" and (2) only gay kids are having anal sex, but the overlap in her words and those of AOUM educators reflects the fact that Come On In! did not directly address the wide-spread heteronormative or homophobic discourses that shaped Emily's need to claim that "it's not who we are" that creates risk, or students' (often incorrect) assumptions about what types of sex are risky and how risk might be reduced.

Conclusion

CSE approaches value universal models of the rational individual and of scientific truth, which lead, conceptually, to a belief that all students should receive the same "complete and correct" CSE programming. What constitutes "complete and correct" information in CSE programs is determined in relation to Enlightenment ideals of rationality, science, and truth. CSE approaches are also shaped by support for universal human rights and progressive and politically liberal ideals related to multiculturalism and respect for diversity, which lead to a desire to acknowledge difference and provide programming that meets the diverse needs of students with different life experiences, language capacities, sociocultural norms, economic backgrounds, and so forth. This tension between starting from a point of people's differences and recognizing diversity, and models of singular scientific truth premised on a particular sociocultural model, was particularly evident at Jefferson high school.

As Reiss, quoted in McKay, says about CSE approaches to sex education, "Pluralism is surely not saying 'just say yes.' If there were a slogan for pluralism, it would be: 'choose wisely'" (Reiss 1992, 219, in McKay 1998). As we see in Emily's and Mrs. Shane's classrooms, the notion that the provision of complete and correct information about sex and sexuality would empower students to "choose wisely" functioned in practice on the assumption that educator and student views of what constituted wise decisions would align more closely as a result of the information students received in class.

The programs I observed largely reflected white, middle-class, adult, liberal, straight mores and sexual norms, and did not question their own beliefs and biases about teen sexuality and its consequences.[13] When students pushed back against these assumptions with claims of different cultural beliefs and practices, Emily and Come On In! tried admirably to negotiate this new territory and provide equitable, effective, and relevant sex education to all students, but they only partially succeeded. For example, Latin@ students' experiences and future plans were not validated as often as those of non-Latin@ students. Nonwhite students experienced more peer policing of gender and sexual identities in sex education classrooms (visible in a comparison of the higher- and lower-track science classrooms), without significant push-back from instructors. Structural inequalities not related to LGBTQ rights—especially those involving gender equity—were reframed as individual hurdles to be overcome, or "cultural" issues that could not be addressed by instructors.

The California research raises questions about how to promote more democratic and socially just sex education approaches, both through addressing tensions within CSE ideals and through addressing the broader inequities within which schools and students operate. In my observations, the experiences of individuals and groups marginalized racially, ethnically, linguistically, sexually, by class, or by gender in every school challenged the assumption that the values underlying CSE were equally inclusive of and responsive to all students.

Students in California enjoyed many more opportunities to talk about sex, raise questions and engage in debate, and question the values underlying CSE programs than did students in Florida and Wyoming. These opportunities to talk are essential to building more democratic schools and classrooms (e.g., Hess 2009), and it must again be emphasized that these opportunities existed only in CSE classrooms—not in AOUME classrooms. Nonetheless, this freedom remained bounded by systems of racial, class, gender, sexuality, and linguistic power and authority that differentially distributed these opportunities. And although California's program and instructors pushed many boundaries compared to the other programs I observed, their strong emphasis on the individual as a rational being who has complete control over her or his own decisions remained unreconciled with issues of inequity and power in sexual relationships and broader social systems.

CSE programs' assumptions of rational individualism and evidence-based decision-making are problematic because sex and sexuality are fundamentally about relationships and the social, economic, cultural, political, and legal systems in which they occur. These assumptions are particularly problematic for students who, for various reasons, are less interested in or able to adopt this rationality, which is itself raced, classed, and gendered/ sexed. Unlike in Florida and Wyoming, students in the Wisconsin and California programs had an opportunity to talk about their diverse backgrounds, experiences, and living situations, and to ask questions about sex. But these realities disappeared when CS educators started providing "complete and correct" information to students. EL students' protestations, and their efforts to get Come On In! instructors to acknowledge, value, and help them think through and transform the relationships through which their sexuality was constituted, were met with earnest rational individualism and concern about respecting diversity.

Ultimately, the ideological underpinnings of CSE require that programs be responsive to, and therefore help address, diverse student needs and experiences. This is a much harder ideal to meet than simply providing the same scientifically rationalized, "complete and correct" information to all students, or for that matter, the same morally rationalized information. It requires instructors to address their own assumptions and biases concerning what counts as important, complete, and correct information and sexual decision-making. It also requires pedagogical approaches that provide more space for students and instructors to debate, discuss, and disagree in classrooms—the kind of pedagogy that, as we saw in Wyoming, takes the most time to foster and is considered the most dangerous for sex education teachers. Jefferson High's programming points to the possibility of CSE policy alignment making this pedagogy possible, but also points to some of the limits of current CSE models.

PART TWO

Macroanalyses of Sex Education

Morality Tales: Adolescent Desire, Disease, and Fertility in Sex Education Programs

All sex education is a morality tale, shaped by the ideology of the official sex education policy and curriculum and the settings and relationships within which the program is implemented. In the United States, sex education's morality tales are most often directed at the "problems" of teen pregnancy and sexually transmitted infections (STIs). This is not surprising, as it was in response to the teen pregnancy and STI (particularly HIV) epidemics of the 1980s that many sex education programs were launched by states. STIs and pregnancy shape both the topics covered in sex education programs and the key outcomes against which sex education programs are evaluated—increased age of sexual debut, increased use of contraception, decreased number of partners, and so forth.

Understanding teen pregnancy and STIs as important problems that can and should be addressed by sex education programs may seem so common-sense as to be unquestionable. But there are three issues concealed by this common sense, which this chapter will explore. First, as Apple (2006), Ball (1990), Cochran-Smith (2005), Stone (2001), and others remind us, there are no purely objective or scientific mechanisms through which policies and their associated practices are determined; all policy is political. STI and pregnancy rates are not the only outcomes that could be measured to judge the worth or effectiveness of sex education, but they are the key outcomes to which both CSE and AOUME programs in public schools are now oriented. This chapter will explore the shared construction of pregnancy and STIs as the most dangerous problems linked to teen sex in all mainstream sex education programs I observed.

Second, the chapter will explore the ascendancy of an effectiveness model focused on individual health outcomes (such as STI and pregnancy rates).

This model marks a shift from earlier debates among CSE and AOUME supporters, which were categorized by scientists and CSE supporters as "fueled by strong beliefs and convictions of right and wrong and . . . [leaving] little room for an impartial assessment of the facts and a definition of pragmatic goals" (Ehrhardt 1996, 1525). Though fierce battles still rage, an "evidence-based outcomes" framework is now taken for granted in the evaluative talk of "liberal" and "conservative" sex educators alike.[1] This framework validates a small list of scientifically rationalized, individualized, easily measured outcomes that are touted by many policy makers and sex educators as the outcomes by which all sex education programs should be judged.[2] As with the identification of STIs and pregnancy as the most significant problems related to teen sex and sexuality, agreement on evidence-based outcomes frameworks as the most appropriate way to understand the effects of sex education should not be taken for granted as the only or best approach. In fact, as discussed in the chapter conclusion, this framework drives sex education programs in directions that may be unwelcome to many CSE and AOUME supporters as well as teens, their families, and their schools.

Lastly, this chapter will explore the effects of these shared frameworks on classroom sex education experiences and school environments, which offer a powerful lens through which to view key components of the differing morality tales CSE and AOUME programs are telling, and to begin to map some of the unintended consequences of these tales on students and schools.

"Official" Sex Education Outcomes

Sex education policies and programs are largely framed as responses to two core health threats to teens: STIs and pregnancy. But the conceptualization of teen pregnancy as a health problem and teen STIs as a serious health threat is relatively new and represents a significant narrowing of the official concerns of sex educators. Many sex education instructors and activists first became involved in sex education because they hoped to accomplish much broader goals. These broader goals are still evident in AOUME programs' talk about the spiritual, psychological, emotional, social, and economic outcomes of teenage sex and sexuality, and in the sex-positive guiding frameworks of some CSE programs and organizations.

PUBLIC HEALTH OR HOLISTIC WELL-BEING?

The shared emphasis in AOUME and CSE programs on STIs and pregnancy as the greatest risks to teen health reflects important similarities across

AOUME and CSE approaches in their framing of teen sexuality as dangerous, teen sexual health as precarious, and teen parenting as an individual failure and social ill. It also raises an important difference. While CSE approaches have largely centered official health outcomes in their understanding of sex education and the problems it is attempting to solve, AOUME approaches have not. The CSE programs and curricula that I observed in public schools largely ignored earlier discussions within the CSE movement about desired moral, social, emotional, relational, and other outcomes, and CSE advocates seldom argued that the effectiveness of sex education programs should be judged by standards other than individualized health outcomes, measured through methodologically rigorous experimental or quasi-experimental studies. Students were understood as rational individuals in need of complete and correct information about teen sexuality, including the skills to learn more about these issues on their own. Individual behavior change would result from teens incorporating this information into their planning and actions and making smarter choices.

[handwritten margin note: this often isn't true teens are emotional not always rational cultural]

In contrast, AOUME supporters who operate in public-school settings have adopted the discourse of sexual health-based outcomes and evidence-based decision-making in their official materials, but AOUME supporters and their curricula continue to understand sex education as a response to a moral, not public health, crisis. For example, while AOUME supporters in Florida publicly rationalized their programs in relation to health outcomes like STI and pregnancy rates, the trainings I attended and curricula I reviewed conceptualized these physical outcomes as the result of teens making *immoral*, not unhealthy or irrational, choices. These negative health outcomes could only be addressed through a transformation of youths' values concerning sex outside of marriage, which would lead to changes in their behavior. Young people were not rational actors in need of more information, they were teens who needed to embrace a belief system that would transform every aspect of their lives, including their sexual health. Indeed, most of the AOUM educators with whom I spoke had been moved to participate in AOUME because they were concerned about the *nonphysical*, particularly spiritual, effects of (premarital) teen sex.

A classroom activity suggested by the trainer in Florida's advanced AOUME educator workshop illustrated this focus on the nonphysical outcomes of sex in AOUME programs:

> So, here is a great way to show kids the danger of condoms, thinking that they will make sex OK. First, open a condom and put it on your thumb. [He does so.] Then hold out your hand. [He does so, fingers up, then begins to address an imaginary classroom.] "So, people say that a condom will protect you. But

how can a condom protect you from the social, emotional, psychological, and spiritual aspects of sex? [He ticks off one uncovered finger for each consequence.] It can't. A condom can't protect your heart or your soul. It's not going to stop kids from whispering about you. They say condoms protect you, at least physically, but actually condoms don't even do that well. [He turns his thumb upside down, and the condom slides off. He then removes a latex glove from his pocket and begins putting it on]. Abstinence is like this glove, though. Abstinence is the only protection for your body, heart, and soul. Abstinence protects every part of you. A condom can never do that.

Florida's "It's Great to Wait" teen rallies similarly decentered the physical outcomes of sex. Speakers talked about the emotional effects of not being virgins when they married, the public shaming faced by sexually active teens, and their own sense of having lost themselves spiritually by engaging in sex before marriage.

AOUME approaches talked about health outcomes only when such talk provided support for their ideological position. For example, every AOUME program I observed emphasized CDC-published condom-failure rates to support their public argument that abstinence equaled "risk elimination," whereas condoms provided only "risk reduction." Reduction of STI and pregnancy rates is not a reasonable concept to AOUME supporters, because it is the sex act itself that is immoral. All sex before marriage is inherently dangerous and wrong, and the moral risk can never be reduced. In contrast, all talk of sex after marriage was glowing and full of pleasure; no AOUME program presented any information about the risks of STI transmission or unwanted pregnancy after marriage because such discussion would be ideologically flawed. Since sex within marriage is morally acceptable, these unwanted health outcomes are not in and of themselves a problem.[3] They may represent additional moral failures (for example, an adulterous spouse), but these failures should be understood as such, not as public health issues best addressed through nonmoralizing, nondirective health interventions and education.

We see, then, that the construction of the problem that sex education is meant to address differs between CSE (teen sexual health) and AOUME (teen morality), as does the type of teen actor assumed (rational individual in CSE, irrational consumer in AOUME).

TEENS AS FUTURE SEXUAL ACTORS

All the AOUME and CSE curricula that I reviewed displayed a similar understanding of teens as *becoming*, rather than *being* sexual actors. This is a common way of thinking about children in Western legal, political, and social theorizing,[4] and is fundamental to understanding why CSE and AOUME classrooms alike consistently downplayed students' experiences, normed a particular ideal of childhood and of families that does not reflect the reality of many teens' lives, and stigmatized teen sexuality and all signs of sexual activity (including STIs and pregnancy), even though such stigmatization might actually negatively affect teens' health and well-being.

Both also reflected the assumption that individual teens *choose* when and how to address these risks. Teens are responsible for their own sexual decision-making, but as people who are rightfully *becoming* sexual actors, there is only ever one responsible decision to make: wait. In both AOUME and CSE programs, STIs and pregnancy were framed as the price teens paid for not waiting.

STIs

STIs constitute one of the key public health arguments used to rationalize the provision of sex education in schools. The AOUME and abstinence-based programs and, to a lesser extent, the CSE programs that I reviewed all adopted what is commonly called a "fear-based" approach to teaching about STIs. The rationale that educators gave for employing this approach was that students were unaware of the risks posed to them by the teen STI pandemic and had to be scared into acknowledging these risks. Indeed, students in every class I observed expressed shock upon hearing that one-fourth of all adolescents have an STI at any given point in time (Forhan et al. 2009), and they were largely unaware of the threat that STIs might pose to their health and reproductive capacities.[5]

The framing of STIs as horrifying diseases resonates deeply for many people around the world. For centuries, STIs have been fearful killers, and even today the effects of some STIs are long lasting and life changing. However, adopting a fear-based approach means that teachers and curricula cannot emphasize three important points: first, that the vast majority of people will have an STI during their lifetimes; second, that most of the STIs contributing to high teen STI rates are not only fully treatable, they have no significant health consequences *if treated in a timely manner*; and third, that stigmatizing STIs and those who have them makes it harder for people to quickly and easily receive preventative care or treatment for STIs. In other words, from a public health perspective, fear-based approaches that do not emphasize prevention *and* treatment and that do not address the negative consequences of stigmatizing people with STIs are likely to be less effective and to have unintended negative consequences.

Although most CSE and AOUME programs are now framed in public health terms, their fear-based approaches to discussing STIs make it difficult for them to reflect best public-health practices. In my research, this was particularly true of AOUME and ABSE programs. While this understanding of STIs may seem like the only reasonable response, it is useful to reflect for a moment on the health outcomes associated with STIs and to compare these to other potential threats to teen health. Chlamydia and gonorrhea, two STIs that are more common in teens than in adults, are both fully treatable with antibiotics, and if treated quickly have no long-term effects. The same is true of syphilis, once a feared killer. It is only if they are *not* treated that these infections may lead to pelvic inflammatory disease, infertility, cervicitis, meningitis, septicaemia, and mother-to-child transmission of the STI.

Other STIs, such as the human papillomavirus (HPV) and herpes, are not curable and are quite prevalent in the US population. For example, one in five Americans over twelve is estimated to be infected with the herpes simplex type 2 virus (National Institute of Allergy and Infectious Diseases 1998). Although the potential effects of HPV and herpes are not insignificant, few people will have long-term negative physical effects if they receive proper treatment and screenings; the number of people who do suffer long-term health consequences would decrease significantly if the HPV vaccine were widely accepted and Pap smears were provided at low or no cost to all women in the United States.

To put the risks that the most common STIs pose to students' health in perspective, HPV is described in AOUME curricula as the most dangerous STI because it is associated with many of the cases of cervical cancer in the United States. The American Cancer Society estimated that in the United States in 2009, 11,270 women would be diagnosed with cervical cancer and 4,070 would die from it. Significantly, most of the deaths would occur in women who had not received a Pap smear in at least five years prior to diagnosis, as cervical abnormalities can often be effectively treated before they become cancerous.

In contrast, from 1999 to 2004, almost 9 percent of young adults reported having had major depression, generalized anxiety disorder, or panic disorder in the previous twelve months. On average, 4,400 teens (aged 15–24) commit suicide each year in the United States (CDC 2011)—more than the number of people of all ages who die of cervical cancer. In 2005–6, 24 percent of young adults (eighteen to twenty-nine years old) were obese, a major cause of later-life diabetes and heart disease. The 2005 Youth Risk Behavior Survey found that almost 11 percent of girls and over 4 percent of boys in a nationwide high-school survey (grades 9–12) reported having been forced to have sex previously (Eaton et al. 2006). In comparison, then, HPV poses a minimal risk to teen sexual health, and its negative outcomes occur largely within and because of systems of structural inequity that negatively affect health prevention and treatment for teens, particularly low-income teens. In 2006, 34 percent of young men and 25 percent of young women reported having no health insurance, which in turn limited their access to services such as Pap smears, mental health care, and STI treatment (CDC 2010b).

No sex educator compared the risks of contracting a STI to the risks posed by other teen "epidemics," nor did they relate these risks to one another (for example, how forced sex, STIs, depression, and drinking may interact). They did not explain the key role that preventive health care plays in significantly lowering the risks posed by STIs, nor did they talk about why many teens cannot easily access such care. Instead, educators focused on categorizing STIs and their symptoms and emphasizing the potentially serious effects of untreated STIs. In CSE classrooms, instructors also emphasized that it was important for individuals to get tested and treated for STIs so that they could avoid these long-term consequences, and in urban areas, they provided students with information about free clinics where they could get tested and treated. AOUME materials and trainings emphasized that condoms do not protect against STIs, only abstinence does. They seldom discussed testing and treatment, and often presented the risks associated with STIs as those of a late-stage, untreated STI. In all cases, educators described the causes and appropriate responses to STIs as individual ones: all teens should make the personal decision to not have sex before marriage, or if they must have sex, they should talk openly to their partners about STIs and seek out testing and treatment.

HIV

HIV is the obvious exception to the argument that STIs could, and perhaps should, be presented to adolescents as infections to be avoided when possible, but that are common and treatable or controllable if teens have access to health care. AIDS significantly shortens people's life spans, and it significantly affects their quality of life. HIV cases are on the rise: in 2009, the CDC reported that there were 48,100 (CDC 2012) new HIV cases in the United States, and in 2009 39 percent of all new HIV cases in the United States occurred in young people under the age of twenty-nine (CDC 2011).

CSE programming on HIV/AIDS differed significantly from AOUME programming in a number of important ways. CSE programs claimed HIV was the most fearsome STI and emphasized that students needed to understand how HIV infection occurs, how it can be prevented (abstinence or consistent, correct condom usage), and which activities do not pose a risk of transmission (sharing plates, tears, saliva, and so on). AOUME programs emphasized the fearfulness and prevalence of HPV and its link to cervical cancer and claimed that condoms were ineffective in preventing HPV transmission because it can be transmitted through skin-to-skin contact. AOUME programs deemphasized HIV, sometimes saying it was an uncommon STI.

CSE, but not AOUME programs and curricula, addressed the stigma and fear that HIV-positive people often face when other people are not aware of how HIV can and cannot be transmitted. CSE programs also tried to have students associate real people with the disease, through videos or by bringing in HIV-positive speakers. This made the disease, the effects of stigma, and the ability to live positively with STIs "real" to students in a way that the paper-based explanations of other STIs likely did not.

These differing programmatic responses to HIV indicate key aspects of the morality tales told by CSE and AOUME programs. CSE responses to HIV were shaped by the health dangers posed by HIV, the public health knowledge gleaned during the 1980s and 1990s about HIV transmission and the importance of minimizing the stigma associated with having AIDS (Ryan White being a key example), and by the campaigns organized by LGBTQ activists and their allies in support of the rights of people living with HIV/AIDS. This response mirrors CSE's dual ideological focus on scientific rationality and universal human rights.

In contrast, AOUME responses to HIV were shaped by their commitment to abstinence as the only morally acceptable response to the dangers posed by sex outside of marriage. Because HIV is quite effectively prevented through consistent and correct condom usage, it needed to be downplayed. Instead, AOUME programs emphasized the dangers of HPV, a disease that is very widespread, can be linked to cancer (but that compared to HIV poses minimum health risks), and is less effectively prevented through condom use. The extent of AOUME's focus on abstinence as a moral stance, regardless of its health implications, is clear in AOUME advocates' rejection and stigmatization of the HPV vaccine, which they feared would make girls more likely to feel they could have sex without negative consequences. The stigmatization of STIs and those who had them is therefore an aspect of AOUME's fear-based curriculum; it is a social consequence that should scare teens into sexual inactivity.

STIGMA

The consequences of a fear-based, individualized approach to teen STI prevention are evident in the public health literature. As Fortenberry (2004) notes in discussing genital herpes,

> Many aspects of sexual behaviour are associated with stigma, the key one being the judgment that sexual behaviour is non-obligatory and volitional, and therefore subject to social attributions of cause and responsibility. For example, sex is considered to be a 'choice', and therefore responsibility for STIs such as genital herpes rests on the person who has chosen to have sex. Personal responsibility is often identified as an attribute of stigmatized conditions—genital herpes is viewed as the 'stain' that links a person to an undesirable characteristic (in this case, irresponsible sexual behaviour). (p. 8)

The stigmatization of "bad" sexual decision-making underlies both AOUME and CSE STI programming. Some AOUME curricula go so far as to encourage this stigmatization; for example, after presenting information about STIs that appears to correlate increased condom usage with increased STI infection, the nationally distributed AOUME curriculum, Project Reality's *Navigator*, instructs teachers that correct student answers to questions about the full range of STI effects include: "[A viral STI] would make it difficult because the person that I would want to marry may not want to marry me because of the herpes. . . ." and "Not only would the STIs cause physical health problems, but they would also affect the way I think and feel about myself. . . ." (Gray and Phelps 2003, 43).

Both AOUME and CSE curricula and instructors validated a narrow spectrum of "good" sexual decision-making. Because they assumed that individuals always choose whether and how to have sex, they validated the assumption that individuals can and should be blamed for behavior that leads to contracting STIs. They elided such issues as gender and social inequities, sexual violence, access to testing and treatment, and the complexities of negotiating trust in relationships, as well as the moral and public health hazards of stigmatizing people who have STIs. For example, I never heard an instructor talk about the rates of forced sex in the United States, despite the fact that in 2002, 21 percent of surveyed US women eighteen to forty-four years of age reported having been forced to have sexual intercourse before they were thirty years old (Chandra et al. 2005). I saw only three efforts to destigmatize STIs in any of the classrooms or curricula that I observed (all three in CSE classrooms and related to AIDS).[6] Having or having had an STI is the norm, not the exception, in the US adult population, and there is a large US and international public-health literature on how stigma affects people's efforts to seek diagnosis and treatment for STIs. By not addressing the stigma associated with STIs, sex educators increase the chances that adolescents, particularly girls and marginalized youth, will not seek treatment for, or speak to others (including doctors) about, STIs.[7]

As a consequence, AOUME and CSE programs decoupled discussions of STI transmission from the following:

1   Issues of choice, negotiation, and control over sexual interactions and relationships.
2   The realities of teens' restricted access to health care services, which in turn greatly affects the chances that an STI will go untreated and have life-changing consequences.
3   An honest discussion about how common STIs are and how damaging stigma and silence about them are to people's well-being.

Lastly, in every sex education class I observed, conversations about STIs were predicated on "traditional," socially conservative sexual norms and social ideals and were fully provincialized to the United States. No effort was made to address global or local trends and consequences of STI epidemics, cultural differences in sexual or gender roles and expectations, or international health guidelines concerning sexual and reproductive health. This was true even in classrooms where many students had recently immigrated to the United States. While sex education teachers might have little interest or time to spend on these broader issues, many students in the classrooms I observed were directly affected by them. By provincializing discussions about STIs, CSE instructors lost leverage to talk to students about what we know is happening and what we know works in the prevention and treatment of STIs around the world. There were no opportunities for students to learn about and debate why there are such different rates of STIs and pregnancy among youth in the United States versus other countries, or how and why STI transmission patterns differ so much in different places for different people.

Pregnancy

PREGNANCY AS A PROBLEM

The construction of teenage pregnancy as a social ill is relatively recent, dating back only to the 1950s–1970s.[8] Nonetheless, as with STIs, teen pregnancy was consistently discussed as a problem across all sex education programs. CSE

and AOUME programs alike assumed that teen pregnancy was usually unwanted and that when it was wanted, this indicated pathological behavior on
the part of the teens in question. The programs assumed teen pregnancy naturally had negative effects on girls, boys, their babies, and society. Though this
may seem like a commonsense argument, presenting pregnancy as a purely
negative health and social outcome does not acknowledge the particular (gendered, raced, and classed) conceptualizations of childhood, adolescence, and
fertility that underlie this construction, the brevity of these assumptions on a
historic scale, or the effects of these assumptions on school, government, family, and community responses to pregnant or parenting teens.[9]

The policy construction of teen pregnancy as a social ill assumes that children are innocent and not sexually experienced, and that "modern" adults
control their fertility until later years (and then have a small number of children living in a nuclear family with appropriate economic-dependency ra-
tios) (e.g., Geronimus 2003; Phoenix 1993). The cultural specificity of these
assumptions is evident when considered in relation to the actual practices of
cultures and communities in the United States and around the world (e.g.,
Konner and Shostak 1986). The assumptions that families will be distraught
and ruined, that teens will "lose out" on their childhood, and that teen pregnancy is socially damaging and a drain on public resources, simply do not
apply in many communities and cultures around the world, including here
in the United States. For example, Geronimus writes,

> Indeed, some evidence suggests that early childbearing among African Ameri-
> cans in high-poverty urban areas mitigates the consequences of the severe
> health risks they face during their reproductive and working age. For example,
> in these populations, early childbearing may act to reduce rates of infant mor-
> tality and the risk of being widowed or orphaned, along with their adverse
> effects on family economies and caretaking systems. Few people are aware of
> this. Well-publicized conventional wisdom continues to hold teen childbear-
> ing to be, in all cases and in every aspect, an antisocial act and an important
> public health problem, *especially* when practiced by urban African Americans.
> Meanwhile, a significant body of reputable scientific evidence has existed for
> more than a decade that casts doubt on the conventional wisdom but does not
> get the same public "air time." (Geronimus 2003, 881)

This quote is the antithesis of the way we usually talk about teen pregnancy in the United States, but as Geronimus says, there is a significant body
of research that indicates that some women and children may be better off
by some health, development, and economic measures if they have babies
while young and unmarried. For example, studies have found that outcomes
such as child neglect, negative schooling outcomes, and negative behavioral

outcomes[10] are statistically no different for the children of some groups of teenage girls than for children born to comparable groups of older women. Teen African American mothers who do not marry are more likely to finish high school than those who do (Fine and McClelland 2006). Other research has examined the correlation between "unintended" pregnancy and poverty rates, and its utility in understanding poor women's decisions about pregnancy, birth, and motherhood (e.g., Kendall et al. 2005). Still other studies indicate that babies born to economically and racially marginalized teen mothers are in equal or better health and cost the state less than children born to mothers in their twenties,[11] that pregnant African American teens may be more likely to complete high school than their nonpregnant colleagues,[12] and that most teen pregnancies are not reported as "unwanted."[13] Taken together, these studies indicate that it is the extent of the teen mothers' (and fathers') preexisting marginalization—the limited resources available to her, her educational opportunities, her socioeconomic status, her race and ethnicity, and so forth—that largely account for these unexpected outcomes (e.g., Levine, Emery, and Pollack 2007; Mollborn 2007). However, as was evident in teachers' responses to pregnant girls in Wisconsin and Wyoming, and as is evident in research conducted with marginalized teens (e.g., Kendall et al. 2005; Burton 1990), marginalized girls and communities that do not respond to teen pregnancy as simply and always a negative (and research that documents these responses) are often dismissed by educators and policy makers.

Not surprisingly, all the sex education programs I observed incorporated data that constructed teen pregnancy as an inherent problem. The observations described above provide insight into why teens choose to parent, the often inequitable health and labor contexts that inform this choice, and the centrality of family and community responses to teen parenting in determining child and parent well-being during and after pregnancy. These insights were similarly absent from sex education classrooms. For example, at one point during my observations in Wisconsin, Mrs. Shane told her class about a time when a girl (whom Mrs. Shane identified to us as Latina) approached her to ask how to get pregnant. Mrs. Shane told the class that she told the girl, "No, you don't want to get pregnant. You are not ready, and there is no way that I am going to help you with that." She also told us that she had observed girls admiring their friends' pregnancies, a practice that she found deeply disturbing. Girls who became pregnant in Teton High mostly dropped out of school or were segregated into the alternative high school largely reserved for students with "behavioral issues." As various studies have detailed, pregnant girls are often discouraged from attending or forced out of mainstream high schools, despite laws requiring that they have equal access to schools.[14]

The alternative schools into which pregnant girls may be tracked often are themselves marginalized in the school system. In Wyoming's alternative high school, for example, most pregnant students were eligible for the free breakfast and lunch programs and counted on this food as a mainstay of their daily calories. The school did not have a cafeteria, though, and received child-sized meals from the elementary school instead of larger meals from the high school. Pregnant students reported being hungry all day.

Though viewed as deeply socially undesirable in all sex education programs, there were important differences in how teen pregnancy was understood in AOUME versus CSE programs. These differences reveal the morality tales underlying teen pregnancy programming.

CSE: Peer education and teen mothering

For CS educators, teen pregnancy indicated a failure of rational decision-making and planning. Pregnancy was viewed as an unwanted, but easily preventable, outcome of sex. Being pregnant signaled a lack of rational contraceptive planning and an end to the middle- and upper-class "bright future" that students were encouraged to imagine for themselves. Though both boys and girls were described as equally responsible for a pregnancy, pregnancy is an embodied experience. Programs emphasized the effects of pregnancy on girls' bodies and futures, and how often fathers did not stick around.

As with their emphasis on bringing teens face-to-face with experts on STIs (from school nurses to HIV-positive role models), CSE programs often brought in teen parents to talk about the daily realities of having a child. In California, Come on In! had a panel of teen mothers talk about their experiences to an assembly of all of the students. The panel members were all Latina or white women, though the coordinator of Come On In! said the panel often included a father. The panelists focused on how much students would lose out on if they had babies while in school and emphasized the economic costs of teen parenting. For example, one presenter had audience members guess how much baby-related items (car seat, diapers, infant formula, and so on) cost, then told them the real cost and the amount of materials needed per week. Many of the girls spoke of their heartache upon realizing that their children's fathers were not, as promised, going to be involved in their children's lives, and they talked about the painful process of obtaining child support from absent fathers.

In Wyoming, Mrs. Curry, who taught the Family and Child Health class, brought in a number of teen mothers, with children of different ages, to talk to her students. These conversations were officially intended to teach students about child development, but Mrs. Curry brought in parents of her students' age group so that they could learn about teen parenting as well. The presenters were all white mothers who brought their babies; in some cases the baby's grandmother was also present. These mothers' conversations often touched on positive and negative aspects of teen parenting (perhaps in part because they were officially there to talk about their children's development—a topic about which many of them showed obvious excitement), and on their efforts to stay in school, work, or both after the birth. Most of the girls talked at some length about their relationships with the fathers during pregnancy and after the babies' births, and in turn how this had affected their and their babies' lives. The mothers also discussed balancing very full schedules with their dreams of fun-filled teen years, and the detailed and complex childcare arrangements that they had to negotiate with family and friends. The students in the class asked a lot of questions and were able to hear how the issues confronting teen mothers changed as their children grew older. They also heard about how having a baby had changed the relationship between the teen mother and her own mother. Grandmothers are often part- or full-time caregivers for children of teen mothers, and their willingness to care for their grandchildren is central to many teen mothers' success in school and work. Despite this, sex education programs usually focus only on the teen mother, not the family and community structures within which she parents. This conversation constituted the only time I witnessed a sex education topic being explicitly linked to broader family, social, and economic relations, and it did not occur in the official sex education class.

Although the central message from both peer panels was that having a baby as a teen significantly limited the mother's freedom, in Wyoming, students learned much more about how having a baby affected panelists' social relations and emotional states and learned much more about the kinds of resources panelists could and did draw on. The effects of teen parenting were therefore presented as much more mixed than in California, and the effects of familial and socioeconomic relations in making the experience better or worse for the mother and child were much more evident.

AOUME: Destructive teen mothers versus joyful, married parenting

AOUME programs downplayed teen pregnancy as an issue while pathologizing single (teen) mothers as a social category. Conversations about teen fathers were limited to occasional comments about the expense of child support and the potential for jail time for men who didn't provide support—the "fear-based" male antipregnancy curriculum. All curricula assumed that the father would not choose to be actively involved in the mother's or child's life, and that the mother and child would be heartbroken by this loss. Teen and non-teen single mothers were discussed in every curriculum, every presentation, and every training I attended as examples of social decay and the cause of their children's negative outcomes.

The generalized stigmatization of single (teen) mothers but silence about fathers, coupled with the relative lack of discussion about pregnancy, may reflect both AOUME's assumption that girls are primarily responsible for maintaining sexual abstinence outside of marriage, and AOUME supporters' concerns that people, particularly women, are becoming too disinvested in getting married, forming families, and having children. For example, one state-funded Florida AOUME service provider, who provided schools with lifelike dolls that the students had to carry around with them twenty-four hours a day for a week in order to literally "bring home" the effects of teen pregnancy, said that only parents whom she called "very religious" had refused to allow their children to participate in these programs. She said of these parents,

> They said that they were really worried that their kids would decide it was too hard! Of course, they didn't want them to get pregnant in school, but they also didn't want them to say "Oh, it's too much trouble, maybe I'd rather not be a parent," especially when that's really common in our culture now.

Although most of the AOUME and CSE programs quoted data about how few teen couples stay together after having a baby (the "fear-based" pregnancy curriculum for girls), there was no discussion in any of the sex education programs about what it means to be a father or what responsibilities fathers bear toward their children.[15] The silence about boys' parenting rights and responsibilities was particularly stark when contrasted with the brief but emotionally charged interactions that I observed in most classrooms between students and instructors concerning boys' right to be involved in abortion decisions.

PREGNANCY OPTIONS

The subject of pregnancy options—that is, what girls can do if they become pregnant—was discussed in all of the classrooms I observed and most curricula I reviewed. This was an area of significant difference between AOUME and CSE programs. AOUME programs presented two options: keep the baby (which was consistently presented as a selfish act on the part of teen mothers) or put the baby up for adoption by a loving, married, financially stable couple. In CSE classrooms, there were three options: keep the baby, adoption, or abortion. Keeping the baby was discussed in the teen panel; adoption was discussed briefly in class, and abortion received slightly more classroom attention, but not necessarily the sort of attention often imagined by CSE advocates or detractors. For example, a conversation in the Wisconsin classroom about abortion exemplifies how ideas abut abortion that would usually be viewed as aligned with AOUME ideology were regularly deployed by teachers in Wyoming's and Wisconsin's CSE classrooms:

> Mr. Kelly starts the class quickly—they have to cover abortion and sexual violence in one fifty-minute class period. He passes out the handout on abortion. As the sheets go around, students begin commenting on the graphic images of partial-birth abortions depicted on one side. Julia says, "I'm going to cry." Another says, "Gross, what is this?" Mr. Kelly says, "Oh, you're getting distracted by the back. Turn it around." He begins the discussion: "What do you know about abortion? That it's gross and terrible?" The students don't respond. . . .
>
> Mr. Kelly says they will take a poll [on when life begins]: "Raise your hand—is it when sperm meets an egg?" Most of the class raises their hands. "So, would you be pro-abortion?" No one answers. Cornell asks, "What about when you're raped? That's different." Theo answers by saying that he knew a girl who had been raped and got pregnant and had the baby. Cornell responds, earnestly, "That's nice." Mrs. Shane adds, "That is nice. Because it's not the baby's fault." The two boys agree with her. "It's hard," she adds. "Some people talk about the baby being a constant reminder of the rape. But it's not the baby's fault. You have to be really strong." Shurita agrees, and she and Mrs. Shane have a brief exchange about being a strong woman and what that entails. At this point, Ellie, who is usually quiet, raises her hand. She says, "It's the woman's choice all throughout, but if she's raped then it's definitely OK." Mr. Kelly responds quickly, saying, "So, if you got pregnant do you think both people should have a say?" "Yes," Ellie says. "But ultimately it's her decision." Another girl says, "I don't think it should be illegal because some women can't raise babies." A boy responds to her, saying, "A bad life is better than no life." Shurita agrees. She repeats what he said and then says that she thinks abortion should be illegal. Julia says, "It depends on the situation. There are many different reasons why someone would have one." Mrs. Shane adds, "What about incest? What if you're raped by your dad?" Theo is shocked. "What?!" he asks. "That happens?" "Yes, it happens," she says. "Young girls who are pregnant, it's often older male relatives. Should she have an abortion?" "Hell yeah!" Theo says.

This conversation touched on a number of debates that emerged across the abstinence-based and CSE programs I observed, including boys' right to be involved in decisions about abortion, the morality of abortion, and women's "culpability" for a pregnancy. For example, in California students were given a list of women and asked to pretend that they were supreme court judges tasked with deciding which of the women would receive the country's last legal abortion. The students' debate about which woman should be chosen touched repeatedly and often stereotypically on the various women's culpability for their pregnancy, and the eventual "winner" in the contest was a woman who had been raped.

In general, instructors skirted discussion of the relational, social, and economic environments that structure girls', boys', and families' decision making about pregnancy and experiences of parenting. None of the AOUME, ABSE, or CSE classrooms I observed or curricula I reviewed provided structured or meaningful opportunities for students to discuss the construction of teen pregnancy as a problem; the social, economic, and cultural drivers of pregnancy and parenting in various communities and at various ages; or the responses to pregnancy that teens found morally, socially, economically, and emotionally feasible. From diseased black bodies shown in the STI presentation in Wyoming, to the teen mothers' panels, to the lack of discussion about who can easily access contraception or abortion in the United States, discussions about STIs and pregnancy were ripe with age, class, race, gender, and sexual-identity assumptions that remained unspoken and unexamined.

Conclusion: The Consequences of Current Sex Education Goals and Outcomes

CONSTRUCTING TEEN SEXUALITY

As a growing number of researchers have pointed out,[16] schools often silence and stigmatize teen sexuality. AOUME and CSE programs appeared to contribute to this trend through their construction of teen STI and pregnancy "epidemics." STIs were discussed as a major short- and long-term health hazard to adolescents, and teen pregnancy was discussed as destructive to mothers, their children, and society. The ideological assumptions about teens and sexuality, and the embedded class, race, gender, and sexual-identity assumptions of these discussions were striking, though they differed in important ways in CSE and AOUME approaches.

Though they may seem commonsense, these ideas about pregnancy and STIs are neither universal nor considered best practice from a public health or social policy perspective. Moreover, they are not the only topics around which sex education can be shaped. Below, I briefly examine how AOUME and CSE programs addressed one of the central topics in sexuality education aimed at adults: desire and pleasure.

While CSE programs styled their approach as "risk reduction" and AOUME programs touted "risk elimination," both approaches emphasized risk, as opposed to safety or pleasure, in their conceptualizations of teen sexuality and sex education programming. From comparing sexually active girls' diseased vaginas to cauliflower heads, to telling students that sex could be "a death sentence," to claiming that girls "lost their power" if they had sex, AOUME classrooms consistently emphasized the danger of sex before marriage to students. Sex after marriage, and waiting for sex after marriage, was consistently described as pleasurable and powerful, particularly for girls. This was a neotraditional understanding of sex—one in which pleasure is a gift from God to married couples and sex guides for Christian married couples abound, but in which sex before marriage poses immediate spiritual, physical, and social danger and threatens to destroy teens' capacity to ever have a healthy marital relationship.

AOUME programs urged students to be active planners for their future sexual agency (for example, buying gifts for their unknown future spouses), and imbued talk of this planning with a great deal of desire and pleasure. Students' desires were appropriately focused on preparing for a (morally) healthy future relationship to a spouse and to God, and longing for the social, physical, emotional, psychological, and spiritual security that they would gain through these relationships. Girls were urged to rein in any current desires in order to assure their and their future spouse's purity; boys were urged to not give in to their animalistic nature by viewing porn or having sex, so that they would be able to properly appreciate sex with their wife.

In some CSE (though not ABSE) classrooms, I heard instructors tell students that sex was natural and should be pleasurable, but this discourse of pleasure was never linked to the present or to students' desires. When instructors talked about sexual pleasure and desire, they did so in a hypothetical manner: "Sex should always be pleasurable for both partners." In contrast, in California students were asked to imagine themselves in ten years; after receiving cards with events such as testing positive for an STI or getting pregnant, they then had to talk about how having sex as teens would derail their desired futures. In Wisconsin, students were given examples of how teen sexual relationships might threaten their friendships, and in Wyoming students were told that school was not an appropriate place to ever "be sexual."

In CSE classrooms, students were told that human sexual desire was natural, but that teens' acting on these desires was inappropriate because of the physical dangers it might entail. "Good" students would rationally calculate the risk and engage in sex only in situations where the risk was minimal, where the disease status of each partner was known, where highly effective contraception was used consistently and correctly, where partners were able to talk clearly to each other about their wants and needs, and where such sexual encounters would not derail their desired futures if they were to get pregnant or get an STI. In other words, when they were older.

It would be incorrect to say that there was no discourse of desire (Fine 1988) in the classrooms that I observed, but these desires were only appropriate if they were future oriented, and they were never "thick" desires (Fine and McClelland 2006) embedded in broader relationally and socioeconomically just relations. In AOUME programs, appropriate desires were tied to marriage. In CSE programs, they were tied to an unknown point in the future when students were responsible enough to address the potential outcomes of having sex in a mature and well-planned manner. Students were *becoming* appropriate sexual actors through sex education, but they could not *be* appropriate sexual actors as teens. Not surprisingly, then, current sexual experiences, questions, concerns, and desires were to be kept secret in the classrooms and schools I observed. Students' current sexual concerns were consigned to the anonymous question box and one-on-one conversations with teachers in CSE classrooms, and were entirely silenced in AOUME classrooms. Future desires were deeply limited by "thin" descriptions of the good life—marriage in AOUME, and descriptions of powerful individuals negotiating exactly what they wanted in a relationship in CSE classes (for example, multiple students in California's high-track classroom said that their desired future included a high-powered job, making a lot of money, traveling the world, and having an attractive sexual partner available as desired). Desire and pleasure, so central to discussions about healthy adult sexuality, were literally unimaginable topics in the classrooms I observed.

EVALUATING EFFECTIVENESS

As with education and state social service provision more broadly, sex educators have faced increasing pressure to define their success in relation to outcomes- or evidence-based approaches that impose a medicalized knowledge and assessment framework on social programs. Within this framework, the success or failure of sex education programs is judged by a small set of outcomes that are defined and measurable in similar, quantified ways across programs and populations. This set of outcomes embeds and reifies the focus on and assumptions about STIs and teen pregnancy described above. For example, in the United States valued measures often include STI infection rates and teen pregnancy rates but seldom include STI treatment rates or teen marriage rates.

Superficially at least, the shift toward the adoption of limited and medicalized evidence-based sex education policy-making and funding appears to benefit CSE approaches: CSE programs are organized around these health outcomes, and "gold standard" randomized trials conducted on the behavioral and physical outcomes of sex education programs have shown no long-term or broad effects for AOUME programs, and some broad effects for some CSE and ABSE programs.[17] If studies of AOUME programs continue to show no significant change in students' reported health behaviors, in time this may significantly undermine public support for them, especially if they clearly display conservative religious values. Furthermore, to the extent that AOUME supporters adopt medicalized evidence-based frameworks to rationalize and evaluate their programs, they run the risk of losing their focus on the cohesive moral framework that has united AOUME programs until now.

But CSE supporters, in their wholesale adoption of evidence-based approaches, face a threat to the values about adolescent sexuality that they hold that go beyond the narrow range of medicalized outcomes. The growing primacy of scientific rationalist ideals in CSE circles has relegated CSE's democratic ideals of equality and diversity to the backseat. For CSE supporters who care about these ideals as much or more than about the ideal of scientific rationality, the current constructions and growing importance of evidence-based frameworks is cause for ideological concern. Moreover, CSE supporters stand to lose public sympathy with these approaches. AOUME's attention to the negative social and emotional effects of sex connected strongly with many of the teens and parents—both liberal and conservative—with whom I spoke. Although fears of pregnancy and STIs were strong, many students and parents were equally or more concerned by the price that students, particularly girls, paid in their social lives for having sex. In Florida I asked Tina (a progressive student activist) and her friend Max to talk with me about friendships and sex in their peer group.

> TINA: You know, everyone always thinks we're all having sex all the time, but in our group, we're girls and boys [who] just hang out all together all the

time. Like going to movies, hanging out at someone's house. Sex screws that up, you know? People start fighting, then they break up, then everyone has this problem: like who's side you're on and who do you talk to and who's in or out?

MAX: Yeah, we all just hang out together. It's not couples, it's just the whole group. We're all really close. Most of us have been friends since kindergarten, so we're like brothers and sisters.

TINA: Honestly, I wish people would recognize there are plenty of us who aren't having sex. But it's so annoying that some people see abstinence as such a bad word. It's like the new insult to say, "Oh, you're a virgin." I've got better things to do than to get all worked up about sex right now. We're all going to be all over soon [when we leave for college], so this is our time together.

Tina's and Max's responses point to the widespread appeal to students and adults of acknowledging how much sex can and often does change social and emotional dynamics among peers. As in Regnerus's (2007) and Cahn and Carbonne's (2007) work, they also point to how students and parents might understand abstinence not as an unyielding religious stance, but as an appealing approach to "keeping things easy" so that teens can focus on their (middle-/upper-class) educational and career aspirations.

To the extent that teens view their own and their friends' sexual experiences as not just physically consequential, and to the extent other outcomes are not addressed by CSE programs, students (and parents) see this as a significant deficiency in CSE approaches. Furthermore, by not addressing these outcomes CSE programs fail to address the inequitable gender, class, race, and sexual-identity norms that underlie many of the "prices" that different students pay for having sex (such as social stigma associated with girls', not boys', sexual activity).

The end result of an adoption of this narrowed understanding of sex education is that many mainstream CSE supporters describe their approach as follows: they wish that teens would not have sex, but because they may do so anyway, they provide them the information they need to protect themselves. This "practical realist" stance is far removed from progressives' calls for a sex-positive understanding of adolescent sexuality, as well as from more conservative calls for an educative approach based on a strong moral stance that does not, as some AOUME supporters have put it, "begin with an assumption of the moral weakness and failure of our youth."

There is an increasing focus on a small number of medically rationalized outcomes (such as STI and pregnancy rates) and highly quantified and methodologically constraining evaluations of these outcomes. All sex education supporters and providers should question the effects that this focus on medicalized outcomes, and experimental and quasi-experimental evaluations of these outcomes, will have on the capacity of sex education programs to address students' holistic experiences, and on educators' capacity to address the moral and ethical implications of different sex education models in students' daily lives.

"Men are Microwaves, Women are Crock-Pots": Gender Roles in AOUME and CSE

"When gender is understood as mattering, questions emerge about power, privilege, and access" (Tolman, Striepe, and Harmon 2003, 7).

Introduction

Halfway through collecting data for this study, I noticed a trend that surprised me and forced me to question my assumptions about the expression of "conservative" and "liberal" values in sex education approaches. The AOUME materials and activities I was reviewing were full of references to gender inequities and the need for girls' empowerment. In contrast, these topics were largely absent from the CSE materials and programs I reviewed. This seemed contradictory, given that sexually progressive, politically and socially liberal organizations historically have been at the forefront of movements that claim to empower women, and New Christian Right groups have not.

A growing research literature addresses the gendered implications of current sex education approaches.[1] Authors note, for example, that girls' and boys' sexual natures and behaviors are often presented differently (for example, girls' pleasure is seldom discussed),[2] that many sex education curricula assume girls are responsible for maintaining sexual innocence and controlling boys' sexual aggression,[3] and that many curricula naturalize inequitable gender roles instead of presenting gender as a social construct (Tolman, Striepe, and Harmon 2003). There is also a growing literature addressing the interplay between sexuality and gender identity and representation.[4] Generally, these literatures point out that all sex education programs reflect social values and norms, including gender norms embedded in models of sexual relationships and social functioning. Because gender ideology is not usually the official focus of sex education programs or evaluations, however, the consequences of these embedded gender norms on teacher-student interactions, classroom functioning, or student outcomes are seldom evaluated. Yet if gender norms and relations are central to social and sexual relations, it is obvious that we should care about and analyze the gender assumptions that shape sex education programs and the consequences of these programs.

Luker's book *When Sex Goes to School* (2006) provides important insights into the often unspoken connections among gender, sexuality, and sex education's hot topics. Building on the categorizations of sexual ideologies by scholars such as McKay (1997, 1998), Seidman (1992), and Weeks and Holland (1996), Luker argues that the core concern of sexually conservative baby boomers is to reinscribe "traditional" gender relations and sexual norms, in which men are family leaders and nonprocreative sex is perceived as a destabilizing force in society. Abortion, contraception, and homosexuality become key issues because their existence challenges the patriarchal model of naturalized gender differences and because they focus attention on topics that should be kept private and sacred (e.g., Fields 2008; Luker 2006; McKay 1998).

In contrast to sexual conservatives, Luker argues, sexual liberals of the same generation view sex as a biological, not a sacred act, and they see sex education as an opportunity to provide teens with developmentally appropriate information and decision-making skills so that teens, as rational individuals, can take responsibility for their own sexual lives. McKay's notion of permissive sexual ideologies is useful here in thinking about the moral model underlying such a view:

> The centrality, within the Liberal approach to sexual ethics, of individual choice and context places individual deliberation, rather than specific sexual acts, at the pinnacle of moral evaluation . . .
>
> While this person-centered approach, with its focus on individual deliberation with respect to making sexual choices, is more permissive than restrictive in nature, it does suggest that sexual behavior does need to be guided by moral principles derived from the Liberal philosophical tradition . . . [for example,] honesty, equality, and responsibility. (McKay 1998, 57)

Below, I describe the gender roles and norms promulgated in the AOUME and CSE programs that I observed and the morality tales about relationships and sexuality evident therein.

AOUME's Neotraditional Gender Model

Explicit discussion of gender differences in AOUME approaches reflects the gender-differentiated model of society upon which AOUME programming is based. In this model, gender differences are naturalized and historicized, and a particular set of "traditional" gender norms are viewed as essential for creating healthy individuals, families, communities, and states. These norms are a central component of AOUME curricula and programming, and they represent the gender relations and ideals that are assumed to structure daily life in the United States, from media representations to romantic expectations.[5] In their more secular form, television, magazines, video games, and other mainstream media quite consistently display some of these norms: men are more often portrayed as leaders, active characters, aggressive, and strong. Females are more often displayed as passive, quiet, sexualized, and weak or manipulative.[6] In their more religious form, these norms are the basis of a broader system of desired family and social relations, in which the man is the head of the household, the wife is his subordinate helpmate, and the children are all under the firm control of the parents.

Though widely evident and promulgated in many of the spaces through which youth move, these gender norms (which are accompanied by sexuality, race, and class norms [Bay-Cheng 2003; Fields 2008]) do not mirror many people's and families' experiences, and are, in important ways, exclusionary in their construction of "acceptable" people, families, and communities. They also no longer reflect the majority of Americans' desires. For example, the Families and Work Institute's 2009 *Study of the Changing Workforce* found that only about 40 percent of men and women agreed that it was better "if the man earns the money and the woman takes care of the home and children." In 1977, 74 percent of men and 52 percent of women agreed with this statement. AOUME programs are actively trying to re-normalize these values, which lie at the core of the neotraditionalist social and moral model they promulgate.

NEOTRADITIONALISM IN THE NEW CHRISTIAN RIGHT AND AOUME

A central tenet of many actors and organizations in the New Christian Right (the historical source of most AOUME curricula, trainers, and activists) is that "the natural family is the fundamental unit of society."[7] The "natural" family consists of a male father, a female mother, and children. This model is rooted in a particular understanding of the Bible and of contemporary Christian texts, which together construct the family as a sacral unit of society. Male leadership and the marital relationship are viewed as mirroring the relationship between Jesus Christ and the church (McCullum and deLashmutt 1996). Within the family, women submit to men (first to their fathers and later to their husbands), and children submit to their parents. This model is referred to by Gallagher and Smith (1999) as neotraditionalism, a term I will use to describe the assumption in many AOUME programs that patriarchy and male-headed nuclear family models constitute the natural and the desired order of the world, and that disruptions to this order are indicative of efforts to undermine God's creation. Neotraditionalism adds an important twist to what would otherwise be a traditionalist understanding with a shift in their framing of women's and men's natures, though not their roles and responsibilities.

Historically, much of Christian literature about men and women has focused on women's secondary position in society and on their lesser status as human beings and as children of God. For example, in the late nineteenth century, Elizabeth Cady Stanton famously said of the women's emancipation movement, "The Bible and Church have been the greatest stumbling blocks in the way of women's emancipation. . . . The whole tone of Church teaching in regard to women is, to the last degree, contemptuous and degrading" (*Free Thought Magazine,* vol. xiv, September 1896).

In contrast, much of the neotraditionalist New Christian Right literature is just as likely to discuss women's roles in families, communities, and the church as better, more natural, or more central than men's roles, particularly with respect to holding relationships together and rearing children.

For example, humans are, in the words of Focus on the Family, "created for connection," and it is in the marriage-based family relationship that adults and children are happiest and best able to fulfill their obligations to one another and to God. Marriage is not easy, however, because men and women's fundamental differences must be acknowledged and addressed in order for relationships to flourish.[8] Smalley and Scott, cited on the website Marriage Missions International,[9] describe neotraditionalist gender differences as shown in figure 1.

Mental/Emotional Differences

Women tend to be more *personal* than men. Women have a deeper interest in people and feelings—building relationships—while men tend to be more preoccupied with practicalities that can be understood through logical deduction. . . .

Men tend to be less desirous and knowledgeable in building intimate relationships, both with God and with others. . . . When a man realizes his wife is more naturally motivated to nurture relationships, he can relax and accept these tendencies and *choose* to develop a better marriage and better relationships with his children.

Do you realize that your wife's naturalized ability for developing relationships can *help* you fulfill the two greatest commandments taught by Christ—loving God and loving others (Matt. 22: 36–40)? . . .

God knew you needed special help because He stated, "It is not good for the man to be alone; I will make him a helper [and completer] suitable for him" (Genesis 2:18). If you let her, your wife can open up a whole new and complete world of communication and deeper relationships. . . .

FIGURE 1. Neotraditional gender roles

Women tend to find their identity in close relationships, while men gain their identity through vocations. Because of a woman's *emotional identity* with people and places around her, she needs more time to adjust to change that may affect her relationships. A man can logically deduce the benefits of a change and get "psyched-up" for it in a matter of minutes . . .

Men tend to express their hostility through physical violence, while women tend to be more *verbally expressive.*

Physical Differences

- Man and woman differ in skeletal structure, woman having a shorter head, broader face, less protruding chin, shorter legs, and longer trunk. . . .

- Woman has several unique and important functions: menstruation, pregnancy, lactation. Woman's hormones are of a different type and more numerous than man's. . . .

- Woman's blood contains more water and 20 percent fewer red cells. Since the red cells supply oxygen to the body cells, woman tires more easily and is more prone to faint. . . .

- On the average, man possesses 50 percent more brute strength than woman. . . .

Sexual Differences

- A woman's sexual drive tends to be related to her menstrual cycle, while a man's drive is fairly constant. . . .

- A woman is stimulated more by touch and romantic words. She is far more attracted by a man's personality, while a man is stimulated by sight. A man is usually less discriminating about those to whom he is physically attracted.

- While a man needs little or no preparations for sex, a woman often needs hours of emotional and mental preparation. Harsh or abusive treatment can easily remove her desire for sexual intimacy for days at a time.

- When a woman's emotions have been trampled by her husband, she is often repulsed by his advances. Many women have told me they feel like prostitutes when they're forced to make love while feeling resentment toward their husbands. However, a man may have NO idea what he is putting his wife through when he forces sex upon her.

  These basic differences, which usually surface soon after the wedding, are the source of many conflicts in marriage. From the start, the woman has a greater intuitive awareness of how to develop a loving relationship. Because of her sensitivity, she is initially more considerate of his feelings and enthusiastic about developing a meaningful, multi-level relationship; that is, she knows how to build something more than a sexual marathon; she wants to be a lover, a best friend, a fan, a homemaker, and an appreciated partner.

- The man, on the other hand, does not generally have her instinctive awareness of what the relationship should be. He doesn't know how to encourage and love his wife or treat her in a way that meets her deepest needs.

FIGURE 1. (*continued*)

In this neotraditionalist framing of gender relations, women are emotional, verbal, and focused on relationships, while men are logical, physically powerful (and violent), and emotionally withdrawn. Men's and women's psychosocial differences are traced to biological differences, which again highlight men's strength and women's relative physical and emotional weakness and need for protection. The psychosocial and biological differences lead, naturally, to sexual differences, which women are largely responsible for understanding and bridging.

Theological debates about issues such as male headship are diverse and often contradictory within and among New Christian Right institutions (e.g., Blankenhorn, Browning, and Van Leeuwen 2004). The description I offer of neotraditional norms necessarily simplifies these debates. For example, women's particular strengths (emotional bonding, community building) may be described as taming and complementing men's strengths which, in modern society, are no longer as needed as they once were for survival; or men may be portrayed as lustful brutes who connect neither to society nor to God until a good woman helps them find their way. In either case, however, there is an assumption that men are less in touch with and responsible for their actions, while women are responsible for managing their own and men's reactions and relations. These neotraditional gender roles are by now well established in our common parlance about gender differences; they reflect a set of ideas about men, women, and their roles in society that bear the weight of millennia of religious, social, economic, and cultural practices throughout much of the world.

NEOTRADITIONALISM IN THE CURRICULUM

Neotraditional gender norms are evident in AOUME programming, in which men and women are regularly portrayed as naturally different. For example, early on in my training to become certified as an abstinence-only educator in Florida, one of the national AOUME speakers told the following (paraphrased) story:

> When it comes to sex, men are microwaves and women are Crock-Pots. Unlike women, men can be ready to have sex in just seconds, without any of the "slow heating" that women need for their emotions to become engaged. Men do not need emotions to enjoy sex. We are visual, and visual stimulus is all it takes for us to be there, ready to go. Women cannot enjoy sex without emotions, though, because it's through their emotions that they become stimulated. For men, the emotional follows the physical. For women, it's the other way around.

The microwave/Crock-Pot analogy provides a powerful starting point for examining the organizing principle of gender relations in AOUME approaches: the biologically distinct (and therefore God-given) bases for sexual arousal and pleasure in males and females, which broaden to distinctions in their physical and emotional lives. These distinctions, in turn, form the basis of the differentiated gender roles that men and women are expected to play in a God-fearing family and society.

Because all sexual activity outside of marriage (and therefore all sex between people of the same gender)[10] is forbidden, girls, who are by their nature less lustful, are responsible for dressing and behaving in ways that minimize the chance of boys' sexual arousal. Activities that reify girls' and women's perceived strengths in shaping relationships are common in AOUME materials. Much has been made of stories found in widely used AOUME curricula that urge girls to put aside their own needs, ideas, or goals in order to manage boys' and men's instincts, and that present stereotypes of male and female capacities, roles, and power.[11] For example, in Sex Respect (Mast 2011), one of the most popular AOUME curricula, Dr. Specter says to students,

> Because they generally become physically aroused less easily, girls are still in a good position to slow down the young man and help him learn balance in a relationship.... Guys can gain self-control for both their actions and their senses when they train themselves to look away from the sensual influences of the culture and try to see young women as people, not sex objects. (Mast 2001, 12)

Such AOUME stories and activities drive home to girls and boys that they are different, and then tie these differences specifically to gender relations and sex acts to argue that girls are, naturally, much less interested in, but more deeply affected by (and responsible for) sex outside of marriage than are boys. For example, in the Florida AOUME training, the speaker followed the microwave/Crock-Pot analogy with a rousing speech about the price that girls pay for sex outside of marriage:

> We need to tell our girls how much they're valued. We need to empower them to understand that it's not fair, but they pay the price for sex so much more than our boys. They are the ones that get pregnant. They are the ones more at risk of STDs. And don't think men will stick around for the consequences.

The neotraditional construction of girls requires the construction of their opposite—boys. Although speakers in the AOUM educator-training workshops, parent workshops, and teen rallies repeatedly said that boys were also expected to remain virgins until marriage, the reasons given were almost entirely spiritual and personal—boys were not at risk of getting pregnant and less at risk of getting an STI than girls, but they would "sully their souls" if they engaged in sex outside of marriage. There was very little discussion of how pregnancy would change boys' lives, other than two comments made to scare boys about child support; there was no boy-specific discussion about STIs, and boys were never presented as having feelings—for the girls with whom they were sexually involved, or in their capacity to be hurt emotionally in a relationship.

A popular teaching activity that the Florida AOUME trainer particularly recommended for middle schoolers, called "Protect Your Heart," provides a clear example of the neotraditional norms AOUME materials reinscribe. "Every time you have sex," the trainer explained, "you give pieces of yourself away. This activity shows that to kids visually." He explained the activity, called "Ms. Tape," demonstrating it with the aid of male audience members:

> You have a boy come up, and [holding up a piece of transparent packing tape] you tell him this is his girlfriend, Ms. Tape. She's thin, tall, a great girl. You think you love each other, you've been together, say, eight months, you wanna get closer, so you have sex. [He wraps the tape around the volunteer's bare arm]. Before you had sex, you baked cakes together, listened to music, all sorts of things. Now, you don't talk as much, you get jealous of each other, it's not working. So you break up. Then you do it with another person. [He pulls the tape off the arm of the first volunteer, to groans of sympathy from the audience. Then he calls up another man and wraps the tape around his arm, then repeats this a third time. He holds the tape up after unwrapping it from the third arm. It's absolutely disgusting, covered with pieces of hair, body oil, and dead skin. He resumes talking.] The adhesive will disappear, and all the body stuff will mingle. Then try to stick the tape to itself. You see it's easy to peel apart. You can show them how easy it is to lose yourself. See, Ms. Tape ain't all that anymore, huh? No condom is big enough to protect your heart.

"Ms. Tape" exemplifies how AOUME programs normalize the notion that boys are largely unaffected by sex and therefore not in need of protecting their emotions, their reputations, or themselves. In contrast, these activities assume that girls will lose themselves, their social attractiveness, and their long-term marital value through premarital sex.

The absence of commentary on or stigmatization of boys who "discard" girls with whom they have had sex in AOUME materials must be understood in relation to girls' assumed responsibility to constrain boys' sexuality and to foster boys' emotional capacity. It is the girl with whom a boy has sex who is responsible for failing to help the boy battle his more sexual, physical nature, and who is therefore responsible for being discarded. As one of the Florida AOUM education trainers explained,

It's wrong for boys to say they have no control, they are not animals. But it's true that boys have a harder time with this sometimes; they don't have as much control. And so it's up to girls to have enough self-esteem and self-control to say no, to resist the boy. And it's the girl who gets hurt the most in the end if they give in.

There are obvious analogies here with Judeo-Christian tales of Eve's responsibility for "tempting" Adam into his downfall. AOUME approaches, as with broader neotraditional New Christian Right debates about family values, sexuality, and gender relations, may no longer always or only describe women's sexuality as inherently dangerous or evil, or simply blame Eve. The stories in AOUME in fact not uncommonly position girls as heroines or leaders, but their acts of valor almost always relate to saving males from their baser nature by constraining female sexuality or emotionality. The onus for personal and social salvation or destruction is reinscribed onto girls in the language of empowerment and self-esteem, and girls' empowerment is encouraged not in order to benefit Eve as an individual or a woman, but in order for her to help Adam control his dangerous natural instincts.[12]

Girls' Empowerment

AOUME references to girls' empowerment were distinguished by two characteristics that the curricula associated with girls' most important choices as sexual actors: how girls lose their power to boys when they have sex outside of marriage, and how girls' sexual empowerment is linked to their presentation of self by means of their consumer choices.

(GIRLS') EMPOWERMENT THROUGH (BOYS') MANAGEMENT

As noted at the start of the chapter, AOUME presenters regularly discussed the need to empower girls. Girls were often described as having "low self-esteem," which led them to engage in sex before marriage in a fruitless attempt to gain boys' attention and love. Speakers were deeply emotional about how unequal the negative consequences of sex before marriage were, and their desire to address these inequities was, I felt, powerful. It acknowledged the realities of current social configurations, from the structured inequities that result in girls being labeled "sluts" and boys being complimented for their perceived sexual promiscuity (e.g., Dunn 2004; Faulkner 2003); to what so many of us have witnessed (in life, perhaps, and certainly in mainstream media representations) as girls' apparent greater emotional investment in their sexual partners than boys'.

AOUME speakers and curricula offered a solution to these inequitable outcomes that naturalized inequities (it's boys' nature to be this way, they can't change) and provided girls a "failsafe" solution: abstinence until marriage. Girls could be empowered only through their resistance to boys' natural demands. If they had sex, they "lost" their power to boys. As one Florida AOUME presenter said,

> Girls, if you are sleeping with a guy, what you want most is commitment and intimacy. Well, you won't get it. Your power lies in your giving of yourself. . . . You're giving away your power with sex.

Such an understanding of girls' empowerment precludes any discussion of power in sexual relationships (particularly forced sex); of sex as anything other than a commodity to be exchanged (discussed further in chapter 10); and of the possibility of variety in girls' desires and needs. It limits models of empowerment to women's capacity to control men, and expunges the possibility of a woman's life not revolving around a man. From this perspective, women are only able to gain power and maintain their rightful place—as beloved wife and mother—by *managing* men correctly. Take, for example, SIECUS's commentary on a story told in the popular AOUME curriculum Choosing the Best Soul Mate, which targets eleventh and twelfth graders:

> Deep inside every man is a knight in shining armor, ready to rescue a maiden and slay a wicked dragon. When a man feels trusted, he is free to be the strong, protecting man he longs to be.
>
> Unfortunately for this knight in shining armor, his princess is not one to sit back and allow herself to be rescued. Instead, she has ideas about how he might best slay the dragon. When the second dragon attacks, she suggests that instead of the sword he uses a noose. This works, and "everyone is happy, except the knight who doesn't feel like a hero this time. He would have preferred to use his sword." The princess's continuing suggestions (for the third dragon she recommends poison) make the knight doubt his own instincts and feel ashamed despite the fact that he continues to slay dragons.
>
> Then one day he hears another maiden in distress. Though he initially doubts himself, at the last minute he remembers how he used to feel "before he met the princess" and uses his sword [to kill the dragon]. He never does return to the princess. Instead, he lived happily ever after with the maiden, "but only after making sure she knew nothing of nooses or poison."
>
> The moral of this story: "Occasional suggestions and assistance may be all right, but too much of it will lessen a man's confidence or even turn him away

from his princess." (*Choosing the Best SOUL MATE*, Leader Guide, p. 51. In SIECUS 2008, n.p.)

Like SIECUS, a number of commentators and reports have described this story as an example of the gender-inequitable traditionalist ideology present in AOUME curricula (e.g., Advocates for Youth 2008; United States House of Representatives, Committee on Government Reform 2004). It is, but the inequities it posits are neotraditional, not traditional. The princess does not lose the prince because she is inherently stupid or evil (older tropes in Christian storytelling); she loses him because she does not *manage* him correctly. The story does not ask her to be less intelligent or to stop having better ideas than the prince. It asks her to be aware of his more fragile ego and of his "natural" need to feel that he is taking effective action. In other words, the princess would still have the prince if, instead of taking on the "masculine" role of decisionmaker, she had convinced him that *he* had had the idea to use a noose or poison to kill the dragons. This framing of girls' capacities questions men's naturalized superiority more than in past tropes. Instead of being *naturally* right, the knight is presented as insecure and limited in his knowledge and capacities.

Though in such stories older discourses of unquestioned male superiority are altered, the newer narratives are best understood not as efforts to transform the traditional gender hierarchy, but to transform the mechanism by which this hierarchy is maintained. As a Florida AOUME trainer said,

> It's a good thing to be a Crock-Pot. Guys are visual stimulators, while girls are relational. Guys have to learn to turn off the visual in their heads. The culture will tell males not to worry, but when it becomes a fantasy in your head, then you want a magazine. Then you want to masturbate. . . . Every day a man battles it, to be faithful in my brain to my wife. Our kids live in a microwave culture. We live in the US, where everything is easy. But relationships are *not* easy. The culture has always got an agenda. *Stepford Wives* and all those shows bash women staying at home. *Desperate Housewives* says cheating and bed-hopping is OK. But it's not. We have to help especially young girls understand they have a lot of self-worth and power. But sex gives your power to him.

AOUME curricular activities and teacher-led conversations in AOUME classes effectively melded older tropes about gender hierarchies with newer discourses of women's empowerment that reflect a neotraditionalist focus on women's responsibility to manage gender relations. A strong woman manages (bestial) men effectively, gaining power through her refusal to hand over her most precious asset (her virginity) to them. If she manages this process correctly, she gains social, emotional, spiritual, and physical security in the present and in the future as a treasured wife and mother, helpmate to a man whose spiritual and emotional life has been vastly improved by her influence. If not, she pays the price now and in the future.

Neotraditional gender norms sound much more empowering than traditional ones to many parents and teens, and both sound more realistic than CSE's "de-gendered" rational actor. But the consequences of nonmarital sex are largely socially constructed, not naturally predetermined. Pregnancy and STI-transmission rates are much lower throughout the rest of the Western world than they are in the United States (Rose 2005; UNICEF 2001), and many of the consequences of STIs and pregnancy for women are less prevalent in other Western countries because basic reproductive health care and other social services (quality day care, job training, and so on) are accessible to all. AOUME curricula center these naturalized (but largely socially constructed) consequences in a new "girl-power" discourse that circumscribes a very specific realm of what females can control (their sexuality, and thus men's naturalized desires), and what they cannot (the potential consequences of having sex outside of marriage, men in any setting where women have not controlled their sexuality). The AOUME model of girls' empowerment does not, in other words, encompass many commonly identified aspects of empowerment. It is not empowering of women's voices, desires, decision-making, or freedom of choice. It is not supportive of structural equity. It restricts women's power, tying it entirely to their ability to control those with greater physical and social power—men—in order to assume their only rightful places in society as mother and wife.

This model of empowerment also denigrates men's capacities and choices, and silences male voices and experiences concerning emotional connections in relationships, responsibility toward women and children, and desires for gender egalitarianism in relationships. Just as it figures women as weak, emotional, and manipulative, it figures men as unaccountable, animalistic, and incapable of deep spiritual or social connection.

FEMINISM, EGALITARIANISM, AND COMPLEMENTARIANISM

The AOUME approach to girls' empowerment should be understood in relation to the tensions that exist in New Christian Right circles around feminism, egalitarianism, and liberalism (in the classical political sense). AOUME organizations and curricula generally adopt a complementary model of gender relations, in which men and women have "separate but equal" roles in the home.[13] While men's role is described as "loving, humble headship," women's is described as "joyful, intelligent submission" (Grudem 2004, 43). As such, AOUME approaches dismiss the evangelical feminist movements that call for equality in gender roles and rights (including in church leadership), which have been pioneered by more liberal evangelical denominations over the past fifty years (Grudem 2004). It is not surprising that these perspectives are largely absent, since more liberal evangelical denominations are not key actors in the AOUME movement.

The perceived danger that egalitarian gender roles—of the progressive political or Evangelical ilk—will transform patriarchy is made clear in statements by supporters of complementarianism. Grudem says, for example, "What then is the doctrinal direction in which egalitarianism leads? To an abolition of anything distinctly masculine. An androgynous Adam. A Jesus whose manhood is not important, just his 'humanity.' A God who is both Father and Mother, and then a God who is Mother but cannot be called Father" (Grudem 2004, 512–513). The need to differentiate and maintain as distinct—and distinctly powerful—male traits and roles is central to this approach, and it is the reason why so much of the AOUME programming actively works to position women's roles and "power" as gained through their "joyfully submissive" relationship to men.

This understanding of the positioning of mainstream AOUME approaches to girls' empowerment within broader doctrinal debates also helps explain why the former tend to emphasize how to create ideal romantic relationships between opposite-sex "soul mates" and strong father-centered families. The curricula teach that the responsibility for creating and maintaining these relationships lies primarily with girls and women. Seen from this perspective, teen pregnancy, date rape, and sexual abuse become, at their core, more female than male failings. Grudem says, for example, while talking about "distortions" that occur to biblical gender roles,

> A wife can also commit errors of passivity . . . She knows her husband and her children are doing wrong and she says nothing. Or her husband becomes verbally or physically abusive, and she never objects to him, never seeks church discipline or civil intervention to bring about an end to the abuse. (Grudem 2004, 43)

BUYING PROTECTION: EMPOWERMENT THROUGH SELF-PRESENTATION

AOUME discussion about empowerment was largely individualized, but group empowerment was occasionally discussed. These conversations revealed an important link between models of empowerment and girls' and boys' roles as consumers. In order to maintain her power, a girl must act in ways that do not tempt boys. This includes her decisions about where to meet and when to be alone with a boy, her behavior around boys, and how she dresses and presents herself. It was in relation to this last point that girls' consumer empowerment was most often discussed, as exemplified by the following story:

> FLORIDA AOUME TRAINING PARTICIPANT: What should we say to people who say that abstinence is discriminating against girls?
>
> SPEAKER: I tell them there is nothing more powerful and nothing more empowering for girls than abstinence. There's a story that I like to tell people about how powerful girls can be. You might want to share it. There was a group of girlfriends in Texas who were getting ready for their senior prom. They were so excited about it, and they were getting all ready, going out shopping for their dresses and shoes and everything. Well, they were just shocked when they went looking for prom dresses, because all they could find were these dresses that were too short, or cut too low, or too flashy. They got really concerned. What kind of message would their dates get if they showed up dressed like this? What would he assume about her? How would they be able to enjoy the prom, worried about how they look?
>
> Well, they were so upset. They were talking about whether they should skip the prom or what they should do, and they decided to write a letter to the president of Macy's, letting him know that they were not happy with their [dress] choices. So they wrote this letter and sent it off, and wouldn't you know it, the president of Macy's read this letter, and he was so impressed with them and their initiative that he called them in to the headquarters, and he called in the designers, and he said, "Let these girls tell you what kind of prom dresses they want, and we will make it happen." And Macy's made a whole line of prom dresses that these girls and other girls like them could wear to their prom, to feel comfortable and beautiful. Isn't that an incredible story? That's the power of fighting for what you believe in. That's the power that these young girls had.

AOUME organizations and the New Christian Right have a complex relationship with the media, consumerism, and commodification. On one hand, every AOUME event I attended was full of disparaging comments about the "liberal media" and its attacks on Christians and their values. On the other hand, many speakers discussed the importance of understanding and using the media to transform teens' ideas and practices. The use of social-marketing techniques, such as the "branding" of abstinence by "It's Great to Wait," was mentioned to me repeatedly as an appropriate and effective way to capitalize on the fact that "teens these days are really savvy about media. You've gotta know who 50 Cent and Britney are. We have to have better, stronger messages than these folks, or our message gets lost" (as a Florida basic AOUME trainer said). Likewise, a private Florida AOUME service provider talked about the importance of receiving federal AOUME funding so that their curriculum could be "updated." When I asked how the materials were to be updated, she said the packaging would be improved, because "if the packaging isn't good, then kids aren't interested." Members of the AOUME movement view teens as powerful consumers; to reach these consumers most effectively, they adopt an individualized, gendered, and demographically targeted approach to behavior change, that is, a consumer marketing approach (e.g., Tadajewski and Brownlie 2008; Pfeiffer 2004).

The literature on the use, costs, and benefits of social-marketing approaches to public health issues is extensive.[14] One important aspect of such approaches is their focus on "branding" a product, be it a message or an object. In order to brand effectively, messages must be simple and widely disseminated. People do not need to understand the product in order to buy it or use it effectively; the primary goal is to change behavior by changing preferences and tastes, not ideas or knowledge. Such an approach fits well with AOUME's adoption of directive teaching approaches and their understanding of children and adolescents as subordinates requiring the guidance of loving, knowledgeable adults, not people who should be seeking knowledge and weighing actions on their own terms (Luker 2006). As one speaker said in closing an AOUME training session, "Teens are looking for clarity and guidance, especially girls. That is what abstinence gives: a clear, easy message for kids to follow to protect their bodies, hearts, souls, emotions, and reputations."

AOUME models thus view teenagers not as rational consumers in need of information to improve their decisions but as emotional consumers in need of guidance and persuasion. By being good consumers of social actions (abstinence) and products (demure clothes) throughout their premarital lives, girls can appropriately fulfill their social roles. They can also assure that boys have fewer opportunities to make "bad" consumer choices. Boys' primary consumer decisions are about girls, and ultimately, about which girl to marry. By removing temptation to stray before marriage, girls assure that boys make better decisions down the road.

Empowerment for girls was tied, then, to girls' capacity to use their individual and aggregate power as consumers to transform the products available to them, be they dresses, television shows, or, potentially, husbands. Their power and their social acceptability and safety is based on their capacity to buy products and ideas that shape an appropriate presentation of self. This is a limited model of power, obviously, directed at controlling their bodies and shaping men's (and thus society's) responses to them. Issues such as sexual violence and people's responsibility to respect girls' physical sanctity no matter their appearance, as well as girls' right to present themselves as they wish without social consequences, are thoroughly undermined by this empowerment model.

CSE's Rational Model of Gender Relations

In contrast to the numerous discussions about gender differences and girls' empowerment that I encountered in AOUME programming, there was very little structured discussion about gender and none about gender-differentiated empowerment in the CSE and abstinence-based programs I observed. CSE programs see themselves as empowering all youth through the provision of information, and view AOUME approaches as actively disempowering. For example, ChoiceUSA, a youth-led advocacy group, compares AOUME and CSE approaches as follows:

> Abstinence-only education assumes that all young people across the country have the same experience with sex and sexuality and disseminates misinformation about contraception, abortion, STIs and pregnancy.
>
> Abstinence-only curriculum [sic] does not respond to the powerful realities we face and stigmatizes:
>
> —those who have already chosen to have sex
> —those who are in or plan to have non-traditional families
> —LGBTQ youth
> —survivors of sexual abuse and
> —those of us abstaining for reasons outside of a marriage model.
>
> Comprehensive sex education programs teach "more than the birds and the bees," empowering young people with truthful information about sex and sexuality. (http://www.choiceusa.org, 2009)

This account of CSE emphasizes the limited range of acceptable social relations propounded in AOUME curricula, and ties empowerment to an expansion of individual and structural choices facilitated through increased knowledge, as opposed to the normalization of a particular gender ideology. But there are serious inadequacies in CSE programming when it comes to gender. What appears to be a formal curricular silence in CSE concerning gender relations actually reflects a gender ideology that is tied to global models of universal human rights and Western liberal feminism. This ideology propounds a gender/race/class-blind equality among all people. Most mainstream CSE programming assumes that society consists of a collectivity of equally agentic, emancipated, and empowered individuals. These individuals are "post-gender/sex/class/race," in that their equality as humans supersedes categorical distinctions that have been used historically to fuel social inequity. This is a liberal (in the classical political sense) model of personhood and social relations that holds the promise of potential social transformation, but in practice, this ideology played out in three unexpected, and ideologically undesirable, ways in CSE classrooms and programs.

First, the nature of this idealized model makes it difficult for CSE programs to engage critically with the realities of social, economic, political, and relational inequities and to connect to students' actual experiences of gender and power. Talking about gender makes visible exactly the categories that the ideology attempts to erase. Not surprisingly, then, most often gender is simply not mentioned in CSE programming, as if by not being discussed, it ceases to exist as a social reality. The questions about "power, privilege, and access" that can be raised by programs that acknowledge and discuss the importance of gender also disappear.

Second, problems translating CSE gender ideology into practice led to teachers often stereotyping and reestablishing neotraditionalist gender norms in their classroom interactions. Finally, teachers and students regularly failed to call each other out on sexist behaviors, so in practice CSE classrooms did not embody gender equal values in conversation or in people's interactions.

By assuming, but not discussing, a de-gendered equality model, CSE programs provided few opportunities for students or teachers to engage with, and potentially adopt, adapt, or reject this understanding of gender and gender relations. Students and teachers often filled this official gender silence with the readily available neotraditionalist gender norms that shape much of our common sense, our gender scripts, in the United States.[15]

GENDER EQUALITY IN THE CURRICULUM

The CSE curricula used in the classes I observed seldom included activities that directly addressed gender. Most activities and written materials assumed that female and male students were similar in their interests, capacities, experiences, and needs. Activities that were likely to raise issues related to gender norms and expectations, such as those that asked students to discuss relationships, families, or life plans, did not structure classroom discussion about gender and did not include follow-up questions that directed students' attention to gender issues. For example, California's curricular materials on abortion, on making a life plan, and on communicating in relationships included not a single mention of gender roles, differences, or inequities. The following excerpt from the Wisconsin curricular unit Building Healthy Relationships shows a similar pattern:

> How to say no
> —Buy time. Say you'll get back to the person.
> —State exactly how you feel. Be direct and honest.
> —Don't apologize for your decisions or values.
> —Use a firm and friendly tone of voice.
> —Use the other person's name.
> — Offer an alternative, healthier, more acceptable-to-you opinion.
> —Avoid compromise if you feel strongly about something. Compromise can
>   be a slow way of saying *yes* when you don't mean to.

The assumption in this exercise is that the negotiation over "saying no" to sex occurs between two rational, equally empowered individuals, and that the individual who wishes to say no can convince the other of her or his position simply by "using a firm and friendly voice" and the other person's name. While these may indeed be useful approaches to "saying no" in some situations and relationships, the activity ignores the power dynamics that shape negotiations about sex, provides no space for students to talk about how to "say no" when the other partner is aggressive about "saying yes," and ignores the copious literature on gender-differentiated social norms concerning sexual gatekeeping (e.g., Tolman, Hirschman, and Impett 2005). Similarly, Fields's study (2008) of sex education in North Carolina found few formal spaces for girls and boys to talk about sexual negotiation, the realities of physical aggression in some relationships, and the power dynamics that shape all relationships. As we saw in the AOUME programs, it is more expected and socially acceptable for women to be handling aggressive sexual demands from men than vice versa, and sexual violence in relationships is largely male-on-female. Eliding discussion about how gender norms rationalize male aggression and female negotiation makes gender categories, but not lived inequities in expectations or in power, disappear.

CSE curricula presumed that all students required the same information and therefore had few or no gender-differentiated activities. It was also assumed that there would be no difference in how females and males used the information they received to make rational and enforceable decisions about sexual activity. For example, while Florida AOUME materials included gender-disaggregated information on pregnancy outcomes and STI rates to highlight girls' increased risk, Wyoming's and Wisconsin's materials contained no gender-disaggregated information, and the curricula and teachers consistently indicated that both boys and girls would "pay" for unprotected sex through potential pregnancies or STIs. Teachers described this as an effort to "not let boys off the hook," but it closed off an opportunity to acknowledge and analyze the social systems that shape many of the gender-differentiated outcomes of teenage pregnancy and parenting, and of STI transmission.

It is understandable that CSE approaches would not emphasize (or even mention) differences based on gender, sexuality, race, ethnicity, age, disability, or any other identity category that has traditionally been used to discriminate against people. Silencing these differences and presenting all people as equal and equally agentic is a powerful discursive move to erase historic inequities in the abstract, and it is a favored approach of universal human rights discourses. Yet as Pollock (2004) demonstrates in examining race talk in US schools, fostering equity by attempting to silently norm it in an inequitable society poses problems in practice. This approach provided few practical opportunities to discuss or to challenge students' experiences of inequities, or to engage students and teachers in a critical analysis of inequities. Instead, students and teachers reverted to the most easily accessible and shared social ideology that explains inequitable realities—one that is based on traditionalist, gender-differentiated norms and that sounded remarkably like the neotraditional ideology promulgated by AOUME approaches. Notably, a parallel silence on homosexuality was used by AOUME supporters to erase acknowledgment of the equal claims—or even existence—of queer people. In both cases, the silence served in practice to stabilize stigmatizing norms.

Even within the presumption of gender equality embedded in CSE curricula, there were contradictions. The curricula generally assumed de-gendered actors, but when girls and boys were represented, examples sometimes reinscribed traditionalist gender norms. The Wisconsin curriculum contained the following exercise for students, which I show in excerpted form:

> Student A:
> You are Josh.
> You've been dating Maggie for three months. You and Maggie have been spending *all* of your time together. You haven't hung out or played basketball with your friends in a long time. Your friends have started to tease you about spending so much time with your girlfriend.
> This weekend they're going to see a basketball game and have invited you to come along. You've already made plans to go to a party with Maggie. You've told Maggie you'll go to the party, so you feel as if you have to go. You're angry, however, because you may be losing your friends . . .

Student B:

You are Maggie.

You've been dating Josh for three months. The two of you spend *all* of your time together. Tomorrow night your best friend is having a party. You're so excited for [*sic*] it. Josh said he'd go with you. Your friends are impressed that you have a boyfriend. You can't wait to walk into the party together. You will look really popular . . .

In this example, Josh is focused on his friends and on sports, not on Maggie. He agreed to go to the party with Maggie, but because his friends don't support him spending time with her, he is now "angry" that he has to go. Maggie, on the other hand, is focused on how her friends will (positively) perceive her having a boyfriend. While Josh will gain status among his friends by ignoring Maggie's needs, Maggie gains status by showing her friends that she is in a serious relationship with Josh. As with AOUME materials, the "Josh and Maggie" exercise reinforces a male-centered social environment in which girls are focused on their popularity, which is gained through their relationship with boys, and boys are focused on physical activities with their same-sex friends where they gain favor by not letting themselves be affected by their relationships with girls. In this example, Maggie's demands for relational attention from Josh result in male aggression (Josh's "anger"), which is another naturalized aspect of AOUME gender norms.

OBSERVED CURRICULA

Beyond the lack of discussion about gender roles, inequities, and differences in formal curricular materials,[16] I observed many instances of teachers and students in CSE schools reinscribing (neo)traditionalist gender relations in the classroom and out. For example, in Wisconsin after male and female students discussed the traits they desired in a boyfriend or girlfriend, Mr. Kelly (the teacher trainee) and Mrs. Shane said the following:

MR. KELLY: As you can see, there is a big difference between how a lot of guys think and a lot of girls think. Lots of guys just think about sex. Everyone is a sexual being, but generally guys care more about the physical relationship. Girls should take care, because lots of times you think he likes you, but he just cared about the physical side. Girls, you need to be careful.

MRS. SHANE: Mr. Kelly pointed out a good thing here. For so many years of teaching, I can't tell you how many times I hear girls say, "But he said he loved me." Dating is to help you find someone that you like!

Likewise, in one of Wyoming's ostensibly ABSE classrooms, Mr. Dean said the following during a lesson on marriage and parenthood, which did not include a formal discussion of gender:[17]

> Turn to page 498; it talks about marriage and parenthood and being together. When you find that person, you make a commitment. What do vows say? [Students say, in unison, "Until death do us part."] There are a lot of things that can almost break this. They might snore. She might be a cuddler—she abstained, she has the perfect life married to the person that she loves more than either Mom or Dad. But now she puts her cold feet on him—that's part of the vows, better or worse, richer or poorer . . . Whoever did that [the vows] is a pretty smart female. Men aren't smart enough to write that! [He laughs.] You know, that's not always happening in society—there's divorce. She keeps putting her feet on me, she keeps spending all of my money! Remember earlier this semester I wrote up here "70/30"? That's about what relationships need to be. The woman needs to give 70 percent, the man 30 percent. [He laughs.] Her job is to wash the dishes, do the laundry, have breakfast on the table. [Kids are laughing, mostly with him.] I'll tell you something, though [gets serious], that is pretty true. Now, the man also needs to give 70 percent. Let her sleep—she's the one having the baby, doing all of the work.

When teachers talked about gender, they regularly reverted to the stereotypes that are deliberately normalized in AOUME curricula and much of US mainstream media: girls want love and connection and are focused on boys, while boys want an easy lay and just don't care as much as girls. Women should care for the home and for children, while men should work outside the home. Contrast the above examples with one of the times that I saw a teacher deliberately discuss gender-equitable norms:

> Students have just finished a quiz from the textbook. Ms. Jeffries has them exchange papers to grade each others' quizzes. She reads the questions aloud, making sure each student answers one of the questions. True or false: It is a developmental task of adolescence to develop intimate relationships? False, answers Megan, "It's a task of adulthood." "Right," says Ms. Jeffries. True or false: Housework is a point of potential contention in marriage. Ms. Jeffries stops and asks, "How many of your dads cook and clean?" Some of the students say yes, most say sometimes. "How many of your moms mow the lawn?" All of the students say yes. Ms. Jeffries then says, "An even distribution is what is important. These things have to be negotiated, you have to really talk about them together so that you don't get this being a point of contention."

I heard relatively fewer statements like the one above, in which teachers deliberately attempted to inscribe gender-equitable norms, than I did of statements that reinscribed neotraditional roles. Students also more often discussed gender relations in an inequitable manner. These conversations often consisted of boys aggressively challenging girls' claims to equality, such as an exchange I heard in Mr. Lauder's Wyoming classroom: Two girls near me were talking to each other about how they felt equal to boys. A boy at the next desk who was listening in shouted, "But who's president?" "Only because a girl hasn't won yet!" one of the girls shouted back. The boy guffawed loudly, and other boys around the two girls joined in.

I never heard a teacher disrupt gender-biased statements or interactions among students. Students only occasionally disrupted each other's or a teacher's gender-biased comments, and as we saw in Shurita's case, these challenges were often ignored. In contrast, when students talked in a way that might be considered threatening to traditional gender norms, other students often silenced them, they were silenced by teachers, or they quickly worked to reestablish these norms and their relationship to social status. For example, in the Wisconsin class, the following exchange occurred between a female student and a male student:

> Theo and Shurita are arguing about food. He says you can live on mac[aroni] and cheese, she says that is not real food. He snarls back, "Oh, and what's real food? Soul food?" "Yes!" she replies. "That's food that [unintelligible] best!" He snarls back an unintelligible response, at which point she says, "Shut up, boy! I mean, girl! I mean, whatever you are . . . I love you, Theo." He tells her to back off, which she does.
>
> A few minutes later, the class is asked to divide up by gender. Theo, adopting a high "girly" voice, first says that he will sit with the girls, then says he will sit between the girls and boys. When he moves over to the boys' group at Mr. Kelly's urging, he tells a lower-status, smaller boy, "Excuse me, Jason, no girls over here."

In this exchange, Shurita challenges Theo's gender identity, and thus his status. Mr. Kelly urges Theo to identify himself "appropriately" as a boy, after which Theo responds by reestablishing his dominance by inscribing femininity on a lower-status, physically smaller boy. Such exchanges showed that talk about gender is charged and potentially dangerous for students; student exchanges consistently indicated that being labeled as feminine or a girl lowered students' status in relation to students labeled as masculine or male. These interactions were often reinforced by teachers.

Students' school experiences outside the classroom also shaped their perceptions of school-validated and socially acceptable gender norms. For example, in Wyoming, teachers were generally uncomfortable with what they perceived as expressions of students' sexuality at school. Their perceptions of what constituted such expressions, however, differed markedly for males and females. While boy/girl couples engaging in public displays of affection were viewed as equally responsible for violating school rules, girls were much more likely to be reprimanded for their self-presentation (particularly for what they were wearing). Many girls complained that their "right to self-expression" through clothing choices was read as sexual by teachers, while boys' was not. Indeed, conversations with teachers supported this view. As one female teacher put it,

> There's this current fashion trend towards sexy clothes for females. On TV, for example, and the shopping options here are narrow. The staff is fighting a valiant effort to have girls cover up. I tell girls that they are gorgeous, but the boys can't get work done, so go home and change for their sake and the school's GPA. Some of the kids debated this, too, saying they have the right to wear what they want. But . . . we are trying to say that sexuality is not OK here.

The district program officer similarly (and unwittingly) echoed girls' concerns that teacher responses to boys and girls were inequitable:

> The school is very nervous. There are girls wearing no underwear and skirts, or thongs and skirts that are see-through. . . . Once they're in our building, boys are making comments, they're distracted in the classrooms, and cleavage seems to be a huge deal, too. . . . We go round and round with the dress code, but we don't talk about sexuality with students. And male teachers won't even get close to the female students, which then makes other [female] teachers uncomfortable. I think they [male teachers] are uncomfortable because of lawsuits; they just don't want to go there.

Some female students' palpable fury over dress codes in Wyoming reflected their understanding that teachers regulated girls' dress as a way of prioritizing boys' needs (in this case, boys' supposed inability to concentrate on schoolwork) over girls' desires for self-expression. Girls who claimed the right to express their sexuality through uncovering instead of covering up were viewed as tempting instead of controlling boys' desires and faced school opprobrium and disciplinary measures. Thus, the type of gender norms promulgated by AOUME curricula was structured into daily educational practices in this officially CSE school.[18]

Schools can address girls' clothing choices in a variety of ways, but Teton's response is perhaps the most common—create a dress code that applies almost entirely to girls (with the exception of boys' pants not showing more than a certain amount of underwear) and enforce the code without further discussion. Levy (2005) argues that girls' states of (un)dress at school reflect norms of sexiness and femininity that are widespread in the United States and that represent a problematic, superficial, and largely negative sexualization of female identity. It is also quite possible that this way of dressing distracts some students and teachers of both sexes. But if a curriculum is premised on a liberal (in the classical political sense) worldview that assumes that teenagers are rational individuals who simply need more correct and complete information to make good choices, then one of two possibilities presents itself. One possibility is that girls are well aware of the potential effect of their clothing on others, but choose to dress as they do for their own well-conceived reasons, in which case, impinging on girls' presentation of self because of boys' responses is utterly inequitable. The second possibility is that girls lack information and opportunities for critical reflection about the decisions they are making concerning their dress. In this case, providing an opportunity for girls and boys to critically explore the effects of advertising, media, and consumer targeting on girls' and boys' identity and sexuality would be in order.[19] In neither case does CSE ideology align with adult policing of student decision-making in the way that occurs in many schools. This practice marks another point of tension, in which teachers' responses to gender differences (in dress) reflect a reversion to neotraditional norms and practices in CSE schools.

I was able to observe teachers' conflicting responses to students' performances of gender and sexuality at a sophomore school dance at Teton High, which was chaperoned by teachers. The dance evidenced the neotraditional gender ideology and heteronormativity that regularly shaped school interactions in both CSE and AOUME schools I observed. Before the dance, students were warned that "inappropriate" behavior on the dance floor would not be tolerated. At one point during the night, a teacher intervened to pull apart a lanky sophomore boy and his petite female dance partner, who were attempting, rather unsuccessfully given the significant height difference, to grind on the dance floor. After the teacher intervened, the boy went to sit with his friends in a chair by the side of the dance floor. The girl walked over to where he was sitting and laughingly drew one of her female friends out onto the dance floor, whereupon the two proceeded to come much closer to grinding than the boy and girl had managed. The same teacher who had pulled apart the boy and girl watched the two female dancers hesitantly. At one point, when the girls were running their hands up and down each others' torsos and pulling up each other's skirts to the tops of their thighs, the teacher seemed ready to step in, but she changed her mind and hung back.

The dance between the girls was performed directly in front of the boy;

this was not, according to teachers with whom I later spoke, a sexual dance *between* the girls, but a performance *for* the boy. As such, though a number of teachers were uncomfortable with the performance, they felt that there were no appropriate grounds to protest the dancing. Since the girls were not "dancing for each other," the dance was not "sexual."

Levy's book *Female Chauvinist Pigs* (2005) speaks to the teachers' understanding of the girls' dance as a "non-sexual" event because it was not performed for the girls' own sexual enjoyment. In the book, she critiques a cultural shift toward widespread support for "raunch culture," in which girls' "sexiness" is predicated on their consumption of clothing, plastic surgeries, and other products that idealize a highly sexualized (as in, based on porn stars) female body and behavior aimed at capturing male attention, not on women's own enjoyment of or pride in their own sexuality.

The teacher's intervention in the first dance, where the boy and girl were enjoying and focused on each other but were not in any danger of attracting much attention from others or of having sex was replaced, following the teacher's intervention, with a *Girls Gone Wild*–style exhibition of girls as sexual objects for boys' enjoyment. It is this tension in adult intervention in students' (but particularly girls') expressions of sexuality in ways that implicitly or explicitly support both neotraditional gender norms and girls' sexual objectification that was a particular ideological contradiction in the hidden gender curriculum at Teton and, to a greater or lesser extent, at all of the CSE schools in which I conducted observations.[20]

EVADED CURRICULA

Although gender was generally evaded in the CSE and abstinence-based programs I observed, teachers, other school personnel, and students identified particular issues that could be addressed to improve girls' and boys' gendered experiences at school. For example, Wyoming's school nurse, guidance counselor, and a number of teachers mentioned their concern with the number of younger girls who were dating significantly older men and the effects of alcohol on both students' sexual behavior and parents' behavior toward their children. California instructors identified similar concerns.

Although these topics were considered key issues in teens' lives by teachers and students alike, they were not openly discussed at school. Other topics such as sexual abuse, rape, and violence in relationships were mentioned as issues by girls in every school in which I conducted observations, but were not addressed in any depth by teachers or curricula.

Unlike in AOUME approaches, where norms about silence, secrecy, and the sacredness of sex made it difficult to discuss even simple sex acts, I heard teachers in California and Wisconsin, and medical personnel in Wyoming, openly and comfortably discuss sex acts that would be considered taboo in AOUME schools. In California and Wisconsin, for example, teachers and students discussed anal sex, and how to make it safer, in detail. But although the "biology" of sex could be openly discussed, I heard gender and power inequities in relationships and relationship-abuse rates mentioned only twice (both times in the course of presenting students with discrete facts about the average age of males and females in teenage relationships). Similarly, I heard no discussion about students' experiences of sexism or other forms of discrimination, nor did I witness a sustained effort by any CSE teacher to disrupt talk that naturalized neotraditional gender norms or to provide students an opportunity to think critically about the gender ideologies that underlay the sex education curriculum or sex education classroom practices.

Teachers also failed to create opportunities to talk about decision-making and sexual negotiation in real relationships. Teachers stuck to hypothetical situations in their examples, and when students challenged these scenarios, teachers tended to revert to a discussion of the laws that govern teen relationships (such as statutory rape provisions), as in Emily's interaction with a student concerning the dangers of older man/younger woman relationships. As described in chapter 6, Emily provided the class with data about the pregnancy and marriage outcomes of such relationships, but she did not have students talk about the topic further, nor did she engage another student's comment about the power dynamics in such relationships.

Conclusion

Too often, evaluations of sex education programs fail to examine the consequences of the neotraditionalist gender assumptions embedded in AOUME and CSE programs alike. This is a failure with potentially significant ramifications for students' formal sex education experiences and for the messages they receive in school about appropriate social relations.

AOUME models draw on a gender ideology that is backed by millennia of religious and social practice. This neotraditionalist model allows AOUM educators to acknowledge and address the effects of socially differentiated gender norms on students' lives, and as such powerfully connects with some teachers', students', and parents' experiences of gender inequity in relationships.

The acknowledgement of girls' more precarious social status in many sexual relationships, and discussion about their need for protection, resonated strongly with many parents and teachers—politically liberal and con-

servative—with whom I spoke. As one politically liberal Florida parent said
to me,

> Look, abstinence [education] really appeals to me more than I thought. Thing
> is, it's *true* that girls get involved more than boys and get hurt more. When
> Jack was growing up, I was worried he would come home and tell me he had
> gotten some girl pregnant. Let me tell you, that's totally different with Emy.
> I'm terrified *she's* going to come home pregnant and it's *her* life that will be
> changed by having an abortion or having that baby. For women, it's the whole
> experience. It's their bodies that go through this. It's on their shoulders to
> make the choices and deal with the consequences.

When it comes down to it, although they identify significant movement
toward egalitarianism in girls' and boys' opportunities and relationships,
parents (and teens) are keenly aware that gender hierarchies still infuse their
daily lives,[20] and that the social, emotional, and physical outcomes of sex,
especially in adolescence, are often in practice inequitable for boys and girls.
Not surprisingly, then, AOUME's focus on these differences speaks powerfully to people's lived experiences, even in cases where parents strongly disap-
prove of the assumption of natural gender differences, are cognizant of the
social conditions that structure the gender-inequitable outcomes of teen sex,
and are themselves thoroughly dismissive of the ideas that sex and childbearing within marriage is always "safe" and leads to positive outcomes, and that
sex outside of marriage always leads to negative outcomes.

Indeed, the gender ideology that underlies AOUME models reflects very
particular social and religious beliefs that are far from universal in the United
States. It does not address what are now most students' and parents' experiences of living in a "nontraditional" family. It shuts out the possibility of
healthy non-heterosexual sexuality, and it reinscribes patriarchy by maintaining a rigid and naturalized hierarchy between men and women, and between adults and children. It is, by Western liberal (in the classical political
sense) standards, inequitable and undemocratic.

The CSE gender model represents an ideal of egalitarianism, and as such,
is conceptually much more inclusive than the AOUME model. In practice,
however, CSE curricula and programs are largely silent about the realities of
gender norms and practices in the United States, attempting instead to create universal human equality by silencing talk about gender. They are thus
often out of synch with teachers', students', and parents' lived experiences
of gender differences and inequities. CSE programs presented students with
an idealized social model consisting of rational, equal individuals engaged
in free choices concerning their sexuality, their careers, their educational fu-

tures, and so forth. While on one hand this can be understood as an empowering message about the equal rights and worth of all students, in practice the lack of engagement with gender inequalities leads to missed opportunities for teachers and students to consider the gendered assumptions that they bring to classrooms and schools, the differences among people's assumptions, and the potential of universal human-rights models to provide an alternate and empowering framework within which to examine and critique existing gender inequities in high schools and US society.

Since CSE's idealized model of de-gendered equality failed to connect to people's lived experiences, and since traditional gender norms are the most readily accessible framework through which to make sense of people's daily experiences with gender differences, teachers and students in CSE classrooms (and even CSE curricula) often reverted to neotraditional gender norms.

CSE approaches embody a particular abstracted model of liberal equality and universal human rights that provides little traction for students and parents to relate to their own lives. Thus, in practice, it ends up providing no real alternative to neotraditional gender norms. The assumption that CSE approaches embody and effectively promulgate more liberatory models of relationships, sex, and sexuality for students and families needs to be questioned.

On the other hand, AOUME models do not recognize that difference does not and should not translate into unequal rights and responsibilities, and in this sense, they are profoundly antidemocratic. AOUME models normalize a traditional family structure that denigrates or denies many of the families in which students live and many of the relationships students want to have, fails to validate the roles that women play as "father" and "mother" in so many families, and does not acknowledge the positive and nurturing roles that many men play in their children's lives.

AOUME gender ideology, visible in every classroom I observed, is fundamentally unaligned with broad liberal democratic citizenship principles as they have been practiced in the United States for the last fifty years, as well as models of politically liberal ethics and social relations. It offers a limited and limiting model of empowerment in which men are naturally chauvinist pigs and women's "empowered" actions support patriarchy. Unless CSE advocates and educators attempt to directly address and transform this hidden gender curricula, this ideology will continue to shape sex education practices in CSE and AOUME schools alike.

"What Are We Doing about the Homosexual Threat?": Scientism, Sexual Identity, and Sexuality Education

There are kids who don't hear as much about sex from their parents as I do. . . . They might learn from sex education [at school]. But there's a lot of students who just don't want to know. Especially stuff about lesbian, gay, bisexual, transgender, and questioning. Like I had a friend who didn't want to know about them at all. I mean all we learned was [the definition of] "homosexual," but she said it made her uncomfortable. Well, I think we should learn this even if its uncomfortable to talk about it. People say "You're so gay" all the time, and stuff like that. Everyone always talks like that, like it's nothing. It's the same thing with the gender stuff we were talking about, there's nothing constant, but teachers will say things about how a girl is dressed but not a boy. . . . that kind of thing. It's just that, really . . . kids are not really accepting of each other. But how they [teachers] treat people, it's not constant, each case is really different. I wouldn't say the teachers or the school is sexist or homophobic, kids get treated differently because of who they are. There are really popular kids who are out, and then there are kids who everyone thinks are just weak and they disrespect them and they are just abused all the time and called names. . . . Teachers don't do anything, and the student council doesn't do anything, and the senior class president doesn't do anything, either. Students aren't ever heard at this school at all. (High school junior, Wyoming, December 2004)

CSE and AOUME approaches share conceptions of sexual and gender identity as fixed in a rigid typology, making it hard for teachers and students to discuss how these identities are overlapping and interwoven in students' daily lives [1] and in our educational, legal, and political systems (Valdes 1995). These fixed typologies contrast with changing and fluid sociocultural constructions of (particularly youth) gender and sexual identity. None of the programs or curricula I observed were able to connect very well to students' lived experiences of sexual and gender identities; to challenge traditionalist assumptions about appropriate (gender and sexual) presentations of self common in school and classroom settings; or to provide a comprehensive, much less progressive or radical, approach to understanding and talking about youth identity. Student self-presentations and responses to one another that I observed wrestled publicly with the dichotomous categories offered by CSE and AOUME typologies. In the case of AOUME approaches, heteronormative and patriarchal assumptions align with the broader religious arguments and sociocultural goals of the New Christian Right movement. In the case of CSE approaches, these assumptions conflict with aspects of their ideology that propound universal human rights and liberal (in the classical political sense) democratic values.

ON (NON-)QUEER TERMINOLOGY

Before discussing the typologies presented in CSE and AOUME curricula, a note on terminology is in order. When discussing a particular sex education curriculum, program, or approach in this chapter, I employ the identity language used by that particular program. If a curriculum names possible sexual identities as "heterosexual" and "homosexual," I use these terms when discussing the curriculum. If a teacher regularly used the terms "straight" and "gay," I use these terms to talk about the teacher's categorizations of sexual identity. When talking about AOUME programs, I contrast "heterosexual" with "non-heterosexual" to reflect AOUME efforts to normalize heterosexuality as the only acceptable sexual identity. Thus, the dichotomous terminology reflects the categorization common to AOUME programs of "heterosexual" as natural and good, and all other possible sexual identities as taboo. When talking about CSE and abstinence-based approaches, I generally use the terms "homosexual," "gay," and "straight" to reflect both the language most often used in the classrooms that I observed, and the silence about transgender and queer identities common to all classrooms I observed. I use the term "LGBTQ" in cases where this term was employed by curricula and educators or students; in these cases, "Q" was defined by curricula and instructors as "questioning," not "queer." I did not have the opportunity to ask students who used the term how they were defining it.

The terms "heterosexual" and "straight" are not meant to include any gender identity or sexual practices that would be viewed in traditional Christian teachings as non-normative; all of the materials I reviewed and classrooms I observed assumed a monogamous male/female couple engaged in a limited range of "traditional" sexual activities (primarily vaginal/penile or oral sex, with occasional mentions of anal sex in CSE classrooms); it would be harder to imagine a class discussion about polyamory or fetishism, for example, than one about "vanilla" gay relationships or desires. For example, all of the gay boys shown in CSE videos appeared to be white, middle class, and conservatively dressed (polo shirts were not uncommon), had hair that was neatly cut short, wore no makeup, had no earrings, and so forth. These were the only images of gay people shown in class, and the limited classroom discussions about gay teens in no way expanded this representation or discussed the class, race, gender, ethnic, and other assumptions about "acceptable" gayness that it embodied.

I use the term "queer" to refer to curricula, classroom practices, and individual identities and presentations of self that do not reflect traditional heterosexual norms, do not reflect a traditional sex/gender binary, and are not heteropatriarchal.[2] The term, then, stands in contrast to "heterosexual," "straight," "homosexual," "LGBT," and "gay" in that it deliberately addresses the interplay between gender and sexual identities, speaks to a broad range of sexual desires and practices, and challenges the essentializing use of terms such as "heterosexual," "homosexual," "lesbian," "gay," "bisexual," "male," and "female" common to all sex education curricula.

Scientism in CSE and AOUME

CSE

Over the past fifteen years, many states have added language to state policies requiring that sex education programming be "scientifically correct," and many curricula now tout themselves as being scientifically "up-to-date." Debates among policy makers and advocacy groups about the relative effectiveness of AOUME and CSE programs almost consistently deploy "scientific" data, particularly data from quasi-experimental or experimental studies of sex education programs, to support their cases. This movement toward the scientific rationalization of sex education is also evident in many of the topics covered within sex education curricula, including sexual identity.

AOUME and CSE advocates and curricula deploy "scientific data" about the biological basis and health effects of homosexuality (almost always assumed to be male) to argue for quite different understandings of the "goodness" or "naturalness" of LGB (and very occasionally T) identities. In the CSE programs, the focus on categorizing sexual identities and using medicalized discourses to explain sexual behavior and identity was similar to the approach CSE programs used to categorize and explain contraceptive types, family types, and STI types. This approach reflects the ideal of scientific ratio-nality central to CSE ideology.

CSE curricula and instructors' reliance on scientific discourse to normal-ize and categorize was evident in the ways that students and teachers talked together about sexual identity. CSE teachers and students most often learned about sexual identity taxonomies by filling out worksheets in which they de-fined and labeled different identities, like "lesbian," "gay," and "bisexual," based not on personal experience but on textbook-based definitions. There were no opportunities to discuss sexual identity in students' daily lives—these taxonomies remained entirely (and deliberately) hypothetical and dis-embodied in almost all activities in CSE classrooms.

While homosexuality appeared in CSE textbook typologies of sexual identities and occasional curricular activities and videos depicting gay male adolescents, it disappeared in discussions about sexual risk and disease. The CSE public health approach deliberately depersonalizes discussions about sex acts and their risks: it is the sexual act—not the person—that is more or less risky. This approach to discussing sex acts has many benefits, not least of which is that it avoids stereotypes and destigmatizes particular sex acts as "gay only." This approach is also more valid from a public health perspective, as it more effectively reflects the realities of sexual practices and STI risks. On the other hand, the abstraction of risk (now associated only with a "sex act," not people involved in a sex act) made it impossible for CSE programs to discuss the different risks that particular students are likely to face, and the social, economic, political, and biological reasons why risk varies so greatly across gender, sexuality, race, and class demographics. As with discussions about taxonomies of sexual identity, CSE curricula and instructors systematically failed to connect the "science" that they presented with students' lived expe-riences and with structured power relations.

AOUME

A reliance on scientific discourse and taxonomies is not surprising in CSE approaches, given their valorization of objective, "complete and correct" information. It is more surprising in AOUME programs and literatures. AOUME is based on a different set of assumptions about what constitutes valid or correct messages; these assumptions are moral, not scientific, ones. Nonetheless, in the Florida trainings and AOUME curricula I reviewed, moral, religiously based judgments of social relations and human behavior were regularly translated into "scientific facts" that lent support to AOUME's underlying ideology. Many programs used public health data to argue that pregnancy and STIs pose more of a risk to girls than to boys, and thus girls are both naturally different from boys and naturally more in need of protection. AOUME programs used survey and demographic data to claim that homosexuality is more risky (emotionally, psychologically, socially, physically, and—unstated—spiritually) than heterosexuality and must therefore be presented as an unacceptable individual health choice. They used CDC data to claim that condoms are unreliable in preventing pregnancy and STIs, and may in fact increase these outcomes by creating a false sense of security; and finally, they used demographic data to claim that the "traditional family" is protective and productive in society, while alternate family structures (particularly mother-headed or gay parent homes) are socially destructive.

The shift toward a rationalization of AOUME approaches as being based on "scientific facts" was a deliberate strategy born in response to AOUME supporters' perception that they were being attacked because of the religious basis of their activities. These attacks were viewed as a threat to maintaining state and federal funding for AOUME and access to public schools. Thus, the scientific rationalization of AOUME positions did not reflect, as it did in CSE, a central aspect of AOUME ideology but instead reflected a deliberate adoption of a way of speaking about sex education that was viewed as powerful in shaping public opinion and access to public institutions. Not surprisingly, the scientific discourses utilized by AOUME and CSE supporters thus presented quite different explanations about the basis of sexual identity, and about relationships among sexual identity, gender, risk, disease, and social relations.

Sexual Identities in Sex Education Programs

SEXUAL IDENTITY IN AOUME

AOUME ideology conceptualizes non-heterosexual, and particularly queer, sexualities as *threatening* or *dangerous* to individuals and the social fabric. This framing of LGBTQ identities is enshrined in the federal definition of AOUME. AOUME approaches to teaching about sexuality rest on a strong insistence that discussion about non-heterosexual identities and behaviors is dangerous and should be silenced. If voiced, the discussion should emphasize that homosexuality is a choice, not an identity, and that it is a dangerous choice. There is an obvious parallel here with AOUME approaches to discussing contraception: it should not be discussed at all, but if it must be, it should be discussed in terms of its failure.

How AOUM educators argued against the validity or goodness of non-heterosexual identities varied based on what they felt would be most effective in persuading different audiences. Strategies for making these claims included using scientific data, incendiary images, arguments for rational choice, and normative propaganda, depending on the site where they were teaching, the ages of the students, the propensities of the instructors, the curriculum writers, and so forth. The most common of these tactics in the public-school programs was to include data from scientific studies that showed different health outcomes for self-identified gay and nongay students. These differences were used to argue that homosexuality is physically and psychologically damaging to the individual and to society. For example, the Florida AOUME advanced abstinence education training included a study comparing drug use and suicide rates of young men who identified as gay versus those who did not to argue that identifying as gay causes these outcomes.

These various strategies all aimed to strengthen support for viewing homosexuality as unnatural, damaging, and dangerous to the individual and the country. In AOUME typologies, there is only one moral and acceptable category of sexual identity and behavior: heterosexuality. By silencing or pathologizing all other sexual identities, AOUME programs attempt to inscribe heteronormative practices as the taken-for-granted "common sense" in schools and society. By doing so, however, LGBTQ students are branded not just as violating sexual norms, but also as destroying society. Just as there are no large studies of the effects of AOUME programs on gender relations and norms, there are no large studies about the effects of AOUME programs on student and school responses to LGBTQ students. Many smaller studies, however, indicate that AOUME, or any school curricula or policies that encourage or do not actively discourage LGBTQ-bashing, make life harder for kids who identify or are identified as LGBTQ. This is particularly true for kids whose queer sexual and gender identities intersect with marginalized class, race, and ethnic identities. For example, Elliott (2010) found in her study of a Wisconsin high school that students who identified as gay or lesbian and were white, middle class, and gender normative faced irregular homophobic behavior from classmates. Students of color who identified as queer or gay faced much more serious abuse, including verbal harassment, physical harassment such as having their breasts grabbed, and threats of rape.

SEXUAL IDENTITIES IN CSE

The CSE curricula reviewed and programs observed in California, Wisconsin, and Wyoming acknowledged and attempted to normalize LGBTQ identities by creating an expanded typology of sexual identities. The expanded typology allowed the CSE programs to recognize sexual identity as a topic worthy of discussion in sex education classes, and to recognize the existence of non-heterosexual identities. These were spaces that did not exist in most AOUME curricula.

Sexual identity is a charged topic in many states and communities in the United States. For many schools that have adopted CSE approaches, sexual identity and condom demonstrations are the two topics about which they face the greatest opposition by AOUME advocates and concerned parents. Efforts to include information on sexual identity in official curricula have therefore often focused narrowly on presenting nonstigmatizing definitions of LGBTQ identities to students. In Maryland, for example, the Montgomery County school district was sued by a group called Citizens for a Responsible Curriculum (CRC) in part for including definitions of "homosexuality," "bisexuality," and "transgender" in a new sex education curriculum.

The CRC, which partnered with the PFOX (Parents and Friends of Ex-Gays, now Parents and Friends of Ex-Gays and Gays) organization and a number of other national New Christian Right organizations, argued that since homosexuality is a choice and not biologically determined, the school was teaching children about alternative lifestyle choices that were unacceptable to the "community." They also argued that the school was presenting only one side of the story about homosexuality by not discussing studies indicating that homosexuality can be "cured." For example, the CRC says on its website that the expanded typology of sexual identities "normalized homosexuality" and "encourages people to label themselves early as to their sexual orientation" (Citizens for a Responsible Curriculum 2011). That is, the CRC claimed that simply presenting a choice of identities to students and defining other terms as if they were as equally valid as "heterosexual" was an attempt to naturalize immorality.

At the time of my research, none of the active CRC members had children enrolled in Montgomery County public schools. The leader of the CRC was a county resident whose children had attended Montgomery County schools decades earlier and who had sued the district a number of times before, without success. The other CRC representatives that I met were either not residents of the county, had sent their children to private (usually parochial) schools, or were homeschooling. Unlike during past legal efforts, during my research the CRC caught the attention of and sought help from groups (like PFOX) outside of the district; the group was discussed on Bill O'Reilly's show on the Fox News Channel, for example. The CRC received assistance from a range of national groups to shape their argument against the proposed curriculum and fund a prolonged legal battle. The district spent years and millions of dollars fighting for the right to implement the new curriculum in its schools. It is because of this sort of activism that the CSE programs I observed generally limited the amount and scope of formal materials and classroom exercises on sexual identity.

CSE typologies attempt to validate the existence and equal rights of people who identify with a number of sexual identity categories, most often heterosexual, lesbian, gay, bisexual, transgender, and questioning (LGBTQ). In so doing, CSE typologies challenge the AOUME assumption of the biological, social, and moral primacy of heterosexuality. However, CSE's understanding of LGBTQ identities is based on a rationalist ideology that claims to eschew values and embrace science as an unbiased and objective standard for categorizing identities. Though this ideology is itself shaped by and reflects a core set of Enlightenment ideals, it views itself as aiming for objective, value-free, complete, and correct scientific information.

As many researchers have now shown,[3] and as this book argues, information about sexuality, because it is always embedded in the fabric of power, privilege, and social structures of society, is never objective or value free. CSE's approach to addressing sexual identity is to present students with a "scientific" typology of sexual identities and then move on to other topics. This approach has moral implications. Because of the form that the typologies take (for example, heterosexual is always the first category in the typology) and the sociocultural environment in which these typologies are introduced (one that is heteronormative), the typologies reinscribe a heterosexual norm and various named and categorized sexual "others." They do not recognize how gender, sexual, and other aspects of identity overlap and intermingle in our daily lives and in social and sexual scripts; and they fail to engage with the needs and experiences (including of school-based abuse) of teenagers who are grappling with gender, sexuality, and identity.

In practice, CSE programs cede the space for discussing complex issues of desire, rights, identities, and values to an ideal of scientific rationalism as a guide for "values-free" sex education. CSE approaches fail to construct a coherent or compelling narrative about the moral and democratic implications of acknowledging diverse sexualities or of heteropatriarchy and homophobia in schools or society. CSE programs seldom explain why the recognition of diverse sexual identities is central to CSE approaches; why abuse perpetrated against students identified as LGBTQ is so harmful to norms of equality, diversity, and participation; or why relegating any group of students to a second-class status undermines social and democratic values that are fundamental to our country. They offer students and teachers few tools to help negotiate this difficult terrain, either in their own lives or in trying to build a more inclusive school community.

In contrast, AOUME approaches are based on and reflect a consistent set of sexual and social values. They offer a coherent explanation of how to make sense of sexual identity and how to understand the questions and feelings that teens are exploring about their sexuality. That this explanation relegates many teens and their families to the category of "outcast" and presents their lives as damaging to society should be of fundamental concern to all educators and society alike, as it poses a serious threat to ideals of democratic inclusion and human equality in the school.

BINARY BIOLOGY IN SEX EDUCATION PROGRAMS

A central "culture war" debate underlies the scientific rationalization of sexual identity in both CSE and AOUME programs. In the CSE activities I observed, attempts to categorize sexual identity drew on limited and often outdated understandings of scientific research to argue for or against a biological basis for being gay. These conversations simplified data and debates about the complex forces thought to influence sexual identity to yet another binary:[4] is homosexuality (and therefore potentially other LGBTQ identities) genetically predetermined or is it not? Teachers argued implicitly that if being gay is biologically determined, then individuals cannot "control" their sexual identity and should not be denigrated or blamed for being gay. Some CSE curricula and the programs in California and Wisconsin continued on to argue that regardless of its roots, individual sexual identity and behavior is exactly that—individual. As long as one person's behavior did not directly or negatively affect others, it was no one's business in what sexual activities that person engaged or with what sexual identity that person identified. This argument reflects the liberal (in the classical political sense) ideology central to CSE models.

In sharp contrast, AOUME programs assume, and often state, that non-heterosexuality is not biologically determined but is instead an individual choice that can be addressed and changed through psychosocial intervention. Because it is a psychologically, socially, physically, and spiritually undesirable choice, it can (and, some would argue, should) be denigrated, and those who choose to be gay are to blame for weakening the social fabric. In other words, a person's choice to "be gay" or engage in same-sex sexual activities affects every other person in the school and the country, and disciplining this choice—through, for example, verbal and physical abuse—is a defense of society. This argument reflects neotraditionalist ideology concerning re-ligiously sanctioned sexual norms and the models of family and society that they support.

Infrequently, CS educators challenged students to think about whether the origins of being gay made a difference to them. The resounding answer from students was yes, and furthermore, they assumed that such a biological basis existed. Classroom approaches and discussions were thus shaped by the arguments about sexual orientation that have characterized mainstream me-dia coverage of the culture wars, including the debate about whether homo-sexuality is a "natural" (that is, God-given) characteristic or an individually chosen identity. This debate is probably familiar to readers. On one extreme, some scientists and queer activists argue that (1) there is a firmly biological basis to sexual orientation (e.g., Burr 1993), and (2) even if there is not, there is nothing wrong with being gay. On the other extreme, New Christian Right activists argue that enacting gay or non-gender-normative identities is not based on biology, but is a freely made choice, and an immoral and unnatural one at that (e.g., Price 2010; Sprigg 2010).

This tired and limiting debate matters in at least two ways. First, quite aside from whether there is a biological basis to sexual identity or not, there is evidence that whether people believe that being gay is biologically based or not affects their stated prejudices. If they believe there is a biological basis, they are more likely to report pro-gay attitudes (e.g., Haslam 2002). (On the other hand, if they essentialize gender and racial/social categories as biologi-cal categories, they are more likely to endorse gender and racial stereotypes [e.g., Martin and Parker 1995].)

Second, the terms of the debate have tended to reinscribe the heterosex-ual/homosexual binary and its mapping onto a gender binary (e.g., Valdes 1995). Curricula that present questioning, bisexual, and transgender catego-ries to some extent destabilize these easy binaries,[5] but as in national debates, multidimensional characterizations of sexuality were largely absent in the classrooms I observed. Teacher and student talk generally re-created bina-ries, and even student movements such as Gay-Straight Alliances (GSAs), consisting of "gay" students and their "straight" allies, reinscribe the binary discourse common in the national debates.

Asserting a biological basis for homosexuality grounds CSE in this dis-course of stable identity categories and the clear divisions among them. Un-like AOUME approaches, CSE approaches place no blame on individuals for same-sex desires and instead focus on minimizing risky sexual behavior in all relationships. However, the assertion of stable identity categories has at least two important effects. First, it sets the terms for sex education in a way that does not capture our best scientific knowledge about sexual behavior and risk reduction. For example, the term "men who have sex with men," or MSM, is widely used in HIV prevention instead of "gay" or "homosexual" because it captures a behavior that prevention activities are trying to target and that can be practiced by a range of people who do not identify as "gay." In other words, public health knowledge destabilizes the essentializing assumption that only people who self-identify or are identified as "gay" have sex with same-sex partners. Such knowledge, which has important implications for risk-reduction efforts, and which reflects the CSE ideal of sex education as a scientifically informed best-practice health intervention, cannot easily be incorporated in curricula that essentialize sexual identity.

Second, these assumptions do not provide opportunities for a more grounded discussion of how sexuality and sexual identity play out in people's lives, how these assumptions are structured in relation to privilege and justice, and how all students (indeed, all people) might consider their own sexualities and gender identities differently if the binaries that have structured mainstream discourses and norms were destabilized.

Despite the fact that CSE approaches reproduced a sexual identity binary by engaging students in discussions about the biological basis of being gay, this engagement also reflected the more progressive rationalist impulse on which CSE approaches are based. By challenging students to question the morality of treating gay students differently, they provided the only space I witnessed in sex education classes that was in some way affirming and protective of LGBTQ students.

Sexual Identity Education in Practice

The rest of this chapter explores how curricula relating to sexual identity were enacted in CSE schools and classrooms. I include the formal activities conducted in class and the informal curricular messages students heard in classrooms from peers and teachers, as well as their conversations among and behaviors toward one another and the messages they felt they received from the school administration about heterosexism and homophobia.

All three schools implementing CSE were located in communities and districts in which public support for some discussion of sexual identity existed, and the schools prided themselves on "welcoming" all students. Two of the three schools were located in politically and socially liberal communities with active gay-rights movements. There is reason to believe, then, that these schools were safer, less discriminatory, and potentially more progressive institutions than many other schools in the United States.

In Wyoming (and eventually, Maryland), school actors had to fight a pitched battle to include definitions of LGBT identities in the official curriculum. While the CSE classrooms differed markedly from the AOUME classrooms and curricula in acknowledging LGBT identities and not always tolerating threats to LGBT group rights, the terms of CSE discussions were definitional and highly rationalized (e.g., "no, that would be bisexuality, not homosexuality"). They did not challenge the socially conservative terms of the culture-war debates, which frame sexual identity as singular and fixed,[6] and they did not engage seriously with the complexity of current scientific knowledge and debates concerning sexual and gender identity.

There were important differences in CSE programs' hidden and evaded curricula, particularly between Wyoming on the one hand and Wisconsin and California on the other. The differences in what schools and teachers did not discuss arose in large part because of the constraints teachers felt they faced from the communities served by the school: the California and Wisconsin schools were located in politically and socially liberal communities in which a number of legal measures had been taken to protect the rights of LGBTQ members, and where there was support for GSAs. Both communities had active gay- or queer-rights movements (or both), and both school districts provided LGBTQ resources to schools and openly discussed the equal rights of LGBTQ teens in their schools. The Wyoming community, in contrast, had already engaged in a heated battle over the inclusion of definitions of non-heterosexuality and a discussion of contraceptives in the curriculum; had no district-level LGBTQ-supportive resources; had no active gay-rights groups; and was located in a much more politically and socially conservative state that is well known nationally for its virulent homophobia.

CSE taxonomies of sexual identity

As in the CSE curricula I reviewed, in CSE classrooms I observed teacher talk generally focused on creating a taxonomy of sexual identities. Some version of the LGBTQ taxonomy, along with a definition of each term, was presented by teachers in all Wyoming, California, and Wisconsin classrooms except for Mr. Dean's. In these presentations, a person could be gay or lesbian, bisexual, transgender, or questioning (though this last category was seldom defined, and even less often discussed), but each category was presented as essentialized and, implicitly, mutually exclusive of the others. For example, the Montgomery County, Maryland, curriculum states, "People can identify themselves as gay, lesbian, bi-sexual, or transgender at any point in their lives."[7] A Wyoming student worksheet asks students to define each term; a separate definition for each was provided in the textbook.

In the Wyoming and California classrooms I observed, this taxonomy was presented by teachers to students as fact and was not discussed in any detail. Both curricula also included video materials and worksheets that talked about gay people, usually, though not always, in relation to HIV/AIDS. In contrast, in Wisconsin's Fontaine High, during the "LGBTQ Issues" class session, outside speakers from a local teen outreach center presented sexual identity as one of five aspects of student identity, each of which has a spectrum along which each individual falls. The other four aspects of identity were: biological sex, gender identity, gender expression, and sexual behaviors. Following this description of identity spectra by the speakers, the class participated in an activity titled "Act Like a Man/Be a Lady," in which students talked about stereotypes they associated with gender identities. Students were then asked what students were called if they violated these norms; responses included "gay," "fag," "butch," "fruity," "dyke," "queer," "freak," and "feminist."

This attempt to talk about identity intersectionality and link it to social scripts and their dangers (for example, students' experiences of verbal abuse associated with not being straight) was the only discussion about identity, intersectionality, and power that I observed in any of the sex education classrooms. But the conversation was short lived. Directly after the activity described above and before the relations between gender norm violations and sexual identities could be explored by students, class ended and the discussion was never taken up again.

In the Wisconsin classroom there was no mention of female sexual identity, aside from students listing words such as "dyke" and "butch" in the session described above. There was no mention of female sexual identity at all in the Wyoming and California classrooms, other than defining the term "lesbian." And none of the CSE classrooms discussed transgender, bisexual, or queer identities beyond a one-line definition. Thus, although CSE classrooms did present a typology of sexual identities that went beyond heterosexuality and male homosexuality, in practice non-heterosexuality was discussed and represented in brief definitions and representations of gay boys. This implicitly parallels the explicit silencing of female and queer sexual identities in AOUME activities.

The efforts in CSE programs to *classify* sexual identities were evident across other aspects of the curriculum as well, including in discussions of contraception, abortion, STIs, and relationships. In the Wisconsin curriculum, for example, the following types of families were defined for students in a worksheet:

- Nuclear family: A mother and father and their natural or adopted children
- Single-parent family: A family consisting of one parent and his or her natural or adopted children
- Extended family: A family of parents, children, and other relatives, such as grandparents or aunts and uncles
- Blended family: A family created by remarriage after the death or divorce of a spouse
- Adoptive family: [definition was missing from the worksheet]
- Foster family: A family formed when a government agency places a child in the temporary care of an adult or couple
- Married couple: A family consisting of two married adults
- Nontraditional family: A group of unrelated people who live together and offer support to one another

As with categorizations of sexual identity, the effort to categorize family types leads to oddly restrictive definitions (for example, would a family not be a "blended family" if a never-married parent with children married a divorced parent with children?). More to the point, the worksheet activity was not accompanied by any discussion about *why* families should be categorized or what such categorizations (mean to) accomplish socially, politically, economically, or legally. The focus on categorization reflects the thread of scientific rationalism that runs through CSE ideology, but because this thread is not brought into dialogue with CSE's concerns for human rights and diversity, the scientific rationalization of sexual identity, family, contraceptive types, and many other topics creates a division between the subject at hand and the messy realities of relationships, emotions, and the everyday experiences of students. Categorization schemes limit discussion of meaning and close off opportunities to discuss issues such as heteronomativity, homophobia, stigma, and discrimination, which might arise if the programs ever asked why categorization is important and how categories have been used positively and negatively throughout history.

The lack of opportunities to discuss the complexities of student identities and experiences in all CSE programs was at least sometimes deliberate. As previously mentioned, simply exercising the right to define multiple sexual identities in the classroom and to acknowledge that there were gay kids at the school and in the community had required a battle for teachers and district officials in Maryland and Wyoming. The battle was among adults, as Mr. Lauder (one of the health teachers in Wyoming) explained:

> Sexual orientation and abortion are issues that parents can opt their kids out of, because this is what adults are most worried about. It's kind of funny, really, when it's now on TV and kids are seeing such a wide range there.

The Wyoming teachers argued that explicitly acknowledging the existence of gay people and their families provided students with opportunities to address discrimination, officially recognize gay students and families in their communities, and learn about sexual identity as a concept. However, teachers were wary of pushing the boundaries of these discussions beyond acknowledging that some people defined themselves as LGBT because of concerns that parents would respond negatively. Not surprisingly, then, the provision of textbook definitions of sexual identities did not create opportunities for broader classroom discussions about sexual identity, heteronormativity, or homophobia. In Mr. Lauder's and Mr. Dean's classrooms, aside from when students worked silently at their desks copying definitions of sexual identity categories from their textbooks into their study guide worksheets, sexual identity was not addressed at all. Ms. Jeffries' class provided a bit more space to discuss sexual identity, although conversations were never prolonged. For example, Ms. Jeffries once led a brief discussion on the topic during an exercise in which students were asked to copy the definitions of heterosexuality and homosexuality from their textbooks onto worksheets:

LUKE: Homosexual means attraction to same sex; heterosexual means attraction to opposite sex. [This is the definition in the book.]

MEGAN: I don't study these things; hold on!

LEXIE: My brother always called people homos, and my mom got tired of it and said, "What if I called you a hetero?" So my brother said, "Well, I'm not!" [People laugh.]

MS. JEFFRIES (J): So what is a stereotype?

PETE: An idea or image held about a group of people that represents an oversimplified opinion, prejudiced attitude, or uniformed judgment. [This is another definition from the book.]

J: So now I'm going to put you on the spot: What kinds of stereotypes of homosexuals have you heard? Is there one you can share with the class?

PETE: I'd rather not.

JOSH: They talk like this. [He lisps.]

JEAN: I know a gay guy and he's not like that at all! I like being with gay guys better. [She and Megan talk about how they like hanging out with gay guys because gay guys don't hit on them.]

J: Are there stereotypes about the kinds of careers homosexuals have?

JOSH: Yeah, they work in hair salons.

JEAN: I just heard one about if a guy is excited about Christmas decorating, he must be gay.

JOSH: Heterosexuals like me like to go shopping because there are cute girls, and I like the atmosphere.

MEGAN: But you're a metrosexual. That's why you like shopping!

Ms. Jeffries provided more opportunities than other teachers at Teton for students to talk, and students made comments about sexual identity with some regularity. In situations where the comments were homophobic (for example, using the term *fag*), Ms. Jeffries generally asked students to not use the word, but did not otherwise take up discussions about sexual identity or students' sexuality. In the class situation above, for example, Ms. Jeffries did not lead the conversation toward a fuller discussion of "metrosexuality" and how it relates to the common categories of "gay" and "straight," "male" and "female," of how stereotypes affect people, or of how such stereotypes play out at the school. Instead, after Megan's comments, the class immediately moved on to the next question on the worksheet, which was about abortion.

In California and Wisconsin, where there was broad community and district support for CSE and active gay- or queer-rights advocacy groups, there was also more classroom talk about sexual identity. Unlike teachers at Teton High, teachers in California and Wisconsin said they felt comfortable talking about the topic with students; they more often disrupted students' heteronormative and homophobic comments; and they even, at times, deliberately introduced sexual identity as a topic for students to discuss. In California and Wisconsin, teachers also occasionally interjected gay (usually male) characters into activities. For example, in California, during a discussion about why boys and girls might choose not to have sex, the instructor (Ginnie) asked students to consider whether reasons might differ for a gay (male) student:

GINNIE: Now, in terms of sexuality, why would a gay teen, why would that boy not have sex?

BOY: He may not want to come out, so meeting people might be hard.

GIRL: He may be teased.

GINNIE: Yes, great. If the teen is lesbian or gay, they can still have sex, definitely. OK, back to why teens might have sex. . . .

While Ginnie opened up an opportunity for discussion, she also, as was common in my observations, limited this discussion to hypothetical situations and did not connect the hypothetical situation to students' experiences. Certainly, sharing anything about students' sexual lives in a classroom setting with a teacher present is fraught. The two students who answered her question, however, brought up two issues commonly mentioned in research on gay teens' school experiences: concerns about how or whether to come out, and the abuse students may face if they are identified as gay. Though Ginnie acknowledged their comments, she did not ask the class to talk about these issues, nor did she ask students to talk about the power dynamics and social relations they reflect. She also separated LGB teens from other teens and limited discussion about their experiences when she told the class that LGB teens can "still have sex" and then told them to return to a conversation about "why [straight] teens might have sex." All of the teachers that I observed avoided discussions about privilege, power, and identity. Ginnie's avoidance of a deeper discussion about gay students' experiences was notable only in that she initially posed a question that was likely to lead to comments about these topics.

CS educators in California and Wisconsin also did not talk about the laws that schools were responsible to implement in response to lawsuits brought by LGBTQ students who experienced abuse in school. In California, a court ruling required schools to discuss bullying and the rights of all students to go to school in an environment free of harassment. At the time of my research, this had recently resulted in the passing of state law SB 719, the Bullying Prevention for School Safety and Crime Reduction Act of 2003. However, only a passing comment was made about bullying and abuse of LGBT students in the sex education class, and the bullying act was never mentioned. Similarly, Wisconsin's *Nabozny vs. Podlesny* court battle,[8] which was the first case to award damages to a student because he was subjected to homophobic harassment, was never mentioned in Mrs. Shane's and Mr. Kelly's classroom, and Matthew Shepard was never mentioned in the Teton High classes. In sharp contrast, in all three classrooms the laws governing rape were presented in detail.

Discussion of sexual identity remained theoretical, not grounded in students' and teachers' actual experiences or in the legal frameworks influencing school responses to sexual identity and violence. This focus on abstract categories versus the lived experiences and political realities of sexual identity was also evident in instructor responses to students. In California and Wisconsin, teachers regularly disrupted student comments that were viewed as challenging abstract group rights. For example, in every case where a student made a comment that assumed marriage to be a necessary aspect of healthy sexuality, their teacher asked some version of the question, "Does [your comment] mean that gay people can never have sex?"[9]

While teachers consistently called out students who appeared to be challenging LGBT group rights claims (such as the right to marriage), they often ignored or even reinforced heteronormative or homophobic comments or interactions among students. The following interaction occurred in the Wisconsin classroom among a high-status student (Theo) who was assumed by his peers to be heterosexual, the teacher (Mrs. Shane), a lower-status student (Jason), and the teacher trainee (Mr. Kelly):

> MRS. SHANE: Boys have more testosterone, and so this is changing a lot at this time in your life. And you can be gay and that's OK. [Theo says something about being gay that I cannot hear.]
> MRS. SHANE: Theo, you don't have to joke about this!
> THEO: OK, OK, I'm gay!
> JASON: Yeah, he's not joking, he is gay!
> MR. KELLY (protectively): All right, that's enough. He was obviously joking. Theo, you're not gay.

Similarly, a straight-identified HIV-positive guest speaker in the Wisconsin class I observed repeatedly discussed the need to understand the effects of systematic discrimination and stigma "on our queer brothers and sisters," but then drew on "joking" homophobic (and sexist) discourses throughout his presentation, such as:

> PRESENTER: OK, what is sex, if you have to define it for your teacher?
> DARREN: Having intercourse.
> JIM: Penis penetrates the vagina.
> COREY: Penis in the mouth.
> KEN: Penis in the butt.
> PRESENTER: There you go, that's what I'm talking about! Well, not really . . . Kind of makes me pucker up. [Makes a fake pain face as (mostly male) students laugh.]

Enforcing heteropatriarchy

Though student comments that challenged LGBTQ group rights claims were relatively rare in my observations, students regularly engaged in homophobic and sexist "teasing" and policing of one another. I found in Wyoming, and Elliot (2010) found in Wisconsin, that some of the more public policing was conducted by straight-identified students on other straight-identified students. For example, during one lunch break at Teton High, I observed a male student who was assumed to be heterosexual let his girlfriend put his shoulder-length hair into two ponytails. After she completed the hairdo, she and he went outside so that the boy could show his new hairdo to a group of male friends. When he first approached the group, he and his male friends laughed and joked about the hairdo, and his girlfriend laughed along when they jokingly called him a girl. In under a minute, however, the mood turned ugly, his friends began to call him "fag" and began throwing plastic drink bottles and food at him with enough force that he and his girlfriend ran back inside the cafeteria to avoid the missiles. Teachers heard the impact of the thrown items through the double doors and came running out to investigate. When I asked students and teachers about this event, they categorically denied that it was an example of homophobia because "no one really thinks [the boy whose hair was put in ponytails] is gay." One teacher added that it was simply a display of "male stupidity" among friends, and nothing to be taken seriously.

Events like this contradicted CSE teachers' classroom messages that homophobic and heteronormative language and actions were not acceptable, and they also contradicted the clean sexual identity typologies presented in the classrooms. They showed clearly that sexual identity was understood, regulated, and responded to as part of a social script in which gender and sexuality are co-constructed. Valdes (1995) uses the term "heteropatriarchy" to refer to the dominant legal and social script in the United States, which conflates gender, sexual identity, and sex. The notion of heteropatriarchy helps explain why a straight guy putting his hair up can lead to jokes about him being a girl, and then rapidly into screams of "fag" and a physical assault. The conflation of gender and sexual identity in these scripts also helps explain people dismissing the event as "not homophobic."

When sexual-identity policing occurred between individuals, it was explained by teachers and students as related to the relationships of the particular people involved. The practical complexities of relationships for the most part silenced teacher and student policing of these acts. For example, can a dance be "too sexual" when the two people involved in it are assumed not to be attracted to each other? CSE approaches to typologizing identities and acts supported a split between responses to individual behavior and responses to abstract attacks against groups. If a person was not "actually gay," could their being called *fag* constitute harassment? If two friends were "just joking around" by calling each other names, could their actions be viewed as reflecting structured homophobia? CSE teachers' common response was "no," while the same actions directed at abstract groups of people generated immediate and consistent opprobrium.

These refusals to interrupt, and not infrequent support of, "joking" interpersonal homophobia and heteropatriarchy in classrooms and informal social spaces are partly a result of CSE worldviews. CSE approaches embody the norms of scientific rationalism *and* universal human rights (e.g., McKay 1998; Meyer 1980). These norms offer a great deal of leverage at the abstract level to challenge language, policy, and laws that disparage universal human-rights claims, and they provide a straightforward rationale for teachers to challenge students who appear to be questioning abstracted group claims to equality. They offer much less leverage in addressing social, cultural, economic, and political relations of power and authority or one-on-one social interactions, particularly when these occur among people whose individual identity is complexly related to challenged group identities.

The scientific rationalization of sexual identity in CSE classrooms led to a depersonalization and movement away from discussions about morality and power. This appeared to increase teachers' comfort with presenting the topic to students in the first place, particularly in Teton, where teachers did not feel they had significant community support to discuss sexual identity. Depersonalization helped control and regulate student conversation about sexual identity and provided teachers with preapproved information that was likely to limit, not create opportunities for, potentially unplanned (and thus potentially dangerous) conversations about the topic. But depersonalization also shut down almost all opportunities for teachers and students to talk about or respond to individual student identities, experiences, and rights.

Wyoming, California, and Wisconsin all had or were beginning to implement antibullying programs, usually because court rulings had mandated that schools address the intense harassment that so many gay- and queer-identified kids faced. Schools and teachers I observed tried to respond to perceived homophobia in their schools, but the personalized, individual interpretations of student identities and interactions meant that homophobia was downplayed as a systemic issue. Take, for example, the following statement by the Wyoming district education officer:

> We had quite a serious case a month ago, with a student making a comment about a gay kid. She said he should end up like Matthew Shepard. I was so disappointed in her; she's kind of attention-seeking . . . There's probably a handful of kids who are out, and usually they are not harassed that much. It really depends on the gay kid's comfort, how they feel.

The officer discusses this serious threat made to another student in terms of the personality of the perpetrator. The girl was transferred to the alternative high school, so her behavior was taken seriously by the school, but the effects of her behavior on the "gay kid" were never mentioned. The officer goes on to say, in fact, that it depends on "the gay kid's comfort" whether they feel that they are harassed at the school. This was a common approach to framing homophobic acts by adults and students alike: instead of focusing on the fact that harassment clearly occurred, speakers talked about individual kids being harassed or feeling harassed depending on their personality and their social status (which was not viewed as being affected by sexual identity). This approach to understanding homophobia assured that antibullying efforts only targeted extreme individual behaviors and actions among students without identifying or addressing systemic homophobia or heteropatriarchy.

Students appeared aware of the ambiguities that surrounded teachers' engagement with teen sexuality and identities, and they were also aware of the constraints they and other students at their schools faced in expressing LGBT or queer identities. They had to resort to riffing on teacher comments, classroom activities, or peer interactions to explore, in a limited and often harassing manner, the ambiguities of teen sexual identity. Students who were exploring these ambiguities also often faced harassment from peers and, as described above, these interactions were not policed by teachers and were generally not viewed by students or teachers as indicative of systemic homophobia.

AOUME: REFRAMING THE "HOMOSEXUAL THREAT"[10]

In most of the Florida training materials and in the larger body of AOUME and abstinence-plus materials I reviewed, sexual identity was most notable in its absence. Most AOUME speakers, materials, and organizations aim to create an unspoken heteronorm by excluding any mention of sexual identities from curricula and activities and enforcing this prohibition broadly in schools, for example through lawsuits like the one filed by the CRC in Montgomery County.[11] In all reviewed AOUME curricula, only heterosexual couples were depicted in textbook activities and the couples fulfilled traditional gender roles. In Florida, sexual identity was discussed only twice in the course of the two abstinence-educator training sessions (both times to emphasize the health dangers of homosexuality), and rarely in any of the state-sanctioned curricula I reviewed. When discussed in AOUME curricula, male homosexuality, the only non-heterosexual identity ever addressed in AOUME approaches, was presented as a personal choice that causes extremely poor health outcomes for the individual and the general deterioration of society. Sexual identity was not discussed at all at the teen rally. Transgender and queer identities were never discussed in any of these settings. Wiley and Wilson (2009) found a similar heteronorming and silence about sexual identity in Texas AOUME materials:

> Sexual orientation is rarely discussed in most of the materials and curricula used by Texas school districts. On one level, the authors of this report were pleased to find that blatantly discriminatory or homophobic materials are relatively rare in Texas sexuality education instruction. The discouraging aspect of this situation, however, is that virtually all curricula, lessons or activities submitted for this study assume that all students are heterosexual. In fact, based solely on materials used in sexuality education instruction, someone might conclude no lesbian, gay, bisexual, transgender or questioning (LGBTQ) students attend public schools in Texas. (p. 36)

AOUME activists offered two arguments to destabilize CSE representations of male homosexuality as a normal and natural identity and to argue for the importance of not acknowledging non-heterosexual identities: first, they argued that homosexuality is physically damaging to youth, citing studies that report higher rates of suicide, alcohol abuse, and STIs among self-identified gay men. Second, they argued that homosexuality can be cured through psychotherapy and religious conversion, and thus could not be biological in origin.[12] The goal of presenting information about homosexuality in AOUME programs, if it had to be presented, was to convince gay students that, with treatment and support, they could choose to be straight. Straight students would in turn learn that gay students were choosing to adopt an unacceptable sexual identity.

Fundamental Religion, Instrumental Scientism

AOUME programs present heterosexuality as the only legitimate, natural, healthy sexual identity for human beings. For New Christian Right advocates of AOUME, a biological basis for non-heterosexual identities is not possible, because it would indicate that such identities were a God-given, "natural" aspect of humanity. They argue that homosexuality stems from a decision that deliberately flaunts the heteronorm that God created as the natural state for humans. This is why groups such as PFOX and NARTH (National Association of Research and Therapy for Homosexuals) have gained stature within the AOUME and anti-gay-marriage movements: they claim to hold proof that, with enough faith in God and a good therapist, gay people can "straighten" out. This is also why conservative Evangelical male politicians and religious leaders who have been caught engaging in sexual encounters with other men can return to the national stage after having been "cured" of their "homosexual affliction." The following statement on human sexuality and homosexuality by the Family Research Council (FRC), a New Christian Right think tank, epitomizes this understanding:

> FRC believes the context for the full expression of human sexuality is within the bonds of marriage between one man and one woman. Upholding this standard of sexual behavior would help to reverse many of the destructive aspects of the sexual revolution, including sexually transmitted disease rates of epidemic proportion, high out-of-wedlock birth rates, adultery, and homosexuality. . . .
>
> FRC does not consider homosexuality, bisexuality, and transgenderism as acceptable alternative lifestyles or sexual "preferences"; they are unhealthy and destructive to individual persons, families, and society. . . . Family Research Council believes that homosexual conduct is harmful to the persons who engage in it and to society at large, and can never be affirmed. It is by definition unnatural, and as such is associated with negative physical and psychological health effects. While the origins of same-sex attractions may be complex, there is no convincing evidence that a homosexual identity is ever something genetic or inborn. We oppose the vigorous efforts of homosexual activists to demand that homosexuality be accepted as equivalent to heterosexuality in law, in the media, and in schools.[13]

The assumptions about the nature of homosexuality articulated in the text above are challenged by several factors: the continued public debates in mainstream media about whether there is a biological basis for homosexuality, the problems that AOUME supporters face with calls to remove religious beliefs from their public school programming, and the force of the gay-rights movement (one of the only well-organized opposition movements to AOUME, according to the New Christian Right).

In part because of these challenges, there is an effort on the part of some AOUME leaders to transform how sexual identity is framed within AOUME programming. This effort was revealed during an exchange between an AOUME presenter and a member of the audience at our basic AOUME training in Florida. During a question-and-answer session, the audience member stood up and asked, "What are we doing about the homosexual threat?" The AOUME speaker responded immediately: "No, no, no! We can't let them drag us off message like that. It's not about homosexuality or heterosexuality, it's about risky sex acts. We can't get into these arguments. Just focus on the sex acts." This exchange was typical of a broader concerted effort in many of the Florida events to convince AOUME supporters to adopt a scientific discourse that would validate AOUME as the only *medically* and *scientifically* defensible sex education approach for adolescents, and that would transform religious arguments about the immorality of non-heterosexuality into scientifically based warnings about the public health dangers of non-heterosexuality.

AOUME curricula and speakers that adopt this approach use science instrumentally, some would claim to the extent of manipulating scientific analysis and conclusions. For example, some studies have indicated that "gay teenagers" (variably defined) are more likely to report having tried to commit suicide, and may have been more likely to commit suicide.[14] The reports' authors usually explain these data as a result of the experience of harassment, stigmatization, and economic and social marginalization many LGBT teens face, and thus argue that their findings should lead, for example, to targeted suicide-prevention activities for LGBT youth and antibullying campaigns in schools (e.g., Ryan et al. 2009; Mays and Cochran 2001). These same data, however, are used as evidence by AOUME supporters to argue that it is gay teens' choosing to be homosexual, and therefore sinful, that causes increased mental health problems and suicide rates (e.g., Socarides 1995; Whitehead, n.d.). In other words, correlations are used to argue for socially constructed outcomes by the studies' authors, and outcomes caused by God's judgment of immorality by AOUME advocates.

A parallel to this framing of homosexuality can be found in AOUME representations of condom efficacy and of single mothers, and in recent mainstream work on welfare recipients. For example, Fitzgerald argues that welfare studies and policies have increasingly emphasized the individual behavioral causes of negative life outcomes for children living in single-parent, especially female-headed, homes (Burack and Josephson 2003). Studies that focus on individual outcomes divorced from social context are used by New Christian Right and AOUME supporters to pathologize single mothers and the harmful effects of their "lifestyle choices" on their children. However, studies that have controlled for contextual factors such as the income level of families have found that the negative effects on child health and well-being were more strongly correlated with income than with single-parenting. In other words, single-parenting did not have significant negative effects on children's outcomes—growing up in a low-income household did (e.g., Mather and Adams 2006; Blum, Beuhring, and Rinehart 2000).

AOUME approaches to analyzing data indicating that gay teens have worse psychological and health outcomes than straight teens individualize both cause and outcome and unmoor them from the social environment in which they occur. As with AOUME conceptualizations of single motherhood, the solution to these "problems" is for the individuals involved to find a moral path back to straight, married life. In this view, good Christians should support these efforts to find the path back to moral living, but they should never accept the behavior that keeps people from living a moral life because it affects all of society. Every person has a stake in policing the sexual identities and behaviors of everyone else, and every parent has a stake in the typologies presented to students in classrooms. Any discussion of non-heterosexual identity that does not pathologize is a de facto validation of immoral decision-making; equivalent, one AOUME activist in California told me, to presenting bestiality or pedophilia as possible lifestyles.

The movement to scientifically rationalize (and thus depoliticize and conceal) the religious basis of the heteronormative positions found in AOUME programming is not without its critics. Other AOUME activists feel that adopting scientific rationales has the potential to undermine their moral position in the long run, for example, if the weight of scientific evidence shows that homosexuality is genetically determined. Though scientific rationalization appears to be "winning" in AOUME public-school curricula and programs right now (largely because of the legal threat posed by previous court rulings upholding the separation of church and state in sex education programs), this rationalization does not currently appear to pose a threat to the central ideological tenets of AOUME, which remain consistently at the core of decision making concerning how and when to scientifically rationalize AOUME programming.

The Consequences of Sexual Identity Categories

The categorization systems of sexual identity in both CSE and AOUME curricula reflect the last decade's culture wars over sexual and gender identities, while the debate concerning the biological basis of homosexuality points to the growing role of scientific discourse in rationalizing all sex education programs (e.g., Sears 1992). Fixed boundaries are a feature of socially conservative categories; the history of race categorization and stigmatization offers a useful analogy. There is a growing recognition that simple categories of race do not reflect biological or lived realities, a recognition accelerated recently by DNA analyses, and perhaps not unrelated to the elevation of racially mixed individuals to positions of leadership and power. This recognition has led to, for example, new census rules that allow individuals to self-identify as belonging to multiple race categories. This is the fastest-growing identification in the census, indicating, at least in part, many people's sense that their identity is not so easily taxonomized. There is also growing official recognition that previously rigid taxonomies do not reflect the reality of human diversity. Similarly, gender and sexuality are increasingly revealed by research as nonexclusionary, fluid identities, challenging many commonsense and legal assumptions about the possible range of gender and sexual identities and the assumption that they can be understood as mutually exclusive.

In CSE and AOUME approaches alike, scientific rationalization and categorization efforts continue to obscure the more central questions about sexual identity for students and schools. As Sears notes (1992, 8), "Decisions about the scope and sequence of [sex education curricula] are *technical,* hiding sexual ideology beneath a veneer of scientism." By focusing the limited curricular time given to sexual identity on typologizing, CSE and AOUME approaches fail to connect with students' questions, concerns, feelings, needs, and experiences; avoid addressing why talking about non-heterosexuality must be controlled and carefully skirted in so many classrooms; and fail to question the uses to which categories may be put.

AOUME approaches, based in a particular understanding of biblical exegesis that renders all non-heterosexual identities and acts immoral and dangerous, deliberately attempt to create a categorical certainty through their programming: the only acceptable and natural sexual identity is heterosexual. All other potential identities are (religious) abominations of personal choice. A scientific rhetoric concerning the effects of non-heterosexuality on individuals and society is increasingly adopted to secularize AOUME's stance concerning sexual identity. This discourse shifts the "problem" of homosexuality from a moral risk to a public health risk. For example, the CRC says of the Montgomery County curriculum:

- The new sections on sexual orientation are added to the health curriculum with no mention of the increased risk of sexually transmitted disease inherent in homosexual sex. Health risks are minimized and only attached to the stress of "coming out."
- Montgomery County is not planning on updating the current infectious diseases section of health curriculum, originally developed in 1999, until 2008. The overwhelming gay sympathetic majority of the CAC does not see this as an issue. To quote the openly gay Matthew Murguía of the CAC: "I could have 100 sexual partners in my lifetime, and if I don't engage in any behavior which places me at risk for infection with HIV, I will remain HIV negative."

    CRC believes that it is irresponsible to discuss homosexuality without discussing the risk of the homosexual lifestyle and the increased Aids [sic] *transmission through anal sex.*[15] (Italics in the original.)

The CRC's conflation of homosexuality with anal sex is common in New Christian Right and AOUME materials; this conflation allows for the argument that being gay *inherently* puts people at greater risk of HIV infection and other negative health outcomes. This is the scientifically rationalized discourse that the AOUME trainer was attempting to get workshop participants to adopt in place of a moralizing discourse about "the homosexual threat." Murguía's comment, in contrast, reflects the general scientific rationalization of CSE programs and of mainstream public-health efforts: it is the act, not the person, that creates risk. There is nothing inherently risky or problematic about being gay, and there is a serious public-health problem in conflating a particular sex act with a particular group of people because then sex education cannot speak to the reality of sex practices. For example, AOUME approaches do not allow for a public health response to the rising rates in the 2000s of anal gonorrhea in straight girls in Texas. Interviews with some of these patients indicated that they were having unprotected anal instead of vaginal sex because they felt that they remained virgins if they did not have vaginal sex. From a CSE advocate's perspective, this simply points to the need to educate every person about the risks and risk-reduction practices associated with every sex act.

The greater openness of the CSE programs and curricula concerning sexual identity creates a tension that does not exist in AOUME approaches. On the one hand, the values that form the core of CSE curricula support individual choice and equality, so the programs refuse (for the most part) to publicly judge sexual actions if they are not illegal or harmful to others. Similarly, CSE ideology provides support for considering multiple sexual identities as equally natural, valid, and valuable, and a matter of individual right to identity and self-expression. This broad ideal was evident in teachers' consistent disrupting of student challenges to LGBT group rights claims.

On the other hand, as with gender, there is no in-depth engagement with sexual identity in CSE curricula, and when materials related to sexual identity do appear, they often reinscribe a homosexual/heterosexual binary. This leaves little room for discussion about sexual and gender identity fluidity, the naturalization of categories in CSE approaches, or the realities of being LGBT or being identified as LGBT at school. The following conversation, which occurred between two students during a Wisconsin sex education class, captures the students' sense that their school was not a particularly welcoming place for LGBTQ students:

> STUDENT 1: I think [this city] is a good place about accepting others [LGBTQ students].
> STUDENT 2: I don't think so.
> STUDENT 1: Yes, it is.
> STUDENT 2: School's not.
> STUDENT 1: Well, no. School's not, but the rest is.

Although CSE classrooms offered many more opportunities than AOUME classrooms for discussions about sexual identity, these opportunities were largely limited to attempts to scientifically rationalize and validate LGBT identities as being equal to heterosexual identity. CSE programs did not address stigma, institutionalized homophobia or heteropatriarchy, or students' actual (often quite complex) experiences of sexual and gender identity in school.

As discussed previously, the model of the abstracted, rational, de-sexualized, and de-gendered individual invested with universal rights and capacities that underlies CSE approaches also supports a public health approach that depersonalizes discussions about sex acts. While this meant that no particular sex act was discussed or stigmatized as "gay," as occurred in AOUME activities, in practice, CSE classroom discussions of anal sex were filled with student-to-student homophobic banter that went unaddressed by instructors and that raised, unchallenged in these "safe spaces," the specter of diseased gay bodies that was raised deliberately in the AOUME curricula to stigmatize homosexuality.

CSE approaches adopt a neutral stance toward "objective" sexual-identity categories that does not acknowledge how sexual politics play out in schools and students' lives. Though CSE approaches represent an honest effort to normalize the existence of multiple sexual identities, they offer little ideological traction for teachers and students to think through what it would mean for schools to no longer be homophobic and heteropatriarchal places.

AOUME advocates, in an effort to appear to remove religion and politics from their approach to sexual identity, have adopted some of the same scientizing discourses as those used by CSE programs, but have remained committed to their ideological and moral position vis-à-vis sexual identity. AOUME approaches engage with the sexual politics that students face in school by actively norming heterosexuality and demonizing non-heteronormative choices, and, intended or not, demonizing kids who identify and are identified as LGBT. This approach raises significant challenges to students' rights to participate equally and safely in public schools.

Conclusion

The scientific rationalization of sexual identity was used in CSE approaches to argue for a biological basis for homosexuality and a resulting rationale that since gay people are not to blame for their sexual identity, they should not be disparaged or harassed. Most CSE programs and curricula failed to mobi-

lize the human-rights frameworks that also underpin CSE approaches to argue for a moral or ethical stance against homophobia and heteronorming in
schools and society. CSE programs pinned their arguments about why queer
and straight students should be treated equally on a superficial presentation
of scientific data and a scientific rationalization of sexual identity, instead of
engaging in deeper discussion about whether and why, regardless of the nature of sexual identity, all students should be respected and treated equally in
public schools and in democratic societies.

The unmet need for deeper discussion and exploration will always be a
struggle in classrooms with limited time and teachers with (usually) limited
training in sex education and diverse personal views. However, the use of
data in CSE and AOUME classrooms to present a simple, "objective" picture
of sexual identity in which there appeared to be no significant social, moral,
or political debate about the topic, no evident application to students' lived
experiences, and no reason for any significant discussion is problematic from
a democratic perspective. There was no opportunity to ask, for example, how
we make sense of people's similarities and differences and what rights and responsibilities we have as fellow citizens to patrol these differences? Such questions draw attention to public schools as democratic institutions that model
and produce both citizenship norms concerning diversity and equality, and
the value of open debate about controversial topics. Instead of providing
rich opportunities for such discussions,[16] CSE approaches connect only in a
narrow way with broader liberal (in the classical political sense) arguments
about equality and citizenship in the United States. AOUME classes do not
connect with these ideas at all. As Hess's work (2009) has shown, these are
more limiting models of classroom conversations and interactions than we
should attempt to create if we want students to learn the value of, and how to
discuss, controversial topics with their fellow citizens.

There is a very important distinction between AOUME's refusal to publicly acknowledge non-heterosexuality and CSE's acceptance and explication
of a multiplicity of sexual and gender identities. This distinction relates to
the fundamentally different ideological stances that the two approaches take
to sexual identity and its relationship to sex education. For AOUME supporters, sexual identity is a central issue in sex education because AOUME is
primarily moral education, and like sex before marriage, non-heterosexuality
challenges the moral doctrine upon which AOUME is predicated. For CSE
supporters, to the extent that they focus on a public health rationale for sex
education and judge their effectiveness by these measures, sexual identity is
not a very important topic. As CS educators say, it's the sex act, not sexual

identity, that determines riskiness. Sexual identity, gender, class, race, ethnicity, language, geography, and other aspects of a student's identity are sub-
sumed by the equally agentic, equally capable rational actor model in CSE
ideology. CSE does care about sexual identity to the extent that people are
being treated differently and unfairly, as this violates the universal human-
rights norms upon which CSE is predicated. The curricular response of introducing a range of sexual identities and norming them all as equal should
be understood as a response to this violation of the equal-rights ideology, as
should teachers' responses to students' challenge of group rights claims.

Because of these frameworks, none of the classrooms I observed or curricula I reviewed gave students opportunities to discuss the scientific and social
ambiguities of sexual (and gender, race, and class) identity; to talk about the
fears and excitement of exploring one's own sexuality or sexual and gender
identities; to discuss the daily interactions predicated on heterosexism and
homophobia that were common in all of the schools and classrooms that I
observed; or to engage in debate about the controversies concerning sexual
identity that play such a central role in our national debates about equality.
Sexual identity was either absent from the curriculum or present as a scientific taxonomy. Nowhere was it a force that powerfully shapes people's lives
or an issue that fuels significant legal and social divisions over the inclusivity
of US democracy and, therefore, public schools.

Rape as Consuming Desire and Gendered Responsibility

Rape and Responsibility

Every sex educator with whom I spoke maintained that the issue that engaged their students most consistently was neither sexual identity ("That's old hat to them," said one) nor abortion, nor contraception, nor teen pregnancy. It was rape. The classroom conversations that I observed concerning rape were contradictory. On one hand, they were boring and bureaucratic (on the sex educators' part). On the other hand, they were the moments in the sex education classrooms when students pushed back the hardest against legal frameworks, curricular materials, and the sex educators themselves. Rape was also a not-infrequent topic of jokes. As with female-bashing and antigay epithets, rape-joking among boys (and sometimes girls) was common in classrooms and schools and consistently went unchallenged by teachers. A closer examination of how schools and sex education programs address rape and culpability for rape, and how students respond to these messages, provides a window into students' engagements with the sexual, social, and consumer norms and ideals represented by and affecting AOUME and CSE programming.

In all but one of the programs I observed, discussions about rape, sexual assault, and sexual violence were minimal and highly legalistic. Given the realities of students' lives and the prevalence of rape and sexual assault in students' experiences (an estimated one in six women in the United States will experience rape, the CDC reports that 12 percent of girls in grades 9 to 12 report having been raped,[1] and over 10 percent of male and female college-aged students report having been coerced into having sex[2]), as well as the strong focus in sex education programs on preventing unsafe sex, the short shrift given rape is a notable oversight. There is nothing more dangerous than forced sex, where there is usually no possibility to discuss or enforce abstention or contraceptive use, and mucous membrane tearing is common.

Despite students' interest in the issue, despite the prevalence of rape and sexual violence in US society, and despite the necessity of understanding and addressing the role of rape and sexual violence in fueling sex education's undesired outcomes (STIs, pregnancy), sex education classrooms were nearly silent on the issue. AOUME and CSE approaches have a hard time addressing these topics for very different reasons, each of which relates to their ideological assumptions about individuals, sex, and society.

There were many similarities between CSE and AOUME programs' approaches to rape. They all used most of the limited curricular time dedicated to rape and sexual violence to review state and national laws that defined rape in each district. This emphasis mirrors broader trends in antirape movements and literatures toward focusing on legal definitions (e.g., Marcus 2002). All of the curricula I reviewed and programs I observed also made clear, in one way or another, that girls were not to blame for rape: that "no means no" and that partners are always responsible for obtaining consent from one another. At the same time, they also all asserted that girls could and should take steps to avoid being raped. They all mentioned only men as aggressors. They were all based on a model of students as consumers, which affected their understanding of sex as a commodity and led them to individualize the causes and consequences of sexual violence. Lastly, none of the programs addressed the larger sociocultural context in which rape occurs, at least in part because they did not conceptualize, analyze, or moralize about the role that men play in rape.

These shared features shaped AOUME and CSE programs and their common failure to address rape as a social phenomenon that affects a significant proportion of children, women, and men in the United States and that is intimately related to power. Notwithstanding these commonalities, there were also significant differences among the programs.

AOUME Programs and Relational Responsibility

The AOUME activities I observed and curricula I reviewed were much less assertive about discussing rape and about the "no means no" message than were CSE programs. AOUME approaches assume that males are easily and naturally tempted sexually, and that it is girls' responsibility to constrain their own behavior so that boys are not tempted. Not surprisingly, then, what discussion about rape did occur in AOUME curricula assumed a situation (such as a date rape) in which a boy was tempted by and "misread" signs from a girl. From an AOUME perspective, if a girl is abstinent and "sending the right messages" through her dress and demeanor, she simply should not be raped. If she is married, she is safe in marriage.[3] So girls who are raped, in the AOUME paradigm, are raped because they are not protected by their own virtue or their faithful relationship to their husband, and therefore "signaled" their availability to others. On the man's side (assuming a heterosexual encounter, which all AOUME curricula do), rape is not really violent or a violation, it's a situation in which a man "naturally" took a woman up on the signals she was giving off. Conceptually, though this was never said directly in any curriculum, if a woman is raped, she is at fault, and the fault lies in her public presentation of self as sexually available. Culpability for stranger rape lies with men's nature (bestial) and women's physical availability (e.g., on streets at night). Other than an occasional aside, there was no discussion in AOUME curricula about forced sex within established relationships, romantic or familial. There was, therefore, no opportunity to address sexual abuse and violence at the hands of family members or "romantic" partners.

CSE Programs and Rational Decision-Making

Although still minimal, there was greater time given to discussions about forced sex and sexual violence in the CSE curricula I reviewed and programs I observed. During these sessions, which consistently discussed rape and sexual violence in depersonalized terms (for example, presenting students with national rape statistics), educators much more strongly asserted that the person who was raped was never at fault, and emphasized repeatedly that if a girl or boy was incapacitated by drugs or alcohol and sex occurred, it was rape whether there was verbal assent from the victim or not. Though they also provided advice about how a girl could avoid dangerous situations (always taking her drink with her into the bathroom so that it could not be drugged, always partying with friends, not walking alone at night) and how she could discourage an overly insistent partner (look him directly in the eyes, use his name, and state her position clearly), the CS educators noted that even if a girl followed none of this advice, it was not her fault if she was raped.

CS educators received a lot of push-back from students when they asserted their claim that the victim (always assumed to be a girl) was never at fault for being raped. Students asked, if a girl was dressed or behaved in certain ways, wasn't she at least in part responsible for the rape? Though this response could be understood as the continuation of old, misogynistic tropes regarding rape and sexual assault, in fact it lays bare a logical flaw in CSE approaches: at every stage up until the discussion of rape, CSE programs focused on students' individual responsibility for and control over their actions. Individual behavior was consistently discussed in relation to individual rational decision-making,[4] and not discussed as shaped by social, physical, economic, or cultural milieus. A core assumption of CSE programming was, in fact, that students as rational actors could fully control, and were therefore fully responsible for, their own decisions and actions. The model of rape presented by CS educators reflects this notion clearly by communicating that rape is a situation in which one person violates the other's right to self-determination. Because this right to self-determination resides in the individual, once it is expressed to others, it should be inviolate. When it is violated, it is always the fault of the other. This is one of the reasons why, in CSE programs, there is so much attention given to "knowing your boundaries and communicating your wants and needs": if a person is not impaired (as impairment makes assent legally impossible) and does not verbalize "no" to the other, their right to control their sexuality is, de facto, forfeit.

This focus on verbalizing boundaries and its effects on students' behaviors, perceptions of rape, and perceptions of coercion and force has been studied and critiqued from many perspectives,[5] and raises important questions about what constitutes open communication concerning sexual wants and needs, and how power, authority, and gender norms affect communicative patterns—none of which were discussed in the CSE (or AOUME) curricula or classrooms.

Students' challenges to CSE discussions about rape were about exactly these issues. From the students' perspectives it seemed that instructors, after talking consistently about people's ability and responsibility to make decisions about sex and sexuality, were suddenly saying that girls' decisions and actions would *not* provide them complete control over sexual situations. This perception, and students' strong response to it, is reflected in field notes taken during one Wisconsin class, in which an outside organization was brought in to talk about rape and sexual assault. The majority of the class time was spent defining the terms based on Wisconsin law; at the end of the class, the presenters shared some data with students on rape statistics in the United States. Note the change in student engagement when the presenter says, "It is never the victim's fault":

> The students are mostly quiet and there aren't very many disruptions. The presenters draw a grid on the board and say that they're going to talk about myths associated with sexual assault. One of the presenters, Jenny, then asks the class to answer the five questions represented on the side of the grid, which she fills in with the first answer they yell out. The filled-in grid looks like this (fig. 2.).
>
> Jenny then says, "OK, is this true? You guys did a pretty good job. Let's see . . ." She goes through each question and gives the national statistics. She explains that the perpetrator is usually male. Mrs. Shane jumps in: "But does

	perpetrator		victim
sex	male		female
average age	24		16
know each other		yes	
weapon		no	
report		no	
who do they tell?			friend

FIGURE 2. Blackboard exercise on rape

this mean that all males are rapists?" "No," the class answers together. "That's right. Most aren't." Jenny continues, explaining that the victim is usually female. She tells the students that one in four girls will experience some form of sexual assault by the time they are eighteen and that one in eight boys will experience it by eighteen. She tells the class that the average age of a perpetrator is twenty-four and the average age of a victim is fifteen to sixteen. She then says, "You seem mature enough for this," and she has the students guess the average age of a male victim. The students call out ages around fifteen or sixteen. "The average age of a male victim is four," she says. The students groan or make sympathetic noises. "What do you see in these numbers?" she asks. Students call out answers. "The perpetrators are over eighteen," "age difference." "Can you see why this is a problem?" she asks. "Yeah," the students answer collectively. There is no discussion about the significant difference in male and female victims' ages. . . .

"Rapes and sexual assaults are usually not reported," she says. "Why?" The students call out: "They can't remember," "they're not sure," "they're scared or embarrassed," "it will ruin their reputation," "threats." Jenny nods and says, "If they do tell anyone, they usually tell a friend." She then emphasizes the importance of being a supportive friend in this situation and asks the students to think about how they would be supportive if a friend came to them after being raped. Students say things like, "Let them talk," "listen to them," "believe them," "tell them to tell someone else." She emphasizes this last one. "Yes. Good." Then she adds, "It's never the fault of the victim."

"But what if the person was being stupid?" a female student asks. "Yeah," others jump in and give situations in which they think the girl would be to blame. What if she's "walking alone," "dressed slutty," "all dressed up," "drunk"? they ask. The class starts talking loudly about situations involving sex and alcohol and it briefly gets a little out of control. There is a lot of laughing around the discussions of girls being drunk. "These situations are not how it usually happens," Jenny says. "But still no. It is never the victim's fault.

There are ways to be safe, but it is not your fault." The students keep pushing back, coming up with more situations that involve a girl being drunk and/ or "in a bad situation" and, therefore, they argue, at least partially to blame. Jenny responds by talking about the ways that girls can be careful, including watching what you drink at parties, never leaving your friends behind at parties, and always taking your drink to the bathroom with you. Then she says, "But being raped is not a natural consequence of being drunk." This seems to get their attention but before the conversation can continue, the class ends.

Indeed, in all of the classes I attended, students pushed back against presenters' claims that victims are never to blame, and their response almost always questioned what they viewed as girls' choices to behave in ways that put them at risk. Given the intense focus in CSE programs on individual responsibility to reduce risk, and the lack of attention to power dynamics in relationships or in society, it did seem contradictory for CS educators and curricula to say that girls had no responsibility for shaping the social interactions in which stranger-on-stranger or date rape occurs. Without opening up to a wider discussion of power, violence, age, and social roles, CS educators could not get students to reflect on the gendered assumptions underlying their expectations that women had to take steps to protect themselves from assault, while (male) responsibility for attack disappears. For example, none of the educators I observed or curricula I reviewed mentioned perpetrator drunkenness as a risk factor. All of them mentioned victim drunkenness. As Filipovic (2008) notes, the greatest number of rapes occur when the perpetrator, not the victim, is drunk, but it is hard to imagine a curriculum that tells boys to be careful and control their drinking so that they can control their aggression.

Given the rational decision-maker model propounded by CSE approaches and the lack of discussion about structural relations of power, I was not surprised that by the end of all of the rape and assault discussions that I heard, the CS educators found themselves urging girls to be careful and providing specific examples of how girls could reduce their risk of being raped. They also frequently reverted to restating the laws concerning what constitutes rape when challenged by students over who is responsible for preventing it, and barely mentioned the responsibility of individual perpetrators or of social norms.

Sexual Commodification and Consumer Responsibility

We can understand both AOUME and CSE programs as being based on models of students as consumers. In AOUME approaches students are consumers of values and moral frameworks (such as that good teens are abstinent) and the goods that identify these values (such as demure prom dresses). In CSE programs teens are rational consumers of information, which they use to improve individual decision-making. Each of these models of students as consumers has embedded in it particular assumptions about responsibility, choice, and accountability; these assumptions in turn played an important role in determining how consent, force, negotiation, and social relations were discussed in curricula and classrooms. AOUME and CSE approaches alike draw on models of sex as an economic transaction and commodify sexual relations in ways that deflect attention from issues of social and relational inequities, interpersonal or structural violence, and the effects of rape on individuals and society.

AOUME PROGRAMS

AOUME speakers and curricula regularly talk about the evils of "the media," including the manner in which female sex and sexuality is displayed in it. Concomitantly, there is a strong focus on girls' responsibility to buck media messages concerning what is "popular" or "sexy," and "empower" themselves by choosing to dress and behave demurely. In the face of female sexuality being used to sell every imaginable product, as well as the widespread messages girls receive that appearing in *Playboy* or in *Girls Gone Wild* is "empowering" and fun (e.g., Siegel 2007; Levy 2005), AOUM educators and curricula send a very different message: choose to behave and present yourself demurely, and you will be truly empowered.

But what, exactly, is entailed by this type of empowerment? Filipovic (2008) argues that because AOUME supporters generally view sex as a commodity, they encourage girls to "get the best deal they can" by saving up sex for marriage. By creating a shortage of the commodity (sex), girls leverage the best possible price for it (marriage, and thus security, happiness, and an established and respected social role). AOUME programs' warnings that girls "lose their power" if they have sex before marriage thus reflect a belief that girls' disempowerment occurs through the low-price sale of the most valuable commodity under their control—their bodies. From this perspective, more than consumers, women are products that lose value rapidly once they are "opened." Girls' desire or potential pleasure not only disappears in this account of sexual transactionism, but if a girl wants to have sex before marriage, she must devalue the only social commodity she controls. Girls' adolescent desires thus actually become anathema to their long-term comfort, protection, or pleasure.[6]

The AOUME programs construct virginity as "priceless," a prize to be given by a girl only to her husband. Girls who have sex, like Ms. Tape, are soiled and disposable. This raises important questions about girls' power, empowerment, and responsibilities. If a girl is out drinking and partying, she is "advertising" herself as available, and at a low cost. If she is known to have had sex before, her value is already low and she is a readily available commodity. In such a situation, who could blame a guy for misunderstanding her market rate? Girls' only option in such a system is to dress and behave in ways that clearly and consistently convey the high price they place on their purity, so that if a girl is raped, everyone agrees that it *really* was not her fault.

Boys fare little better in AOUME curricula's constructions of rape and sexual transactions. Boys' natures lead them to want to consume as much sex as possible, at as low a price (they are good consumers!) as possible. But such behavior is not healthy for them. Left to their own devices and limited self-control, they become addicts of a low-cost commodity (for example, pornography or sex with non-virgins), and this addiction renders them incapable of valuing the high-cost commodity (their wife-to-be's virginity and lifetime sexual availability). Men then suffer because they cannot find contentment in their marital relationships or in their relationship with God. Women suffer because the husband for whom they traded their most precious commodity is, it turns out, a bad deal. Society as a whole suffers because men's dangerous and violent natures have not been effectively controlled through marriage to a woman whose "better" nature connects him to family and to God (e.g., Lehr 2003).

Less cynically, the notions that real men will "naturally" want to have sex with any woman, that women use sex primarily as a commodity that they withhold until a good enough bargain is reached, and that having sex therefore is a matter of two consumers reaching agreement on the price of the commodity, has important implications for our understandings of rape, consumerism, and relationships in AOUME curricula and US society more generally. This model of male-female romantic relationships, as extreme as it may sound, is taken for granted in many popular movies, video games, TV shows, books, and magazines,[7] in studies of relationships and sexuality (e.g., Regnerus 2007), and in many students' descriptions of social relations in and after high school (e.g., Tolman, Striepe, and Harmon 2003). Taken to its logical extreme, a commodified conception of sex and a consumerist model of relationships assumes that (1) the commodity is available for purchase if the right deal can be struck; (2) however wonderful the product, there are likely going to be better models arriving in the future; and (3) therefore, the commodity will always be viewed as disposable by the consumer unless the transaction has transformed the commodity (that is, men will always keep looking for more and better sex unless the act of being married effectively transforms their view of sex, God, family, and responsibility).

CSE PROGRAMS

In CSE programs, the assumption that each individual is an equal and equally rational consumer leads to an understanding of sex as an equally distributed exchange commodity: both boys and girls control their own sexuality. What sexual actors, as rational beings, should be looking for is an even exchange of goods and services. Rape is not the outcome of the victim misrepresenting her value and the aggressor therefore misreading the price of sex; it is the outcome of a consumer taking by force what he or she cannot bargain for in good faith. As rational, equally empowered individuals, people involved in negotiations over sex should be able to express their needs, wants, and desires clearly. When these do not align, sex should not happen. When they do, sex should. Conceptually, there is no space for partners to be unsure about or unable to clearly explain their wants and needs, nor is there space for communication issues or differential power relations to affect this negotiating process.

While this model theoretically places the blame much more squarely on the shoulders of the perpetrator, by failing to address issues of power and of relational dynamics, it reinforces the need for an individual to be a certain type of communicator and actor: clear on her own wants and needs and articulate in presenting them, direct and firm with potential partners, and able to negotiate a mutually beneficial arrangement in sexual interactions in order to avoid blame. When students questioned the instructors' assertions that girls were not responsible for dressing and behaving in certain ways and that they did not have absolute control over the final outcome of a sexual encounter, they were pointing to the contradiction between these statements and CSE's implicit assumptions about the kind of actor who could avoid sexual coercion.

What's Missing?

Both AOUME and CSE approaches were limited by their assumptions of students as consumers and sex as a commodity. Though their models of consumerism and consumption were markedly different, the missing discourses in both approaches were remarkably similar. In none of the discussions that I heard or curricula that I reviewed was there any serious discussion about the roles and responsibilities of male and female aggressors involved in committing rape, nor of rape as a fundamentally antisocial and scarring act of violence. While female ability (and students argued, responsibility) to reduce risk was front and center in the discussions I heard in every classroom, none of the educators linked the presence of risk for rape victims to the absence of responsibility, morality, or intelligence on the side of individual rape perpetrators, or to social and institutional arrangements (such as prison systems) that in practice support sexual abuse and rape. The focus in all programs on presenting the legal definition of rape resulted in abstracted classroom discussions largely dominated by boys questioning when a situation might be called rape. These discussions ignored what rape does physically, emotionally, socially, psychologically, and spiritually to both victim and perpetrator. There was no conversation about outcomes or consequences for rape victims, and there was only brief discussion about the threat of jail time for perpetrators.

In AOUME and CSE classrooms alike, the silence about outcomes and consequences, the focus on victims' responsibility to reduce risk, the assumptions about victim (straight woman) and perpetrator (straight man) identities, and the resulting assumption that sex is a commodity did nothing to disrupt the "commonsense" gender norm that boys are just naturally sexually aggressive. Further, it positioned rape as a sexual interaction gone a bit off-track, not an attack or a violation. Since men are assumed to always want to consume sex, it placed responsibility for avoiding sex (desired or not) on women. And, because of the gendered assumptions underlying the sex-as-commodity model (in which the encounter is not one of differential power and force, but one about the terms of the exchange of a commodity), neither AOUME nor CSE programs destabilized the assumption that rape "naturally" involves a male aggressor and female victim.

Both AOUME and CSE programs also avoided anything more than passing comment about male-male rape, although some studies in the United States estimate that up to one in six men in the general population will experience rape. Male-male rape and its consequences are intimately tied to the prison system in the United States, a system through which a growing percentage of the US population cycles. Robertson (2003) warns that

> criminologists have yet to reach consensus on the prevalence of male inmate-on-inmate rape. The leading prevalence studies found that 7–12 percent of the responding male inmates had been raped an average of nine times. With a national jail and prison population of 2 million at mid-year 2002, the U.S. likely exposes tens of thousands of male inmates to rape, and consequently, to HIV/AIDS and other sexually transmitted diseases (STDs). The release of inmates from jails and prisons—estimated at 11.5 million persons in 1998—

transforms the consequences of male rape from a correctional matter into a public health crisis.

Likewise, though it was mentioned occasionally as a statistic, there was no sustained discussion of adult-child rape, and there was no sustained discussion of rape perpetrated by strangers. Instead, all of the programs focused their attention on date rape situations, especially those where teens were out drinking and partying. With the exception of the classroom conversation described previously, none of the presentations focused on age differences among actors in these situations. This focus reflected, said instructors, an effort to talk with students about the "statistical reality" of teen sexuality and rape, but it also made it easier to avoid talking about power and inequity by focusing on a rape situation between two "peers"—the scenario most likely to be understood by students as a "he said/she said" assault situation. Indeed, it appeared natural and easy for students to assign responsibility for a rape to the victim in such a situation. The ease with which blame was assigned in the classrooms I observed was important. In most, if not all, of those classrooms, there were students who had been raped or affected by the rape of someone close to them, or who will experience sexual violence in the future. These realities were not acknowledged, and there was no sustained discussion about what a person should do or where a person could find support if raped.

The most remarkable omissions in the classroom conversations about rape were force, coercion, fear, and morality. In most of these classrooms, rape appeared to consist of boys misinterpreting girls' cues, possibly because everyone was drunk, or, in the case of statutory rape, of adults interfering in consensual relationships. The majority of students' questions, particularly those of boys, were about when boys could be charged for rape in situations where the boy did not think he was "doing something wrong" (e.g., when the girl lied about her age, when both partners were drunk).

Teachers' focus on legal definitions of rape and assault in response to student questions signaled a shift away from honest discussion of the conundrums of assigning female responsibility for sexual security despite clear social, and sometimes physical, power disadvantages vis-à-vis (particularly older) males. It also signaled the evasion of personal responsibility for aggressive and overpowering sexual actions, with an implicit link to "traditional" constructions of masculinity reinforced by constant consumer and entertainment images of desirable male power exerted over women (for example, the Axe deodorant ads). Lastly, it signaled a shift away from the complex realities of rape and sexual assault, across ages and genders, and within very different institutional and social settings. In other words, the statistically striking gender and age/power disparities involved in who has the right to (try to) have sex and who has the responsibility to avoid unwanted sex in "date rape" situations were not discussed at all, nor were power dynamics in other rape scenarios.

The other important silence in all of the curricula was noted above: at no point did programs discuss the consequences of rape for individuals or communities. Most other sex education topics were discussed in terms of their physical outcomes (CSE curricula) and physical, spiritual, social, psychological, and emotional effects (AOUME curricula). But the consequence of rape most often discussed was jail for the perpetrator. Some of this silence stems from the lack of attention given to power and violence in rape. I think it likely, however, that a central reason that none of the instructors talked about STIs or pregnancy, or psychological or emotional consequences, was because all of the sex education approaches assume that individual choice and volition lie at the heart of sexual encounters. This assumption affected how all of the programs talked (or failed to talk) about STIs, pregnancy, and stigma, as we saw in chapter 7. In the case of rape and sexual violence, if the victim is really not at fault, a discussion of the (unfair) negative outcomes that can still result would challenge the moral assumptions behind all models' conceptions of the consequences of sex. For AOUME programs, if a girl behaves appropriately, she should always be protected from rape. For CSE programs, if victims are effective rational consumers who make the right kinds of decisions about their behavior, they too should be safe from abuse. The notion that a person can make all the right individual decisions and still experience rape or sexual violence undermines the central arguments being made about how people should behave as "good" sexual citizens in all sex education programs. The conversation among Mrs. Shane, Theo, Cornell, and Shurita about how brave and good a woman was for having a baby conceived from rape points to this notion of whether the unintended outcomes of sex are "deserved" or not, and the difficulties students and teachers faced in making sense of the moral conundrum posed by an "undeserved" consequence.

To circle back to the earlier discussion about AOUME and CSE models of commodification, consumption, and sex, to the extent that sex is conceptualized as a commodity, and sexual interactions are thus exchanges of a commodity, and to the extent that teens are viewed primarily as consumers in a market of sexual practices, rape becomes (1) more a violent act against a supplier of a commodity in a free-market interaction, less a personal assault or a violent act against a person; (2) more the responsibility of the supplier, who should be protecting their goods against theft (in a more violent environment, the supplier is held even more responsible for installing alarm systems, hiring guards, and so on); (3) more regulated by the reality of legal enforcement than by the morality of the act; and (4) more open to interpretation, as negotiations between buyers and sellers can get heated, thus, the male concern that girls will "cry rape" because of "buyer's remorse."

Students are not passive, but rather critical consumers of sex education information. When they heard something that seemed to directly contradict the otherwise consistent message that they had the responsibility and capacity to control their own sexual decision-making, they responded by questioning the instructors. Students were not given the opportunity to reflect on or talk about the social and structural constraints in which rape occurs, how different students faced these constraints, and how these constraints should and should not shape students' attitudes, sexual experiences, and decision making. Because their sense of themselves as individual, empowered consumers was not challenged at any other point, none of the sex education curricula I observed could engage students seriously in a discussion about force and violence, either from the perspective of consumer interactions or from the perspective of human rights and values. Instead, students' discussions about rape remained highly gendered, did not destabilize the assumption that rape "just occurs" (Marcus 2002), and were infused with comments about girls' responsibility to avoid the trouble in the first place.

Students as Disempowered Consumers

CSE and AOUME programs are based on implicit models of students as consumers. In Florida, CS educators expressed their disgust with AOUME programs' focus on "flashy" materials, and appeared at times to almost take pride in dry, straightforward "fact sheets." CS educators felt it was disrespectful to treat teens as irrational consumers who could be easily swayed by advertising ploys and bells and whistles. Florida AOUM educators sometimes expressed a similar disgust with focusing on the "packaging" of their messages and materials, but felt it was a small price to pay to connect with students, whom they described, not always admiringly, as "savvy consumers."

In the limited interactions I had with students on these issues, it certainly appeared that they judged sex education programming, messages, and outside educators at least in part based on their "packaging." In the Wisconsin classroom, for example, students said that although they thought the information in a video on HIV/AIDS was "probably good," they were less likely to believe it because the video appeared "outdated." When asked how the video could be improved, they said it should be remade with people who looked like they were "from this decade."

Given this focus on products' external appearances, should one be surprised that students judge each other on these terms as well? And that, therefore, girls in particular face deeply contradictory messages about how more or less sexualized presentations of self will affect their social standing? Rape programming in sex education helps to uncover some of the unexamined but inextricable links between students' senses of themselves as consumers of sex and relationships. AOUME and CSE approaches are engaged, at least in part, in a battle over the kind of consumers they want students to be. Most CSE supporters, if pushed hard, would say they do not actually believe that students are Spock-like rational decision-makers when it comes to sex and sexuality, and most AOUME supporters were intensely denigrating of "consumer society" and "the media" and said they did not want students to act as passive consumers of products, ideas, or values (indeed, they called abstinence the antimedia message).

At the same time, AOUME supporters concentrated on understanding how youth interact with each other, media technologies, and "consumer culture." Though denigrating of it, AOUME supporters were generally comfortable using consumer approaches, even ones that they otherwise opposed, in order to reach the higher goal of re-creating a moral (Christian) society. The adoption of consumer-culture approaches in church life and Christian outreach has created its own literature and counterliterature (e.g., Jethani 2009; Miller 2003); AOUME approaches to consumerism reflected this larger tension within the New Christian Right.

The lack of extended discussion in all of the sex education programs about responsibility, violence, and rape is linked to the lack of discussion about consumerism, responsibility, and sexuality. The discomfort with mass consumerism shared by all sex educators with whom I spoke was not used as a platform on which to build a cross-generational discussion of how female sexuality is used to drive the consumption of goods, and what this does to girls' and boys' ideas about a woman's "value" as a sexual commodity or a person, and men's roles in "setting the price" by consuming this sexuality.

There are many conversations about consumerism, sexuality, and relationships that could occur in sex education programming about rape and sexual violence, but that did not. For example, a discussion about gender and media images might have led to questions such as the following: If girls follow the styles marketed to them and dress in ways that fit right in with TV commercials, but that are perceived by some as trashy or overly sexy, are they responsible for putting themselves at risk and sending inappropriate signals to potential sexual partners (or predators)? If girls resist style consumerism, what are the social consequences? Are they viewed as less feminine? As a different kind of feminine? As a different or less-valuable commodity? If boys respond to sexual stimuli and consumer marketing with the consuming sexual desire implicitly expected of them, will they be date rapists? What message is sent about the nature of masculinity when males are not expected to be thoughtful and responsible (and fearful) consumers to the degree that females are? If men are positioned as the primary consumers of women's sexuality, how does this change the boundary between rape and consent? These questions may not have easy answers, but the students in the classrooms I observed made it clear in their comments to sex educators that they wanted to explore them. By not linking consumerism, sexuality, gender, and power, the sex education programs lost the chance to provide students opportunities to voice their questions, concerns, and ideas, and to begin these conversations that linked sexual violence to students' actual social experiences.

Adult concepts of sexuality, public health, individual choice and behavior, and morality frame sex education to the virtual exclusion of student perceptions, needs, and priorities. The lack of student voices is related to an absence of dialogue in sex education programs on all topics, but is perhaps most evident in discussions about rape and the rights and responsibilities of girls and boys, men and women concerning unwanted sexual acts and sexual violence. The links between choice, gender, sexuality, and consumerism appeared to underlie many of the students' own formulations about sex and responsibility. The complexity of the links among these phenomena posed a challenge for students trying to navigate social relations, physical security, and sexuality. Though this challenge was very real for students, it was off-limits as a conversational topic for virtually all of the adults who shepherded them through their days in high school.

Finally, students struggling with issues of rape or sexual violence in their own lives were unacknowledged in all of the sex education programs I observed. There was no discussion of the broader social drivers of sexual violence, nor were students presented with statistics or personal stories of family abuse, abuse within marriage or long-term relationships, or child abuse. This is a troubling finding that points to the silences, inequities, and continued stigmas that shape AOUME and CSE approaches alike.

Concluding Thoughts:
Sex Education as Civics Education?

Power, Social Relations, and Enacting Democracy

In the introduction to this book, I asked whether the United States is at a point where the culture war between CSE and AOUME approaches could be transformed by asking a new set of questions. I argued for a shift from our current focus on sex education *content and public health outcomes* to a new emphasis on the *sociopolitical consequences of sex education approaches*.

AOUME and CSE approaches, in their most divergent forms, embody two distinct models of students, schools, society, and sex education. The morals and values most readily apparent in national sex education debates relate to teen sex, religion in schools, and sexual orientation. These debates shape the "hot topics" identified by teachers and adults: homosexuality, abortion, and contraception. But the critical issues at play in sex education practices are bigger and run deeper, right to the core of power, social relations, and the enactment of democracy at this time in US history.

The previous ten chapters examined how states, communities, teachers, and students influence the shape and scope of sex education programming in their public schools, how AOUME and CSE approaches function in a variety of schools and communities across the United States, how these sex education approaches connect (or fail to connect) with students' lives, and if and how the assumptions embedded in sex education curricula and practices align with the democratic ideals and practices that public schools should, in theory, be promulgating. I have shown how decisions about sex education are made in different communities, schools, and classrooms, and I have demonstrated the dearth of student or youth involvement in these decisions. The analysis of sex education practices in four states provides insights into how new understandings and analyses of daily sex-education practices might serve as the cloth from which we could cut new approaches to supporting students' health, well-being, and education as democratic citizens, and to involving students, parents, teachers, and communities in decision-making processes concerning controversial issues such as sex education.

I have argued that AOUME and CSE approaches embody different ideologies concerning individuals, society, truth, information, and morality, and that, not surprisingly, their community mobilization and educational programming approaches reflect these differing ideals. For all their divergence, however, I have also argued that AOUME and CSE programs share some fundamental similarities in worldviews, including their general agreement on teen sex as a problem and their understanding of individuals as consumers, their concern about the negative role of the media on adolescents, the neotraditional gender norms that in practice underlay all of the programs I observed, and the scientific rationalization of sexuality increasingly evident in both approaches. These similarities and differences offer potential opportunities to reformulate the sex education debates.

CSE and AOUME Approaches

CSE programs take an approach that is more about information-sharing and is more sex-positive than AOUME approaches. The CSE approaches I observed were less fear-based than AOUME approaches (for example, CS educators regularly commented that sex is natural and not something that students should be afraid of) and were more "sex-positive" (for example, CS educators said that sex should be pleasurable for females and males, and sometimes discussed how to make it more pleasurable). However, these messages were generally abstracted and disconnected from students' actual sexual experiences, desires, and fears. CSE curricula and instructors focused a great deal of their time and evaluative energies on the physical consequences of sex (pregnancy and STIs), not infrequently reflected sexually restrictive or conservative values in the classroom (for example, about abortion or gender roles), and, when discussing many topics, but particularly "hot topics" such as homosexuality, abortion, or contraception, focused on introducing, defining, and categorizing terms, and thus scientifically rationalizing emotion, relationships, embodied experience, and power out of sex education.

AOUME curricula and activities were premised on the benefits of gender hierarchies, the moral supremacy of heterosexuality, and the goodness of all people being organized into traditional family units. These values did not reflect the real-life experiences or desires of most students in classrooms I observed. AOUME's stance that students choose to sin by having sex, being queer, not submitting to their parents, or not supporting neotraditional gen-

der norms reinscribed responsibility for social, economic, and political inequity onto the individual sinner/student. AOUME efforts to normalize this
model of the family and society and to socially sanction others (for example,
their consistent references to single-mother families as a sign and cause of
social decay) represented attempts to normalize a particular masculinist,
heterosexual, middle-class, and white ideal of social organization that would
require the majority of students to "joyfully, intelligently submit" to a hierarchy in which they could never be on top. The ideology underlying AOUME
approaches is thus fundamentally oppositional to liberal democratic ideals of
equality, respect for diversity, and participation in governance.

Sex education in each school and state in which I worked was shaped
by distinctive social, economic, political, and cultural norms and practices.
Different people and organizations were involved in debating and shaping
school curricula and practices in each research setting, and in some cases significant conflicts among teachers, parents, communities, policy makers, and
students ensued. In response to these pressures and their own discomfort
with teaching sex education, all of the teachers and schools that I observed
had privatized some or all of their sex education programming. Every teacher
and policymaker with whom I spoke said that they were more concerned
about backlash from AOUME supporters than from CSE supporters; this informed the risks they were willing to take, the conversations they were willing to allow in their classrooms, and sometimes the selection of the private
groups they invited in. A number of teachers and students noted that this
meant sex education was driven by adult concerns with no opportunities for
student voice.

CORE IDEOLOGY

AOUME and CSE approaches are based on very different core ideologies.
CSE approaches are informed first and foremost by a scientific rationality
arising from Enlightenment ideals about truth, justice, and individual rights
(e.g., Meyer 1980). A valuing of quantified public-health (e.g., Morris 2005),
medical, and scientific data grounds the curricula, approaches, and programming decisions viewed as "best practices" in CSE, so that if "gold standard"
research showed that AOUME benefited some or all children more than CSE,
no small number of CSE supporters would urge the adoption of AOUME
approaches for these populations. For example, the report by Jemmott et al.
(2010) concluded that an abstinence-only (but not AOUME) program resulted in statistically significant reductions in sexual initiation in a certain

population of teenage girls and boys. In a *Washington Post* article, Rob Stein reported that

> longtime critics of the [AOUME] approach praised the study, saying it provides strong evidence that such programs can work and might merit taxpayer support. "One of the things that's exciting about this study is that it says we have a new tool to add to our repertoire," said Monica Rodriguez, vice president for education and training at the Sexuality Information and Education Council of the U.S. (February 2, 2010)

Rhetorical as this quote may have been, it is something that AOUME supporters would never say, regardless of the preponderance of scientific evidence supporting CSE approaches. On the other hand, as this book has also highlighted, CSE curricula and educators do propound values beyond scientific rationality. They are supportive of abstract universal human rights, equality, and diversity; liberal (in the classic political sense) approaches to mediating social and sexual issues; and democratic political processes. CSE classrooms in Wisconsin and California actively supported group rights, particularly gay rights and, in California, a woman's right to abortion. As was evident in these classrooms, however, the values of (individual) scientific rationality and of universal human rights and equality in practice sometimes conflicted. These tensions and the politics of sex education provision in public schools combined to create classrooms where a range of student opinions and ideas were aired and acknowledged, but the ideals of teaching students to think critically and to engage actively in democratic discussions and debates based on analyses of data and opinion were not reached. For CSE supporters, this creates a conundrum related to balancing CSE ideals of universal rights and equality, with ideals of scientific rationalism. Most of the AOUME curricula, providers, and activities I observed actively violated the human-equality ideals supported by CSE approaches. AOUME providers in Florida were engaged in an active and heated debate about the potential moral effects of adopting a medicalized rationale for AOUME approaches. In contrast, CSE supporters did not appear to be debating or talking about how to resolve tensions within and among central tenets of their approach. If a study appeared to indicate that AOUME approaches work well for certain student subgroups, would the effectiveness of the program in reducing age of sexual initiation be more or less important than exposing students to the kinds of antidemocratic homophobia and sexism evident in many mainstream AOUME programs?

AOUME approaches are based on a biblical foundation that offers one clear moral framework through which to judge sexual topics, curricular materials, pedagogical approaches, and social relations in the classroom. Most of the curricula, speakers, and programs come out of the New Christian Right, and AOUM educators with whom I spoke discussed the difficulties they faced with "removing religion" from their public school activities, a reflection of their clarity about the ideas and beliefs that shaped their programming. AOUME supporters appeared to be more cognizant of and able to adopt multiple approaches to achieving their ends, such as using consumer marketing techniques with which teens were familiar and to which they appeared responsive; sometimes appropriating "scientific data" as a tactic to support their cause, and other times dismissing such data; or silencing voices and topics that represented or called for alternative social orders. AOUME approaches also directly addressed relations of power and social inequalities in ways that, while stereotypical, "rang true" for some students and parents.

AOUME interpretations of biblical exegesis included a valuing of hierarchy and of social and sexual laws that conflict with US constitutional values of equality, individual rights, diversity, and democratic political processes, and that conflict with many students' lives, desires, and ideals. These conflicts are visible in AOUME representations (or lack thereof) of gender roles and sexual identities, their approach to "keeping secret and sacred" information about sex and sexuality, and their active pursuit—to the point of bringing legal suits against schools—of what they view as the appropriate relations of power and authority between males and females, and sex educators, schools, and community members. For public schools, parents, and policy makers, AOUME approaches should raise important questions about the shared values that public schools can and should promulgate; about how community norms and values should be measured, incorporated, and addressed throughout the sex education policy-making process in public schools; and about what lessons AOUME programs have to teach all sex educators about the importance of recognizing and talking about relational and social aspects of sex and sexuality.

HEGEMONIC NORMS

Despite ideological differences, all of the sex education classes and most of the curricula I reviewed made assumptions about healthy teen sexuality and individual sexual behavior that reflected hegemonic class, race, gender, and sexual norms. In AOUME approaches, these norms represented core neotraditional ideological assumptions. CSE approaches theoretically valued diversity and equality, but in practice their model assumed all high school students were white, middle-class, straight, rational individual decision-makers who had the right and the responsibility to control their environment and their sexual encounters (Sears 1992). These approaches failed to engage with structural inequities and students' experiences of desire, dependence, poverty, caring, insecurity, violence, and interconnection—from Wyoming students who had no private or public transportation to and from home, to Latin@ students who had recently made physically and emotionally perilous border crossings from Mexico, to queer students facing daily harassment, to girls doubtful of their ability to demand condom use once in a relationship. Instead, this model inscribed responsibility for healthy sexual outcomes onto each equally agentic individual.

In its reliance on scientific rationality, CSE approaches failed to provide opportunities to enact or debate their ideological assumptions concerning universal human rights and equality, the value of diversity, and the central role of scientific evidence, human reasoning, and individual decision-making in teens' well-being. Without such discussions, which might have provided opportunities for students and teachers to think through how these ideals might be translated into daily practices, students and teachers tended to revert to conservative and consumerist social scripts and norms (such as neotraditional gender norms).

CONSUMERISM AND DIVERSITY

I have argued that AOUME and CSE approaches both rest on socioeconomic models of teens as consumers; these models reflect aspects of each approach's core ideology. In CSE approaches, the student-consumer is a scientist, gathering information, weighing evidence, and making the most rational health choice. The goal of sex education is to provide "complete and correct" information and to teach students how to be better consumers of information throughout their lives. All CS educators and curricula also, however, had deeply held beliefs about what constituted science and rationality, and therefore what would constitute good sexual decision-making and behavior. In theory and practice, these beliefs conflicted in various ways with the support for human rights and diversity in which CSE approaches are also rooted. For example, despite evidence about the potential benefits of teen versus later pregnancy for some women and children, CSE instructors and curricula could not conceive of teen pregnancy as ever being a good outcome for students. These conflicts reflect some of the underlying tensions in liberal (pluralist) approaches to diversity, recognition, and inclusion (e.g., Mayo 2006; Taylor 1994.).

AOUME approaches, on the other hand, which rely more heavily on models of teens as consumers of culture and peer norms, assume that student decisions are based on consumer desires, peer trends, and teens' perceptions of the social acceptability of messages and products. Teens' consumer identities are naturally gendered (and raced, classed, and sexed); by marketing ideas (such as abstinence) and products (such as silver rings) to different identity groups, AOUME programs aim to achieve their goal of the moral transformation of teens and society. The goal of better marketing is to figure out how to get a diverse set of teens to buy the same "product," so differences between groups become marketing niches and target groups, not valued as diverse ways of knowing, seeing, or living in the world—they are a means to the same moral end for all students.

GENERATIONAL AND SOCIOCULTURAL GAPS IN SEX EDUCATION

The state studies revealed generational and sociocultural gaps among actors in schools. As others have reported (e.g., Luker 2006; Irvine 2002), the responses of most teachers and parents with whom I spoke about sex education reflected their experiences of the culture wars that raged in the 1980s and 1990s. They felt that the "hot topics" in sex education were contraception, abortion, and homosexuality, and it was around these topics that they focused many of their energies and concerns. For teachers, this usually meant that they had outsiders come in to talk about these subjects, they approached conversations about these subjects warily, or they limited or avoided conversations about them entirely.

Students, on the other hand, were generally blasé about contraception and sexual identity. They actively debated abortion, but on terms that differed from their instructors', and were conflicted but relatively silent in class about their experiences with gender roles and social identities. Students were extremely concerned about instructors' framing of sexual violence and rape, and this was the only arena in which they consistently and actively pushed back against the sex education programming I observed. Their concerns were generally not addressed by teachers, who seemed unable to recognize or rationalize the apparent inconsistencies in their lessons on rape.

There were important differences among classrooms and students, within and across schools. For example, the California students in the high-track science class were some of the most blasé about discussions of sexual identity, while students in the English Learner classes were actively disruptive. These differences in student responses to adult "hot topics," their own sexual experiences and concerns, and their own "hot topics" reflected their own positionality and identity vis-à-vis sexuality, gender, race, class, ethnicity, and citizenship. This was not addressed in a serious way in any of the programs or curricula I observed, in part, perhaps, because of what appeared to be an underlying desire by all the teachers in all of the programs to avoid conflict in classroom conversation. The effort to silence potentially "uncontrollable" student voices should in turn be understood in light of teachers' deep-seated concerns that parents and other community members would mobilize against teachers, the sex education they provided, and their schools.

Values and Governance

Schools did not only fail to solicit or listen to students' voices, they also failed to model or practice participatory democratic decision-making processes. In most of the research settings described here, as well as in my work in Maryland, a minority of adults in the community shaped decision-making concerning sex education. This is not in and of itself surprising, as parental involvement in school decision-making is usually uneven, but sex education is often particularly controversial, and most of the schools in which I worked quite deliberately took steps to minimize parental concern around their sex education programming. Data based on nationally representative samples of US adults show consistently high support (over 80 percent) for sex education programming in which abstinence is prioritized but information about contraception is provided (e.g., Bleakley, Henessy, and Fishbein 2006). Yet a growing number of schools and teachers report that they are mandated to present abstinence-only programming to students. These mandates arise not only in response to federal and state policies, but also in response to community organizing. Community groups organized in support of AOUME are much more common than those that support CSE, and teachers and district officials consistently reported that schools are much more scared of mobilized AOUME supporters than of mobilized CSE supporters. The result is that schools are more conservative in their approaches than is warranted by either the evidence about people's support for CSE, or the evidence about different sex education approaches' efficacy as it is currently measured. This is a policy dilemma for schools, and one that relates directly to listening to, incorporating, and addressing both adults' ideas and ideals concerning sex education, and student needs and desires in this arena. Teachers and schools have not, to date, received effective support in navigating these issues.

Sex education represents and reproduces a public debate about the shape of US society and the shared values that a democratic society should support. I agree with McKay (1998) that "the ideological debates around sexuality education in the schools are the wider social and moral conflicts related to sexuality in our culture writ large" (47) and that these debates have been intensely contentious and divisive in our recent history. McKay also argues that "because of its role in molding us as individuals and social actors, education may be an ideal template for exploring reasonable and democratic approaches to sexuality in our society" (9).

CSE and AOUME curricula represent two different ways of resolving tensions among values concerning sex, gender, society, diversity, individuality, equality, parenting, participation, consumerism and commodification, and religious and scientific rationalities. AOUME approaches teach us about the importance of acknowledging that all people operate within relational webs of power and authority; the centrality of social relations in people's daily lives and sexual experiences; and the consumer rationalities that increasingly drive teens' and adults' sexual, political, social, and economic engagements.[1] CSE approaches, on the other hand, teach us about the central role that schools could play in fostering democratic ideals concerning the dignity and equal rights of each individual and in supporting students' development as citizens who can participate effectively in political and social decision-making processes, in part by inquiring and deliberating about knowledge, facts, opinions, and forces (such as marketing) that aim to influence how they see the world. *A sex education approach that supports the broader democratic goals and responsibilities of public schools in the United States would draw on both of these models to fundamentally transform current school-based sex education and citizenship-education practices.*

Citizenship Education?

Public schools have a particular role to play in US democratic society. American adults claim a right and responsibility to guide and shape the next generation of citizens through public schooling. Teens are denied full adult political rights, and in exchange, the state, through schools, are tasked with training teens for their adult roles and responsibilities as citizens (McKay 1998). Sex education provides a rich opportunity to engage teens in discussions and debates about the nature of US society and democracy, the ethical and moral frameworks that Americans, as groups and as a collective, choose to uphold, the tensions that everyone faces engaging with ideas, people, and institutions with whom they disagree, productive avenues for engaging in local and national debates about these issues, the rights and responsibilities of the individual and the various collectivities of which each individual is a part, and the mechanisms through which Americans may legally and ethically debate the value of various ideals.

In my research, sex education programs in US public schools failed uniformly to engage in this type of democratic training. At the official policy-planning and policy-implementation stage, schools tend to be responsive to the demands of vocal minorities who claim a right to be heard in public-school curricular debates because they are "taxpayers," but who may not have children in the schools and may not even live in the school district area (e.g., Kendall 2008a.). Schools are responsive to these groups in part because of the serious costs they can incur if such groups undertake legal action, as we saw in the case of the CRC. While in the past courts and parents tended to be protective of school autonomy and teachers' professional expertise, this has changed significantly over the past decades (e.g., Hursh 2003).

Parents who are not vocal, perhaps because of language barriers, other demands on their time, or a less-intense interest in the topic, are generally not heard in current sex education policy-making processes. Take, for example, a PTA meeting I attended in Maryland, where a number of parents, many of whom were Latin@, came to school on a weeknight to meet with the school principal and teachers and review the proposed sex education curriculum. A volunteer translator was present, and the parents, who had received a flyer from the CRC, expressed concerns about some parts of the curriculum. There was a long discussion between the parents and school officials about various topics and materials, including a review of sections of the curriculum that were mentioned in the flyer. In the end, the parents agreed that the curriculum was adequate and, although they disagreed with some of the topics being included, said that they trusted their children's teacher to be conscious of diverse family values and realities and to handle them in ways that would be age appropriate. This engagement between parents and teachers was lost entirely in the ensuing federal court case brought forward by the CRC—a group of people who did not have children in the school and who received support, including legal representation, from national New Christian Right organizations.

Student voices played no role in selecting the sex education curricula or in shaping topics or approaches in sex education classes and were generally absent from debates about sex education policies in all of the schools I observed. Although student voices are often front and center in debates about the formation of student Gay-Straight Alliance (GSA) clubs, these groups are not part of the formal curriculum and often represent the only instance in which students' voices are systematically attended to in relation to sex and sexuality in public schools. As in the case of AOUME supporters, schools may pay more attention to GSA supporters because they have been involved in a series of very public court cases around the country that schools have consistently lost. In their day-to-day experiences in schools, however, most students' engagement with and concerns about sex and sexuality were routinely silenced or ignored by adults.

Within schools, teachers expressed a general discomfort with students' sexuality and an unwillingness to engage in discussion when students had concerns about how the school was addressing their sexuality (such as student dress codes). In CSE classrooms, which are predicated on the ideal of open and complete communication of information, some teachers deliberately silenced student voices and questions for fear that they would provoke controversy. Teachers who were themselves supportive of sexually liberal values tended to not directly state their opinions, while those supportive of sexually conservative values were more vocal about their beliefs.

As has been noted in research on other school subjects, this research also indicated that teacher training, content knowledge and comfort level, personality, and perceptions of students mattered in how teachers managed sex education classes and engaged various students (e.g., Darling-Hammond 1999; Cooper and Tom 1984) and in turn how students engaged with them (e.g., Skinner and Belmont 1993). The particular group of students that constituted the classroom visibly affected the teacher-student dynamics in classrooms where students did have the opportunity to speak. While all student voices were generally silenced in discussions about sex education, certain students faced greater directed silencing efforts from teachers. The groups of students or individual students who were systematically silenced differed in each school, but they consistently included queer students; racial, ethnic, or class minority students; those who were pregnant or parenting while staying in school; and those who had or were experiencing sexual violence in the home or in a sexual relationship. These students and their experiences were not represented in sex education activities, and students received strong messages that such experiences were a private matter that could not be discussed in public settings.

DEMOCRACY-BUILDING SEX EDUCATION

Given these community, school, classroom, and curricular realities, what might a more democratic approach to sex education look like? First, sex education might address its democratic charge, and likely better fulfill its official goals, by involving students more fully in determining curriculum content, pedagogical approaches, and school policies related to sexuality. Though CSE approaches do this to a limited extent through their use of anonymous question boxes,[2] my research, along with other studies (e.g., Skinner and Belmont 1993), indicates that CSE and AOUME classrooms alike do not readily take up students' concerns and experiences, particularly when this would require a discussion about relations of power and the structural inequities that affect students. The "hot topics" in the observed classes and the pedagogical approaches employed by instructors were far more representative of adults' concerns and experiences than of teens'. For example, I never heard a discussion about how students might protect their privacy while using new technologies to learn about and explore sex and sexuality (such as the Internet and cell phones), despite teachers' and parents' self-professed concerns about online predators, child pornography, and so forth. I never heard a conversation about self-presentation, consumerism, and the media, although students were furious about school dress codes and teachers were scandalized by girls' choices about what to wear to school. I never heard about desire, excitement, or sexuality as an embodied experience. I never heard a discussion about what it feels like to belong, or not belong, to various social groups, and how group sexual norms can differentially affect students' sense of identity and sexual behavior, yet this topic was consistently raised by those students whom I was able to interview.

Second, instead of having teachers, students, and community members view each other as minefields that can be defused only through tight control, sex education classrooms might be arranged to foster new kinds of deliberation and debate.[3] One study found that in situations where social-science teachers made their views on controversial issues known, teachers' opinions influenced students less than those of their peers (Hess and Posselt 2002). This research raises questions about the common fear that what teachers say (or indeed, what textbooks say) will singlehandedly sway students, and concomitant efforts to control teachers' utterances and curricular materials. In the observations conducted for this book, teachers' opinions affected the topics of conversation and raw data that were formally made available for students, but teacher utterances about various topics did not seem to affect students' opinions, if students' vocal disagreement with teachers was any indication.

In situations where family and peer influences are particularly powerful in shaping students' beliefs, where topics are publicly discussed outside the school if not inside, where other public influences (such as television) significantly shape students' perceptions, and where teacher and student opinions and biases are diverse, sex education could explore pedagogical approaches that destabilize straightforward presentations of "the facts." It could do so by having teachers and students examine and debate the arguments made about particular topics by a range of people and from a range of perspectives. This would require a discussion about the epistemological and ideological claims (scientific rationality, religious, consumerist) underlying different perspectives, and the evidence each perspective brings to bear in arguing its position. Although these lessons might initially focus on a narrow topic, such an approach could more readily lead to students exploring linkages among problems and between "sexuality issues" and the wider social, economic, political, and cultural systems in which students operate. For example, a unit on the Internet and adolescent sexuality might initially explore online representations of men and women, talk about the Internet and pornography, bring in a police detective to talk about online predators, or visit popular teen chat rooms. From there, the class might explore different personal, family, and public arguments concerning protecting children through filtering Internet searches versus allowing students complete access to the Internet in order to honor their right to information or free speech. Students might then engage in critical debates about new technologies and their effects on sexual identities and experiences, conduct an analysis of consumer messages about health and sexuality on medical websites, compare various databases concerning students' use of technologies to access health information, or research child exploitation on the Internet. In other words, such a classroom approach would link sexuality topics both to students' daily experiences and to a critical examination of how broader social structures impact their lives and sexualities. This approach draws on models of inclusive, deliberative democracy (e.g., Fraser 1997; Young 1997) and on the rich literature that exists on teaching for understanding or critical thinking[4] and teaching for critical scientific literacy (e.g., Gross 2006). It would place critical analyses of data, opinions, structural inequity, and social diversity at the center of sex education classrooms and task students and teachers to develop their own opinions in dialogue with others in the classroom and with the complex and contradictory body of evidence that exists for most sexuality topics. It would foster deliberative practices concerning controversial issues that we know can be powerful drivers of democratic engagement (Hess 2009).

Some of the topics that might be examined in such classrooms are evident from existing sex education curricula, such as the effectiveness of condoms against HIV. Others would be developed with students through conversations about their questions, needs, and experiences. For example, a class might debate the role of sex education in informing student sexual decision-making, raising questions about the comparable role of family, media, religious institutions, and peers in influencing students' sexual attitudes and actions; providing opportunities for students and teachers to learn about each others' concerns, questions, and educational needs; debating the "STI epidemic" and its relationship to adolescents' access to preventive health care and health insurance; mapping differences in health-care access rates across groups of teens and exploring the effects of these differences on long-term sexual health outcomes (including the United States' shamefully high infant mortality rates); exploring the linkages among health education topics; or discussing student and teacher perceptions of the relationship between drinking, sexual behavior, and "serious" versus less-serious relationships.

In order to achieve such changes in classroom practice, dialogue between sex and sexuality researchers and curriculum specialists, teacher educators, local policy makers, and teachers would need to change significantly (Sears 1992). In Wyoming and Wisconsin, health, science, and PE teachers are often asked to teach a subject for which they have little training or support, and about which they have not had much opportunity to reflect. The distribution of classes, the positioning of sex and sexuality in the curriculum, and opportunities for teacher training (content, pedagogical, managerial) and reflection would all need to be centered and expanded in the school's mission in order for the classroom environments described above to be realized.[5] Open dialogue with parents and community members about classroom management and classroom discussions as learning opportunities would be a prerequisite for community support.

Were such an approach adopted, it would still be feasible (though, I would argue, not desirable) to corral teacher-led discussions about adults' "hot topics" into curriculum-based units that parents could review and approve. For example, in an abstinence-based sex education classroom, the type most adults in the United States say that they favor, teacher-led discussion about condom efficacy could be textbook-based, but followed by student projects examining current debates about the topic. In other words, such an approach would allow parents to continue constraining teacher talk, if they so desire, while still opening up opportunities for students to explore, talk about, debate, and interact around sex and sexuality topics that affect their daily lives. Current sex education practices often place the power to shape programming in the hands of the teacher (or their supervisors writ large). But they also increasingly place the onus on teachers to constrain dangerous student conversations. This not only places teachers in an extremely difficult position, often stifles their voice (not to mention their creativity), and encourages the privatization of sex education, but it also is bad educational practice. Instead of authorizing teachers to stifle student and adult engagement with the issues students are facing, this approach would authorize teachers to shape teaching and learning experiences in which students are deeply engaged, but in which the "sex ed debates" are clearly framed and discussed. Instead of trying to stifle debate, it would build curricula around it.

In an ideal world, teachers would receive professional development support to develop and become comfortable with such an approach to sex education. Most teachers receive no training on sex education content or pedagogical approaches and therefore feel more uncomfortable teaching than they might otherwise (e.g., Pawlowski 2011). Though perhaps equally unlikely to receive funding, were an approach to sex education like the one described above adopted by a school system, the pedagogical professional development that would accompany it would support improved teaching practices across many disciplines.

By providing opportunities for students to express their beliefs and opinions and to discuss the reasons for their beliefs, classrooms could meet *some* of the needs of *diverse* constituents. They would give voice to teachers and students and their concerns. They would provide more conservative parents with assurances that their students would understand these issues are fundamentally linked to morals and values, though such a classroom would foster the understanding that there are multiple moral frameworks. It would provide more liberal parents with assurances that their students are learning to critically engage in scientific research and debate. It would do all of this by adopting not sex education models, but citizenship education models, which speak directly to the goal of socializing students as democratic citizens.

In addition to changes in classroom practices and professional development opportunities, community-school decision-making processes would also need to be significantly democratized. Regular student involvement in policy-making processes, even in an advisory role, could be one important step toward ensuring that teens' needs are addressed in sex education classrooms and that schools introduce and teach students about participation in democratic processes. But the question of who should have a say in public schools' policies and practices is critical here. Who does and should constitute the community to whom a public school is responsible? Much of the literature on accountability, for example, assumes that the parents of students in a school can and should play the central role in holding a school accountable. But, in practice many of these models offer parents only two venues through which to hold the school accountable: leave, or come to meetings and speak up. Yet relationships between parents and schools are diverse and gendered, classed, and raced. Not all parents can readily hold schools responsible by opting out of the school or attending meetings, not all parental participation can or should take these forms, and not all schools facilitate parental involvement. At the same time, because of wider political pressures, schools are often quite responsive to individuals or groups that are vocal, organized in support of some goal, and threatening a lawsuit.

Schools are increasingly stuck between a rock and a hard place in official sex education policy-making. Most have neither the time nor the energy to determine why some parents are not engaged. Many want to be responsive to the full range of students and parents that they serve, but often hear from only a minority of their constituents. And many schools and school boards face increasing questions about whom, exactly, they serve (and who should have to pay for public schools), particularly as practices such as homeschooling increase. Teachers' professionalism is increasingly under attack, sometimes making schools more defensive and less willing to talk openly with parents about struggles they face in determining their mandate.

In order to serve their entire community, schools need to foster democratic debate, consensus, and trust between and among members of the communities they serve. For example, what do community members feel are and should be the rights and responsibilities of parents with children in the school? How about parents whose children attended the school previously? How about people who pay property taxes to support the school? How about people in the district or county? In the state? Outside the state? What decision-making processes and approaches will help to strengthen the compact between schools and parents, so that parents trust the school and the school trusts that they have active and widespread parental involvement in and support for their decisions and their decision-making processes? How might schools foster more open discussion about why they teach sex education, reconciled with the efficacy of school-based sex education versus the much greater importance of family-based sex education? For example, could and should schools support sex education programming for parents, a mechanism for affecting students' sex education experiences that offers potentially greater promise than school-based sex education, that involves parents engaging in meaningful ways with the schools' sex education curricula and teachers, and that offers the possibility of multigenerational sexual health improvements? And, were schools to try to take on such an initiative, where would the time and additional resources come from?

School personnel would need to determine how to avoid tasking already overburdened teachers, parents, and community members with additional responsibilities; demands for participation always carry the possibility of further marginalizing those who cannot afford to participate. And notions of participation would themselves most likely need to shift in order to more fully engage parents who do not or cannot regularly participate in current school-community processes. As Rayner says,

> To create a governance discourse, we might begin by contrasting the concepts and practices of participation with a term that seems to have fallen out of favour in the last 30 years, that is "mobilization." A discourse of mobilization . . . suggests a very different approach. It begins with social issues of identity and emergent solidarity rather than technocratic ideas of risk. It seeks to destabilize taken-for-granted knowledge. Since it is explicitly values-based, it is inevitably conflictual. (2003, 169)

Schools often face a situation where one group of (typically AOUME-supportive) parents have adopted a mobilization approach while the school and other parents have not. Fostering new modes of engagement and dialogue among more parents and with the school might reconfigure the democratic calculi that shape sex education policies and practices, while also building a more solid relationship between the school and its parental constituents.

Though these are very brief sketches of the types of changes that might lead to more youth-responsive sex and civic education and a deeper engagement and trust between schools and communities, they provide a conceptual starting point for building on the strengths of existing sex education approaches and addressing some of their weaknesses. Sex education presents an opportunity to engage students in critical learning and thinking activities, as well as to discuss and practice democratic citizenship. Importantly, such approaches actively seek to understand differences in opinion about various topics, while emphasizing the necessity in a democracy to tolerate, and perhaps even recognize and respect, others' perspectives.

Invoking Evidence

The model of improving sex education outlined above stands in contrast to current directions in sex education policy-making and funding, which are increasingly driven by ideas about evidence-based practice that rest on very specific notions about what constitutes "gold standard" scientific evidence (e.g., Sandler 2008). Despite concerns about the limited number of quality sex education evaluations (e.g., Silva 2002; Oakley et al. 1995), there is a small but growing number of sex education programs based on models of "what works" derived from randomized experimental findings that recombine aspects of AOUME and CSE programs in new ways, based not on the moral or consumer frameworks laid out above, but instead on medicalized and scientized models of behavior change, learning, and adolescent sexuality (e.g., Jemmott, Jemmott, and Fong 2010; Wight and Abraham 2000).

Proponents often claim that such approaches are "value free" and that they allow schools to leverage our best scientific knowledge about how to prevent teen pregnancy and STIs to improve students' health. The experiences of students, teachers, schools, and communities in this book make plain that no approach to sex education is value free. There is an important place for scientific evidence gathered about sex education programs and their effectiveness in reducing particular negative health outcomes. But by measuring only the effectiveness of prepackaged curricula in relation to a limited set of outcomes, randomized experiments provide no information about either how curricula are used in classrooms or which topics or pedagogical approaches would have been more useful for students. Moreover, the results of comparative experiments indicate that different programs often affect different health outcomes for different populations (for example, the Jemmott, Jemmott, and Fong study).

The policy implications of these findings are unmanageable at the school level, unless they are positioned within the broader learning goals of the school and the communities it serves. A number of authors have noted that evidence-based practices of the type described above do not engage with the politics of school- and district-level sex education policy processes. They thus face significant hurdles in terms of schools' ability to adopt programming that does not address sex education (or student behavior change) in established ways, or that requires sometimes quite different pedagogical approaches or evaluative processes than are common in education programming.[6]

A reexamination of sex education as citizenship education may be in order across levels of policy practice. A number of researchers have analyzed the damaging effects on queer students of the limited notion of acceptable citizenship that underlies liberal theory and public schools (e.g., Rhoads and Calderone 2007; Mayo 2006); I have argued in this book that current sex-education efforts are limited as well by the models of rational individualism and consumption upon which they are based. Sex education offers a powerful arena in which to rethink the liberal (in the classic political sense), neoliberal, and neotraditional norms that shape the current messages about citizenship and belonging that students experience in schools. For example, assumptions about "good" sexual decisions mean that STIs are presented in a stigmatized and stigmatizing fashion in all sex education classrooms. Stigma affects people's sense of self and belonging, as well as their health-seeking behavior, and positions those who have STIs as falling outside of the "good" sexual body politic. This is not only problematic from the perspective of the democratic values of mutual respect, equality, and diversity, it is also bad public-health policy. By reconstituting these approaches, we might create much more valuable and effective sex education programming for students.

Repurposing Sex Education

Sexuality is central to our identities. It has for too long been marginalized in schools as an aspect of self that lies outside of student and teacher roles. Conceptually, sex education remains at the margin of most schools' interests and curricula. But it has the potential to sit at the center of school engagement with student experiences, well-being, and development. It offers an opportunity for school officials, students, and community members to rethink and establish new norms concerning fuller community participation in decision making, and it offers an easy (though certainly charged) space in which to engage students and teachers in critical teaching and learning activities. As a number of studies have argued previously, very few current sex-education programs examine teen sexuality within the social, economic, political, and cultural relations of power and authority that shape teens' identities, sexual practices, and long-term emotional and physical health. They likewise, as with broader sexual-health models, often ignore gender relations (Tolman, Striepe, and Harmon 2003). In this sense, sex education programs largely reproduce established and inequitable gender, sexual, social, economic, racial, health, age, and educational orders in the United States through both their silences and their assumptions about healthy sexuality.[7] Current efforts to more fully medicalize sex education provision through the adoption of outcomes- and evidence-based frameworks will make it more difficult for sex education to attend to the broader social, political, and economic relations that structure sexuality and to recognize and evaluate the consequences of the moral frameworks being propounded by various curricula.

School-based sexuality education is only one of many mechanisms (and not, by most indications, the most important) that can be used to improve students' sexual health. More importantly, the purposes and intended outcomes of sex education should also be to improve US education efforts to engage students in critical thinking and reasoning; to provide a safe space for students to reflect on their own and others' sexual values and experiences and the relationship of these experiences to the social, political, and economic systems in which they live; to educate students about democratic processes; and to strengthen the relationships among school officials, students, and communities. These are certainly not the usual goals for sex education propounded by policy makers, but they represent students', and more than a few teachers and parents', desires for a space where students can ask the questions that really affect their lives, critically examine the diverse relationships and information flows that shape their beliefs concerning sex, and engage in thoughtful debate and action to align school and classroom practices with the democratic ideals we propound as a society and a country.

Appendix 1

TABLE 2. Information on federal AOUME funding

	Florida	Wyoming	Wisconsin	California
2008 Total AOUME funding	$13,101,054[3]	The state of Wyoming received no federal funding for AOUME in fiscal year 2008.[4]	The state of Wisconsin declined federal funding for AOUME in fiscal year 2008.	The state of California has never accepted federal funding for AOUME.[6]
TITLE V Section 510[1]	$2,521,581			
CBAE[2]	$10,279,473	No Wyoming organizations received CBAE or AFLA funding.	$2,728,219[5]	$5,134,064 (2007)
AFLA	$300,000		$152,000	$2,248,214 (2007)

1. Title V abstinence-only-until-marriage grants require states to provide three state-raised dollars or the equivalent in services for every four federal dollars received.

2. Community-Based Abstinence Education (CBAE) and Adolescent Family Life Act (AFLA) funding may be provided directly to nongovernmental organizations, so organizations based in states such as California, which refuse Title V funds, may still receive CBAE and AFLA funds.

3. http://siecus.org/_data/global/images/FL%20Report%20-%20Sex%20Education%20in%20the%20 Sunshine%20State.pdf.

4. http://www.sexedlibrary.com/index.cfm?pageId=868; http://www.siecus.org/index.cfm?fuseaction=Page .ViewPage&PageID=1155.

5. http://www.siecus.org/index.cfm?fuseaction=Page.ViewPage&PageID=1154.

6. http://www.siecus.org/index.cfm?fuseaction=Page.viewPage&parentID=487&grandparentID=478& pageId=825.

TABLE 3. Information on key state policies

	Florida	Wyoming	Wisconsin	California
Sex education guidelines	The law in 2005 required students to complete 0.5 credit of coursework in "Life Management Skills" in order to graduate high school. These courses were required to include instruction in the prevention of HIV/AIDS and STIs, family life, the benefits of sexual abstinence, and the consequences of teen pregnancy.[1,2]	There are no state requirements for sex education. If school districts choose to offer sex education, they may decide whether to follow suggested guidelines in the health framework and standards developed by the state.[3]	At the time of research, there were no state requirements for sex education or policies regarding what should be taught if schools choose to offer sex education.[4]	There are no state requirements for sex education. If schools choose to offer sex education, they must follow certain guidelines. These include that all instruction be age appropriate and medically accurate.[5] A number of legal rulings compel schools to address particular issues often considered "sex education" issues. These include homophobic bullying and gender identity.
HIV/AIDS education guidelines	Instruction in the prevention of HIV/AIDS and STIs is required.	A mix of sexually conservative and liberal guidelines advocate that HIV education be taught at every grade, use methods that research has found effective, be consistent with community standards, follow guidelines set by the CDC, stress the benefits of abstinence, address students' own concerns, be taught by trained instructors, and involve parents, families, and communities.[6]	The state encourages instruction in HIV/AIDS prevention in high school, but does not mandate it.	HIV/AIDS education is required at least once in middle school and once in high school.
Health education guidelines	Until 2007, students were required to receive health education as a graduation requirement.	A rigorous state health framework, the *Wyoming Health Content and Performance Standards*, includes the *HIV/AIDS Model Policy for Wyoming Public Schools*.	The Department of Public Instruction (DPI) can create guidelines but school districts are not required to follow them.	The state's *Health Education Framework* emphasizes the need to address HIV/ AIDS, STIs, and pregnancy prevention and provides suggestions for curricula.

Antibullying policies	None at the time of study[7]	None at the time of study[8]	None at the time of study.[9] Legal ruling has held adults in school settings culpable for not stopping public bullying.	Schools are encouraged to incorporate antibullying strategies, such as a safety plan. No definition of bullying or harassment is given.[10] Legal ruling has held adults in school settings culpable for not stopping public bullying.
Gender identity policy	None	None	None	California law states, "Instruction and materials shall be appropriate for use with pupils of all races, genders, sexual orientations, ethnic and cultural backgrounds, and pupils with disabilities."[5]

1. As of the 2007–8 school year, school districts now have the option to require students to take 0.5 credit of coursework in PE and 0.5 credit in Personal Fitness, or to complete one 1-credit course titled, "Health Opportunities through Physical Education" (HOPE), which integrates personal fitness and life management skills.

2. http://www.siecus.org/_data/global/images/State%20Profiles%202005/Florida.pdf.

3. http://www.siecus.org/_data/global/images/State%20Profiles%202005/Wyoming.pdf.

4. http://www.siecus.org/_data/global/images/State%20Profiles%202005/Wisconsin.pdf. Laws governing sex education have changed three times in the past three years, as political power has shifted.

5. http://www.siecus.org/_data/global/images/State%20Profiles%202005/California.pdf.

6. Wyoming Department of Education 1998, 14.

7. Antibullying law passed in 2008.

8. Antibullying law passed in 2009.

9. Antibullying law passed in 2010.

10. http://www.bullypolice.org/ca_law.html.

Appendix 2

TABLE 4. Data collection activities by state

Data collection period	California 2004–2006	Florida 2004–2005	Maryland 2004–2005	Wisconsin 2004–2009	Wyoming 2005–2006
	Semistructured interviews				
State officials	Yes	Yes	Yes	Yes	No
State-level NGOs	Yes	Yes	Yes	Yes	No
State policy review	Yes	Yes	Yes	Yes	Yes
District officials	Yes	Yes	Yes	Yes	Yes
District/local NGO/ actors	Yes	Yes	No	Yes	Yes
School board/PTA representatives	No	Yes	No	No	Yes
Private sex-education providers	Yes	Yes	No	Yes	Yes
Teachers	Yes	Yes	No	Yes	Yes
Parents	No	Yes	No	Yes	Yes
Students	No	Yes	No	Yes	Yes
	Observations				
Classrooms	Yes: 3-week program	No full program	No	Yes: 5-week program	Yes: 5-week program
Schools and classrooms	Yes: 4 classrooms in 1 school; 1 classroom in a second school. Schools were in different districts.	1 class session in 1 school	No	Yes: 1 sex education program in 1 classroom in 1 school; research conducted over multiple years	Yes: 5 classrooms in 1 school in 1 district; visits to middle schools that serve the high school
Conferences, teacher training	No	Yes	Yes	No	No
School board meetings	Yes	No	Yes	Yes	Yes
Other					
Document collection (including curricula)	Yes	Yes	Yes	Yes	Yes
Review of legal cases	Yes	Yes	Yes	Yes	Yes

Notes

Chapter 1

1. Hunter (1991) argued that there were two evident ideological camps in the United States in the post-1970s culture wars: progressivism and orthodoxy. Researchers on the culture wars in the twenty-first century, particularly after Obama's election, have argued that this clear delineation has been complicated by identity-group and regional distinctions and a move toward "moral pragmatism."

2. New federal funding for the Teen Pregnancy Prevention Act requires sex education programs to have scientific evidence of improving students' health outcomes. This favors CSE programs, which by and large are the only programs that have shown such outcomes. At the time of writing, it is not clear whether Congress will maintain funding for teen pregnancy prevention.

3. For example, Wisconsin's SB 237 abstinence-only bill, passed in the Wisconsin senate on November 2, 2011, which overrides a CSE-supportive bill (the Healthy Youth Act, or AB 458 and SB 324) that was passed the previous year.

4. Because the book only addresses school-based sex education programs, from here on, I will use the term "sex education" to refer to school-based sex education. I note in the text any time I refer to sex education programs or approaches that are not school based.

5. STIs: A note on usage. Although the term "STD" (sexually transmitted disease) is more common in daily parlance and is often used in sex education programs because of concerns about students' familiarity with the term, "sexually transmitted infections" (STIs) is the more correct and preferred term in public health, since many infections have no apparent symptoms (and are therefore not "diseases"). I use the term "STI" to refer to the body of common sexually transmitted infections that are labeled as either STDs or STIs in various curricula.

6. Though certain characteristics unite all federally funded AOUME programs, there is still significant variation in content and pedagogical approaches. For example, programs vary in how much information they give students on particular subjects. Some programs reflect the belief that providing any information about a subject validates it, and therefore do not mention topics including contraception, homosexuality, and abortion. Some mention these issues, but only in terms of their failure and socially destructive outcomes. So, for example, some programs mention anal sex to clarify that having anal sex does not constitute abstinence; others believe that mentioning the practice will encourage students to try it. Some emphasize the joys of mar-

riage and the promised sexual and emotional freedom it will bring, while other programs focus largely on scaring teens into abstention.

7. Federal funding for abstinence education began during the Reagan administration and played an important role in providing early support for key AOUME organizations and individuals (SIECUS 2009). However, in part because of court challenges to the funding (see Perrin and DeJoy 2003 for this history), federal resources did not increase significantly until 1996. After 1996, they increased rapidly and through multiple funding mechanisms until the Obama administration. At the time of writing, the fate of AOUME federal funding is unclear, but it is likely to remain reduced from its early 2000s levels because an increasing number of states have now refused to accept such funding, because of the economic downturn, and because of the increasing evidence that AOUME approaches do not delay initiation of sex or decrease adolescent STI rates.

8. See, for example, the Advocates for Youth report at http://www.advocatesforyouth.org/index.php?option=com_content&task=view&id=89&Itemid=161.

9. I conducted research in Maryland as well, but because of confidentiality issues arising from a court case filed in the district in which I was working, I do not report on that ethnographic research here.

Chapter 2

1. E.g., Bleakley, Hennessy, and Fishbein 2006; Bowden, Lanning, Pippin, and Tanner 2003; Dailard 2001; Kaiser Family Foundation 2000.

2. For example, compare Kalina 2011, diMauro and Joffe 2009, versus National Abstinence Education Association 2007, Sheffield 2010.

3. E.g., Lee, Donlan, and Paz 2009; Kirby 2002; Franklin and Corcoran 2000.

4. E.g., Waxman 2006; Whatley and Trudell 1993; Trudell and Whatley 1991; Whatley 1988.

5. E.g., Tolman, Hirschman, and Impett 2005; Tolman, Striepe, and Harmon 2003; Tolman 2002.

6. I was particularly interested in this topic because of previous research I had conducted in Malawi on HIV/AIDS education and adolescent sexuality. In that research I tried to understand how teens made sense of and responded to adult efforts to shape their sexual identities in an era of HIV and neoliberal economic and state reform. The Ford Foundation's Sexuality Research Fellowship provided me with two years of funding to do similar research on this subject in the United States. These resources, so essential to conducting comparative ethnographic work, are very seldom available for sexuality or sex education research.

7. See Shore and Wright 1997 for a review of the increasing importance of policies.

8. See Raymond et al. 2008 for a discussion of state-level shifts, and see Burch 2009, Apple 2006, Deem 2001, and Ball 1998 for discussion of these shifts in other school arenas.

9. E.g., Deaux 2006; Vavrus and Bartlett 2006; Sutton and Levinson 2001; Shore and Wright 1997; Marcus 1995; Reinhold 1994. Burchell, Gordon, and Miller (1991) provide examples of this approach in other fields.

10. See, for example, Dyer 1999, Fox 1990, Sabatier 1993, and Rhoten 1999 about the historical emphasis on unilinearism in policy studies.

11. The research that I began conducting in Montgomery County, Maryland, in 2004 came to a halt when the school district and its proposed sex education curriculum were taken to court by a New Christian Right group called Citizens for a Responsible Curriculum (CRC). Because of

the court case, I could no longer guarantee confidentiality to research participants. I have therefore chosen not to use any of the data I collected in Maryland. When I discuss it as an example of the types of community-school confrontations that AOUME supporters have undertaken, I use data that are publicly available, and situations in which the CRC approached and confronted me—that is, times when I was not officially conducting research.

12. See Tolman, Hirschman, and Impett 2005 for a parallel approach to analyzing gender inequities across studies.

13. E.g., R. Parker, "Collier school board fires Gulf Coast sex ed teacher," *Naples Daily News*, Jan. 31, 2005. Retrieved from http://www.naplesnews.com.

14. E.g., Segura 2005, about the funding for Maryland's CRC.

15. The primary result of these bureaucratic fears is to make researchers work around school and university perceptions of teen sexuality and sex education as minefields by limiting their capacity to speak directly to students. This forces researchers to rely on stories told about teens by adults, to rely on particular subsets of students (e.g., those over age eighteen), or to conduct research outside of the public education institutions in which almost 90 percent of US teens spend a significant amount of their lives. This re-creates in the research the silencing of their voices that students expressed such concern and anger about when I could speak to them, and is a significant ethical problem.

16. Pruitt (2007) describes a similar process of learning what he "really learned" from conducting research on AOUME in Texas.

17. The studies cited by MISH were generally not included in peer-reviewed meta-analyses of sex education programs because they were deemed to be scientifically invalid.

18. See diMauro and Joffe 2009 for a review of some of the Bush appointments that had the greatest effect on officially sanctioned funding for and knowledge about reproductive health.

19. E.g., Gibson 2005, and the 2006 "War on Christians and the Values Voters" event, at which Tom DeLay was a speaker.

20. Research on teen sexuality within school settings has become difficult and restricted enough that some researchers have moved out of schools to conduct research on adolescent sexuality and sexuality education (e.g., Fields and Tolman 2006). I decided to locate my research primarily in schools precisely because I wanted to focus on the institutional cultures and personal interactions around sex and sexuality that occur in the institutions in which most teens spend a significant portion of their days, and the site in which community- and state-sanctioned sex education is provided. The cost of this decision was that I could hear and see students but not interact with most of them. I was able to interview only a handful of students in each school and state, and they were not representative of the student populations at the schools in which I worked: some were over eighteen but still in high school, others were very recent graduates who were still living nearby or who were home for holiday or summer breaks, still others were among the tiny group that got the permission slip to talk to me signed by their parents. I cannot assert how these students relate to the student populations on the whole, and therefore use the information collected from student interviews only in cases where I feel confident that the information I heard in the interviews supports my observations of students and the conversations I heard among them.

21. The role of institutional review boards in silencing marginalized people's (and particularly youths' and children's) voices is a significant problem that is being addressed in a growing qualitative research literature. See Bledose et al. 2007 for a discussion of the IRB's effects on faculty and student research at Northwestern University.

Chapter 3

1. In this chapter, I present a fuller analysis of the AOUME approach than may be warranted by the data that I can immediately provide, in order to draw parallels and distinctions among AOUME and CSE approaches from the start. Many of the points that I make about AOUME approaches in this chapter are supported by additional data and analysis found in chapters 4 and 8 through 11. I ask for the reader's patience in laying out my case in this more divided manner.

2. http://www.greattowait.com/program.html; accessed June 1, 2009.

3. Quotes are based on field research and interview notes. Wherever possible, they include exact quotes written down during interviews or transcribed from tape recordings of interviews.

4. There is a growing literature (e.g., Burch 2009; Apple 2006; Apple 2005; Simkins 2000; Strathern 2000; Shore and Wright 1997; Whitty, Power, and Halpin 1998) on managerial ideologies and audit cultures in schools, which provides important insights into how state involvement in social services has been reshaped by neoliberal economic and political rationalities (for example, the idea that private services are always more efficient than public ones).

5. A similar process was occurring internationally during this time, as President Bush's President's Emergency Plan for AIDS Relief (PEPFAR) began funding a growing number of faith-based non-governmental organizations—some with no public health programming experience—to transmit an AOUM message to 40 million of the 66 million people who received PEPFAR-funded AIDS prevention messages (Dietrich 2007).

6. Observational data were collected by the author without the use of tape recorders. Quotes are therefore near-approximations of what the speakers said, based on extensive field notes that often include sections of exact speech.

7. As was the case for state personnel, the trainer uses the term "grassroots" to refer to a group of like-minded people who work together within and across geographically identified communities toward a common goal; this notion of "grassroots" reshapes notions of locality and interest, and therefore notions of who has the responsibility and right to engage schools in discussions about how they should teach sex education.

8. DiMauro and Joffe (2009) chronicle how the Bush administration and the New Christian Right used political appointments in a range of government offices to transform public scientific discourse (such as information on the CDC website) concerning reproductive health and STI prevention. A similar effort occurred around climate change.

9. Though these gender norms might sound extreme, young women around the country have reported that they experience similar constructions of appropriate (inequitable) male and female teen sexuality in sexual relationships. See, for example, Tolman, Hirschmann, and Impett 2005 for a review of four such studies.

10. The AOUME presentations and curricula I reviewed consistently downplayed STIs such as HIV, for which condom use is particularly effective in decreasing transmission rates, and played up those, such as herpes and HPV, that are spread through skin-to-skin contact. See chapter 7 for further discussion.

11. http://www.cdc.gov/condomeffectiveness/latex.htm#HPV.

12. See chapter 8 for further discussion.

13. Pruitt (2007) found a similar use of directive approaches in AOUME programming in Texas.

14. http://group5advertising.com/portfolio-study.php.

15. Similar individual stories have been used recently in legislative meetings as evidence of the effectiveness of AOUME. As Tolman, Hirschman, and Impett (2005) note, though there are serious problems with the use of such testimonials as scientific evidence, their persuasive power was evident in these settings as well.

16. It is not unimportant that politically and sexually conservative efforts to transform US morality are regularly linked to welfare reform acts. As a number of researchers have noted (e.g., Fields 2008), political constructions of immorality and declining family values are raced, classed, and gendered. Because the nonwhite, poor women who are the target of the "family values" efforts are perceived to be (but are not) the primary recipients of welfare, welfare reform acts are viewed as appropriate places for legislators to tie these women's and their children's survival to changes in their "moral" status. This is discussed in greater detail in chapter 7.

17. http://www.acf.hhs.gov/healthymarriage/about/mission.html#goals, accessed July 2011. The goals of the Healthy Family Marriage Initiative, as listed on its website in July 2011, included the following:

- Increase the percentage of children who are raised by two parents in a healthy marriage.
- Increase the percentage of married couples who are in healthy marriages.
- Increase the percentage of youth and young adults who have the skills and knowledge to make informed decisions about healthy relationships including skills that can help them eventually form and sustain a healthy marriage.
- Increase public awareness about the value of healthy marriages and the skills and knowledge that can help couples form and sustain healthy marriages.

18. SIECUS 2009 reviews the use and amount of TANF and MCHBG funds that the state of Florida used to support AOUME activities.

19. I use the terms "Hispanic," "Asian," and "African American" in this section because these are the terms used by the presenter. These choices speak to the presenter's apparent sense that "Asians" and "Hispanics" were not Americanized in the same way as African Americans, as well to a particular set of race, ethnicity, and identity politics surrounding the use of the term "Hispanic" instead of "Latin@".

20. Parker, R. 2005. "Collier school board fires Gulf Coast sex ed teacher." *Naples Daily News*, January 31.

21. See, e.g., Hutchens 2009 and Nahmod 2008 concerning the effects of *Garcetti vs. Ceballos* on public employee freedom of speech and its potential effects on teachers, and Lima 2008 for its extension through *Meyer vs. Monroe County Community School* into teachers' speech.

22. See, for example, Goertz 2005 and Goldhaber and Hannaway 2004, for discussion of some of these differences.

23. A similar process of privatization of accountability has been noted for NCLB-mandated tutoring services; see, for example, Burch 2009.

Chapter 4

1. All places and people in the Wyoming, Wisconsin, and California chapters are composites, developed from my research with multiple teachers, students, parents, and schools in each state. Data are presented as composites to assure confidentiality of individuals and locations. All quotes attributed to individuals were said by a person that held the core composite characteris-

tics (for example, AOUME-leaning teacher in a CSE school in the identified state), but quotes cannot be attributed to one individual. Composite names are, of course, pseudonyms.

2. This perspective has been identified in other rural areas of the United States as well, where communication and negotiation between the school, school board, school district, churches, and parents was the dominant feature in determining the formal sex education curricula (e.g., Blinn-Pike 2008).

3. A similar environment was created in the Wisconsin CSE classroom, as discussed in chapter 5.

4. Ms. Jeffries and the other PE teachers were regularly absent (for trainings and sports events); while Ms. Jeffries's students spent class periods with the substitute teacher speaking with each other, including about the class content, when the same teacher substituted for Mr. Lauder or Mr. Dean, the classes stayed almost entirely silent. Thus, the environment of comfort and camaraderie that Ms. Jeffries created when she was present was quite evident when she was not, and the silence created by Mr. Lauder and Mr. Dean was similarly evident when they were absent.

5. Ms. Jeffries told me that she did not usually allow as much conversation as I heard in her class; it was only because the class was so small that she said she felt able to allow students to talk as much as they did. Usually, then, her classes may more closely resemble Mr. Lauder's.

6. Schalet's (2004) work comparing US and Danish parents' conceptions of adolescent sexuality, healthy relationships, and parental control over children's behaviors provides a similar account of how cultural values associated with sexuality and adolescence, parental relations with students, and socioeconomic structures interact to create quite different environments in which parents make sense of and try to influence their children's sexual behavior.

Chapter 5

1. Classroom observations were conducted jointly with Kathleen Elliott; I conducted the interviews with organizations and individuals at the district and national levels reported on in the chapter. Kathleen's research with students and at the classroom and school levels was much more extensive than the observations that I conducted, and is reported on in her dissertation. When I use the pronoun "we," I am referring to observations that we conducted jointly. When I use the pronoun "I," I am referring to comparisons I (Kendall) am drawing between our shared research in Wisconsin and the research I conducted in other states.

2. Kathleen also observed Mrs. Shane in 2008 and 2009; in comparison to past years, the 2009–10 class had a more vocal group of students that directed the shape of most conversations, but the classroom ambience, the relationships that Mrs. Shane developed with her students, and the content of the sex education class (including invited speakers) were similar.

3. Discussed further in chapter 8.

4. There are interesting parallels here with studies of science teachers in districts and states where there are strong anti-evolution movements.

5. Discussed further in chapter 9.

6. E.g., Bernal 2002; Ladson-Billings 1999; Sadker and Sadker 1995.

Chapter 6

1. The year that I conducted my observations was the first year the school allowed Come On In! to work with EL students. The program was hoping to recruit a Spanish-speaking trainer

in the future, but because of the organization's tight budget, Emily agreed to try to do extra research and work to ensure the students received the information they needed that first year. Emily not only did a great deal of work to identify additional resources and materials in Spanish for the EL classes, but also, despite the occasional language barriers, created a warm and positive relationship with most students in the EL classes.

2. Gilbert in Rasmussen, Rolfes, and Talburt 2004.

3. Emily's answer reflects California laws, which define a minor as anyone under eighteen and require that there be no more than a three-year age difference between minors, or between a minor and an adult, who have sex in order for no crime to have been committed.

4. Cahn and Carbone note the deeply problematic class and race implications of this family model, given current job opportunities for less-educated people (particularly men), increased educational costs, and marital and childbearing patterns in the United States.

5. I combine my discussion of the two EL classes because student responses to the curriculum and student interactions with Emily were quite similar across the two classes. I speak Spanish relatively fluently; my observations in the classrooms thus reflect students' comments in both Spanish and English.

6. E.g., Pearson 2006; Tolman, Hirschman, and Impett 2005; Holland et al. 1998.

7. See Mitchell 2002 and Ferguson 1990 for a discussion of the reframing of international development issues into problems that have techno-rational solutions. This parallels the construction of sex problems that can be resolved through the expert's provision of complete and correct information to the rational, empowered individual student.

8. For example, Hokoda et al. (2007) found differences in perceptions of the acceptability of domestic violence between more and less acculturated (measured by language preference) Mexican American adolescents. This study points to some of the complex issues related to individual and social identity and to individuals' capacity to "choose" safe sex in relationships that students in the Jefferson classrooms referred to during the classes I observed.

9. Student comments are translated from Spanish.

10. M. Talbot, "Red Sex, Blue Sex: Why Do So Many Evangelical Teen-Agers Become Pregnant?," *New Yorker*, November 3, 2008, 64–69.

11. Since I could not speak directly to students, I could not collect data to help me determine whether the apparently greater alignment in instructor and student expectations regarding sex and sexuality arose because the students in the high-track and EL classrooms had different sociocultural norms and experiences (as Regnerus's research [2007] might indicate), or whether the high-track students simply "did school" in a way that led them to respond to Emily in a manner that more closely aligned with her expectations (as Pope's research might indicate [2003]).

12. See chapter 7 for further discussion.

13. The limits of liberal theory in recognizing and validating a range of identities, evident in the Jefferson High classrooms, is reflected as well in the literature examining how queerness and queer identities are invalidated in many liberal frameworks (e.g., Rhoads and Calderone 2007; Mayo 2006).

Chapter 7

1. Fitzgerald (in Burack and Josephson 2003) notes a similar shift in welfare policy debates.

2. Outcomes- and evidence-based models of program evaluation increasingly underpin this agreement on the intended outcomes of sex education. These models constitute "an assemblage of rationalities, strategies, technologies, and techniques that allow 'government at a distance'"

(Larner and Butler 2005, 83) to define, measure, and provide a rationale to act upon objects of government interest (e.g., STI rates) through indirect managerial approaches. The shift toward a reliance on these evaluation models to judge the effectiveness of social programs is not, of course, unique to sex education in the United States; these models are increasingly used to judge the effects of a range of public services around the world (e.g., Sandler 2008; Trinder and Reynolds 2000).

3. This stance caused an uproar in AOUM programming for HIV/AIDS education in Africa, where the greatest risk for HIV infection for women was posed by being married. From an AOUM perspective, the problem here would not be the need to reduce people's risk of becoming infected in marriage, it would be the need to strike at the root (moral) cause of infection in marriage—infidelity and sex before marriage.

4. E.g., Prout and James 1990; Qvortrup 1994; Jenks 1996; James, Jenks, and Prout 1998.

5. Sterility was consistently mentioned as a potential health effect of STIs.

6. In one case, the teacher brought in an HIV-positive speaker; in the other two, a video shown in class included people talking about how they never thought they could become infected and what it was like to live with the virus.

7. E.g., Lieber et al. 2006; Fortenberry 2004; Cunningham et al. 2002; Fortenberry et al. 2002.

8. E.g., Luker 1997; Irvine 1994; Furstenberg 1991; Vinovskis 1988; Murcott 1980.

9. See Cahn and Carbone 2010 for a discussion of the class and race effects of this framing of teen pregnancy on poor women and families.

10. E.g., Levine, Emery, and Pollack 2007; Geronimus 2003; Massat 1995.

11. See Geroniums 2003 for a review of the literature.

12. See Pillow 2004 for a review of the literature.

13. E.g., Driscoll et al 2001; Frost and Oslak 1999. The findings from these various studies indicate the complex interactions of social relations, economic realities, and community and cultural perceptions in teen pregnancy outcomes. For example, pregnant African American girls are just as (or more) likely to graduate from high school as their nonpregnant peers, but pregnant Latinas are more likely to drop out. Latinas are more likely to report that their pregnancies were intended than other groups, and are more likely to be in a positive relationship with the father. Any blanket statement about the effects of teen pregnancy does damage to these complex and quite different realities.

14. E.g., California Latinas for Reproductive Justice 2010; Pillow 2004.

15. This was a strong emphasis in the AOUME "healthy family" activities, but because teens were constructed as "children," they were to be the target of directive parenting approaches, as opposed to potential parents being taught about this approach to raising children.

16. E.g., Bay-Cheng 2003; Epstein, O'Flynn, and Telford 2003; Weis and Fine 1993.

17. A recent randomized trial (Jemmott, Jemmott, and Fong 2010) comparing the effects of abstinence-only (not AOUME; the program deliberately linked abstinence to discussions of students' readiness and removed "moralizing" discussions) and CSE programs found that an eight-hour abstinence program resulted in a significant delay of sexual initiation among twelve-to fourteen-year old inner-city African American youth, whereas a CSE program tested at the same time with the same population resulted in a significant increase in safer-sex practices. In other words, each positively impacted the behaviors they aimed to change.

Policy makers can draw a number of different conclusions from this study: that different students can benefit from different programs, that CSE and abstinence-only programs may both be successful at achieving particular outcomes, that none of the programs makes a tremendous difference in students' sexual behaviors. An early newspaper headline reporting the results of the study read, "Abstinence ed, minus moralizing, may just work" (*Salt Lake Tribune*, February 1, 2010; retrieved from http://article.wn.com/view/2010/02/02/Abstinence_ed_minus_moralizing_may_just_work/). The article reported,

> An experimental abstinence-only program without a moralistic tone can delay teens from having sex, a provocative study found. Billed as the first rigorous research to show long-term success with an abstinence-only approach, the study differed from traditional programs that have lost federal and state support in recent years. The classes didn't preach saving sex until marriage or disparage condom use. Instead, it [*sic*] involved assignments to help sixth- and seventh-graders see the drawbacks to sexual activity at their age, including having them list the pros and cons themselves. Their cons far outnumbered the pros.

Chapter 8

1. E.g., Doan and Calterone-Williams 2008; Luker 2006; Kehily 2002a, 2002b.

2. E.g., Fields 2008; Levy 2005; Fine 1988.

3. E.g., Doan and Williams 2008; Waxman 2006; Weis and Carbonell-Medina 2000.

4. E.g., Anyon 2008; Pascoe 2008; Whatley and Henken 2001.

5. Regnerus's (2007) work provides an example of this common explanation of gender norms and "realities." Other research, however (e.g., Gerson 2009; Families and Work Institute 2008), has indicated that these explanations and assumptions may not represent women's and men's feelings, desires, or marriage and family patterns very well. This may be particularly true for women and men born in the 1970s and later.

6. E.g., Dill and Thill 2007; Miller and Summers 2007; Witt 2000; Peirce 1993.

7. Howard Center, quoted in Buss and Herman 2003.

8. Foster, D. "The divine marriage: Divine order in creation and covenant." http://pureintimacy.org/piArticles/A000000406.cfm.

9. http://www.marriagemissions.com.

10. Theoretically, if US state laws were to allow for gay marriage, AOUME arguments against homosexual sex would shift significantly. Given, however, that AOUME frameworks do not allow for the possibility of valid marriage between two people of the same sex, in practice such a shift in laws would more likely lead to a discursive reframing that again would render sex between two people of the same sex morally forbidden.

11. E.g., Waxman 2006; Whatley 1991; Trudell 1993.

12. See also Lehr in Burack and Josephson 2003.

13. It is from this model of gender difference that the discourse on homosexuality as narcissism arises.

14. See, e.g., Lefebvre 2011; Guidotti et al. 2009; Hanson et al. 2008; Shive and Morris 2006; Pfeiffer 2004; Hastings 2003; Moore, Raymond, Mittelstaedt, and Tanner 2002; McDermott 2000; Frankenberger and Sukhdial 1994; Bertrand, Stover, and Porter 1989; Lefebvre and Flora 1988; Kotler and Zaltman 1971.

15. An important aspect of this common sense is the double standard applied to female and male sexual activity. See Crawford and Popp 2003 for a review of thirty studies indicating the pervasiveness of, and individual, relational, cultural, and ethnic variations on, the double standard.

16. According to the website for Come On In!, the program recognized that gender issues

needed to be more directly addressed and critiqued in their curriculum, and a new set of activities and discussions focus on exactly this issue. This book is based on my observations before these changes occurred, but the program's acknowledgment points to a potentially very positive movement toward more directly addressing these issues in some CSE programs.

17. As I have noted previously, Mr. Dean is best understood as an AOUME teacher in a CSE school. Nevertheless, I think it is important to note that this information was presented in a CSE classroom with no response by parents or teachers.

18. See Tolman 2002 for a discussion of constructions of female versus male desire, and the opprobrium teenage girls often face if they express sexual interest and desire.

19. I do not mention a need to talk with boys about their decision to be distracted or not by girls because I did not, in my observations, observe boys being distracted by girls' clothing. In fact, boys seemed generally rather oblivious to all but the most extreme states of undress at the school. It was teachers, not students, who responded so strongly to girls' dress.

20. Students' interactions with one another and how these interactions reflect gender norms and expectations could fill an entire book; in my observations, gender norms and expectations functioned in a variety of ways that were complexly interwoven with sexual identity. In this sense, students' interactions around gender were often either less heteronormative than teachers' or appeared to function as deliberate efforts to reinscribe masculinist heterosexism. Though this is an area of research of great interest to me, constraints on my ability to talk with students limit what I can say in this book about these interactions.

Chapter 9

1. In an earlier observation of Mrs. Shane's sex education class (when Mr. Kelly was not present), Elliott observed a presentation by an external group that talked about sexual and gender spectra and allowed for greater discussion about fluidity. I do not discuss it in detail in the present book because the group did not present during our observations, and Elliott's notes on the presentation were not focused on this issue of typologies.

2. Valdes (1995) coins this term to describe the "conflation of sex, gender, and sexual orientation" in legal and political arenas in the United States.

3. See, for example, Fields 2008; Fine and McClelland 2006; Irvine 2002; Moran 2000; McKay 1998.

4. See, for example, "Part VII: Sexual Orientation" in Moore, Davidson, and Fisher 2009 for some examples of a wide range of studies that have been and are being conducted on the genetic, biological, and familial influences on sexual identity; and sociocultural and survey studies examining sexual identity fluidity.

5. See, for example, Paul in Rust 2000.

6. CSE approaches most commonly argue that people's public sexual identification may change, but sexual identity is inherent to the person. AOUME approaches are based on the belief that there is only one valid identity, and all others are a willful choice to disobey this natural order.

7. Cited on the Citizens for a Responsible Curriculum website, http://www.mcpscurriculum .com/curriculum.shtml.

8. This landmark court case was the first in which a court ruled that school officials could be held responsible for failing to stop students from engaging in antigay actions targeting other students. Nabozny was mock-raped, urinated upon, beaten up so badly he required surgery,

and consistently verbally abused by other students in his high school. He attempted to commit suicide and eventually ran away after school officials told him he should expect such treatment for being gay.

9. These challenges were particularly striking because I observed them only in response to heteronormative talk, in the same classrooms where sexist and xenophobic comments regularly went unchallenged.

10. This section draws on several kinds of materials: participant-observation notes, printed materials distributed by the state of Florida, interviews with Florida state personnel and sex education service providers describing their efforts to strengthen AOUME supporters' religious position on homosexuality using a scientific rationale, and popular AOUME curricula used around the country.

11. See also Fields and Tolman 2006 for additional examples.

12. See the Citizens for a Responsible Curriculum website (http://www.mcpscurriculum .com/curriculum.shtml) for examples of these two arguments.

13. Sprigg, P. 2010. "Top ten myths about homosexuality." Washington, DC: Family Research Council. http://www.frc.org/brochure/the-top-ten-myths-of-homosexuality.

14. See Remafedi 1999a and 1999b for an overview of studies.

15. Citizens for a Responsible Curriculum (CRC). 2011. "Citizens for a responsible curriculum." http://www.mcpscurriculum.com/curriculum.shtml.

16. See, for example, Hess 2009 for one model of such discussion and its potential effects on students and schools.

Chapter 10

1. CDC in Fine and McClelland 2006; similar rates are reported in Tjaden and Thoennes 1998.

2. See Struckman-Johnson, Struckman-Johnson, and Anderson 2003 for a review of some of these studies.

3. AOUME curricula focused on the safety, security, and joy of marriage. There was no discussion in any curricula or program I observed about potential dangers within marriage. There is some recognition in broader New Christian Right teachings that abuse can occur in marriage or in the family, but this was not a conversation that ever made its way into any AOUME curricula I reviewed.

4. Sears (1992) discusses the centrality of rational decision-making in current sex education approaches.

5. E.g., Struckman-Johnson, Struckman-Johnson, and Anderson 2003; Albury 2002; Sawyer, Pinciaro, and Jessell 1998.

6. Regnerus (2009) provides a similar argument about sex-as-market. He concludes that women should marry younger, to older men, in order to "cash in" best on their assets.

7. See, for example, Raymond 2009 for a discussion of the commodification of sex in a number of PG-13 and mature video games.

Chapter 11

1. E.g., Schor 2004; Quart 2003; Kilbourne 2000.

2. But cf. Fields 2008 on the role of anonymous question boxes in silencing student voices.

3. See Parker 2006 for a discussion of inclusionary conversational approaches for classrooms.

4. E.g., Kasl and Yorks 2002; Pithers and Soden 2000; Mintzes, Wandersee, and Novak 1998; hooks 1994.

5. See Fields 2008 and Alldred and David 2007 for discussions about the marginalization of sex education classrooms, classes, and teachers in the United States and United Kingdom respectively.

6. E.g., Schaalma et al. 2004; Greenberg et al. 2003; Wight and Abraham 2000.

7. E.g., Fields 2008; Connell 2008; Bay-Cheng 2003; Wyatt 1997.

References

Advocates for Youth. 2007. *Abstinence-only-until-marriage programs: Ineffective, unethical, and poor public health.* Washington, DC: Advocates for Youth.

———. 2008. *Illinois abstinence-only programs: Disseminating inaccurate and biased information.* Washington, DC: Advocates for Youth.

Albury, K. 2002. *Yes means yes: Getting explicit about heterosex.* Australia: Allen and Unwin.

Alldred, P., and M. David. 2007. *Get real about sex: The politics and practice of sex education.* Berkshire: Open University Press.

American Social Health Association (ASHA). 2005. *State of the nation: Challenges facing STD prevention among youth; Research, review, and recommendations.* Triangle Park, NC: ASHA.

Anderson-Levitt, K. 2003. *Local meanings, global schooling: Anthropology and world culture theory.* New York: Palgrave Macmillan.

Angelides, S. 2004. "Feminism, child sexual abuse, and the erasure of child sexuality." *GLQ* 10 (2): 141–78.

Anyon, J. 2008. *Theory and educational research: Toward critical social explanation.* London: Routledge.

Apple, M. 2005. "Education, markets, and an audit culture." *Critical Quarterly* 47 (1/2): 11–29.

———. 2006. *Educating the "right" way: Markets, standards, God, and inequality.* New York: Routledge.

Ball, S. 1990. "Markets, inequality and urban schooling." *Urban Review* 22 (2): 85–100.

———. 1998. "Big policies/small world: An introduction to international perspectives in education policy." *Comparative Education* 34 (2): 119–30.

Bartkowski, J., and X. Xu. 2000. "Distant patriarchs or expressive dads? The discourse and practice of fathering in conservative Protestant families." *Sociological Quarterly* 41 (3): 465–85.

Bay-Cheng, L. 2003. "The trouble of teen sex: The construction of adolescent sexuality through school-based sexuality education." *Sex Education* 3 (1): 61–74.

Bernal, D. 2002. "Critical race theory, Latino critical theory, and critical raced-gendered epistemologies: Recognizing students of color as holders and creators of knowledge." *Qualitative Inquiry* 8 (1): 105.

Bertrand, J., J. Stover, and R. Porter. 1989. "Methodologies for evaluating the impact of contraceptive social marketing programs." *Evaluation Review* 13 (4): 323–54.

Bettie, J. 2003. *Women without class: Girls, race, and identity*. Berkeley and Los Angeles: University of California Press.

Blankenhorn, D., D. Browning, and M. Van Leeuwen. 2004. *Does Christianity teach male headship? The equal-regard marriage and its critics*. Grand Rapids, MI: Eerdmans.

Bleakley, A., M. Hennessy, and M. Fishbein. 2006. "Public opinion on sex education in US schools." *Archives of Pediatrics and Adolescent Medicine* 160 (11): 1151–56.

Bledsoe, C., B. Sherin, A. Galinsky, N. Headley, C. Heimer, E. Kjeldgaard, J. Lindgren, J. Miller, M. Roloff, and D. Uttal. 2007. "Regulating creativity: Research and survival in the IRB iron cage." *Northwestern University Law Review* 101 (2): 593–642.

Blinn-Pike, L. 2008. "Sex education in rural schools in the U.S.: Impact of rural educators' community identities." *Sex Education* 8 (1): 77–92.

Blum, R. W., T. Beuhring, and P. Rinehart. 2000. *Protecting teens: Beyond race, income and family structure*. Minneapolis: Center for Adolescent Health, University of Minnesota.

Bowden, R. G., B. Lanning, G. Pippin, and J. Tanner. 2003. "Teachers' attitudes towards abstinence-only curricula." *Education* 123 (4): 780–88.

Bowe, R., and S. Ball. 1992. "Subject departments and the 'implementation' of National Curriculum Policy." *Journal of Curriculum Studies* 24 (2): 97–115.

Bullough, V., and B. Bullough. 1994. *American sexuality: An encyclopedia*. New York: Garland.

Bully Police USA. n.d. "California." http://bullypolice.org/ca_law.html.

Burack, C. 2008. *Sin, sex, and democracy: Antigay rhetoric and the Christian right*. Albany: State University of New York Press.

Burack, C., and J. Josephson. 2003. *Fundamental differences: Feminists talk back to social conservatives*. Lanham, MD: Rowman and Littlefield.

Burch, P. 2009. *Hidden markets: The new education privatization*. New York: Routledge.

Burchell, G., C. Gordon, and P. Miller. 1991. *The Foucault effect: Studies in governmentality*. Chicago: University of Chicago Press.

Burr, C. 1993. "Homosexuality and biology." *Atlantic Monthly* 272 (3): 47–65.

Burton, L. 1990. "Teenage childbearing as an alternative life-course strategy in multigeneration black families." *Human Nature* 1 (2): 123–43.

Buss, D., and D. Herman. 2003. *Globalizing family values: The Christian right in international politics*. Minneapolis: University of Minnesota Press.

Cahn, N., and J. Carbone. 2007. "Red families v. blue families." GWU Law School Public Law Research Paper 343, George Washington University, Washington, DC.

———. 2010. "Family classes: Rethinking contraceptive choice." *University of Florida Journal of Law and Public Policy* (forthcoming), GWU Legal Studies Research Paper 504, George Washington University, Washington, DC. http://ssrn.com/abstract=1598361.

California Latinas for Reproductive Justice. 2010. "Young women speak out! Perspectives and implications of reproductive health, rights & justice policies." *CLRJ Research Report* 2 (1): 1–19.

Centers for Disease Control and Prevention (CDC). 2004. *STD Curriculum for Clinical Educators: Genital Human Papillomavirus* (HPV) Module. Washington, DC: CDC.

———. 2010a. "Condoms and STDs: Fact sheet for public health personnel." http://www.cdc.gov/condomeffectiveness/latex.htm#HPV.

———. 2010b. "Health stats." http://www.cdc.gov/nchs/products/hestats.htm.

———. 2011. "HIV among youth." http://www.cdc.gov/hiv/youth.

———. 2012. "HIV in the United States." http://www.cdc.gov/hiv/topics/surveillance/resoures/factsheets/us.overview.htm.

Chandra, A., G. Martinez, W. Mosher, J. Abma, and J. Jones. 2005. "Fertility, family planning, and reproductive health of US women: Data from the 2002 National Survey of Family Growth." *Vital and Health Statistics* 23, no. 25.

Chapman, L. 2004. "No Child Left Behind in Art?" *Arts Education Policy Review* 106 (2), 3–20.

Cochran-Smith, M. 2005. "The new teacher education: For better or for worse?" *Educational Researcher* 34 (7): 3–17.

Connell, E. 2008. "Expelling pleasure? School-based sex education and the regulation of youth." In *Probing the problematics: Sex and sexuality*, edited by M. Kohlke and L. Orza, 119–31. Oxford: Inter-Disciplinary Press.

Cooper, H., and D. Tom. 1984. "Teacher expectation research: A review with implications for classroom instruction." *Elementary School Journal* 85:77–89.

Crawford, M., and D. Popp. 2003. "Sexual double standards: A review and methodological critique of two decades of research." *Journal of Sex Research* 40: 13–26.

Cunningham, S., J. Tschann, J. Gurvey, J. Fortenberry, and J. Ellen. 2002. "Attitudes about sexual disclosure and perceptions of stigma and shame." *British Medical Journal* 78 (5): 334.

Dailard, C. 2001. "Sex education: Politicians, parents, teachers and teens." *Guttmacher Report on Public Policy* 4 (1): 9–12.

Darling-Hammond, L. 1999. *Teacher quality and student achievement: A review of state policy evidence.* Seattle: Center for the Study of Teaching and Policy, University of Washington.

Deaux, K. 2006. *To be an immigrant.* New York: Russell Sage Foundation.

Deem, R. 2001. "Globalisation, new managerialism, academic capitalism and entrepreneurialism in universities: Is the local dimension still important?" *Comparative Education* 37 (1): 7–20.

Demerath, P. 2009. *Producing success: The culture of personal advancement in an American high school.* Chicago: University of Chicago Press.

Dietrich, J. 2007. "The politics of PEPFAR: The president's emergency plan for AIDS relief. *Ethics and International Affairs* (21) 3.

Dill, K., and K. Thill. 2007. "Video game characters and the socialization of gender roles: Young people's perceptions mirror sexist media depictions." *Sex Roles* 57 (11/12): 851–64.

diMauro, D., and C. Joffe. 2009. "The religious right and the reshaping of sexual policy: Reproductive rights and sexuality education during the Bush years." In *Moral panics, sex panics: Fear and the fight over sexual rights*, edited by G. Herdt, 47–104. New York: New York University Press.

Doan, A., and J. Calterone-Williams. 2008. *The politics of virginity: Abstinence in sex education.* Santa Barbara, CA: Praeger.

Driscoll, A., M. Biggs, C. Brindis, and E. Yankah. 2001. "Adolescent Latino reproductive health: A review of the literature." *Hispanic Journal of Behavioral Sciences* 23:255–326.

Dunn, J. 2004. "'Everyone knows who the sluts are': How young women get around the stigma." In *Readings in deviant behavior*, 3rd ed., edited by A. Thio and T. Calhoun, ch. 30. Needham Heights, MA: Allyn and Bacon.

Dyer, C. 1999. "Researching the implementation of educational policy: A backward mapping approach." *Comparative Education* 35:45–61.

Eaton, D., L. Kann, S. Kinchen, J. Ross, J. Hawkins, W. Harris, R. Lowry, T. McManus, D. Chyen, S. Shanklin, C. Lim, J. Grunbaum, and H. Wechsler. 2006. "Youth Risk Behavior Surveillance—United States, 2005." *Morbidity and Mortality Weekly Report* 55 (55–5): 1–33.

Ehrhardt, B. 1996. "Our view of adolescent sexuality: Risk behavior without developmental context." *American Journal of Public Health* 86:1523–25.

Elia, J. 2000. "The necessity of comprehensive sexuality education in the schools." *Educational Forum* 64 (10): 340–47.

Elliott, Kathleen. 2010. "Gender, sexuality, and social change in high school." PhD diss., University of Wisconsin–Madison.

Emihovich, C., and C. Herrington. 1997. *Sex, kids, and politics: Health services in schools.* New York: Teachers College Press.

Epstein, D., S. O'Flynn, and D. Telford. 2003. *Silenced sexualities in schools and universities.* Stoke on Trent, UK: Trentham Books.

Families and Work Institute. 2008. *Times are changing: Gender and generation at work and at home.* New York: Families and Work Institute.

Faulkner, S. 2003. "Good girl or flirt girl: Latinas' definitions of sex and sexual relationships." *Hispanic Journal of Behavioral Sciences* 25 (2): 174.

Fausto-Sterling, A. 2000. *Sexing the body: Gender politics and the construction of sexuality.* New York: Basic Books.

Ferguson, J. 1990. *The anti-politics machine: "Development," depoliticization, and bureaucratic power in Lesotho.* Cambridge: Cambridge University Press.

Fields, J. 2008. *Risky lessons: Sex education and social inequality.* New Brunswick, NJ: Rutgers University Press.

Fields, J., and D. Tolman. 2006. "Risky business: Sexuality education and research in US schools." *Sexuality Research and Social Policy* 3 (4): 63–76.

Filipovic, J. 2008. "Offensive feminism: The conservative gender norms that perpetuate rape culture, and how feminists can fight back." In *Yes means yes: Visions of female sexual power and a world without rape,* edited by J. Friedman and J. Valenti, 13–28. Berkeley, CA: Seal Press.

Fine, M. 1988. "Sexuality, schooling, and adolescent females: The missing discourse of desire." *Harvard Educational Review* 58 (1): 29–53.

Fine, M., and S. McClelland. 2006. "Sexuality education and desire: Still missing after all these years." *Harvard Educational Review* 76 (3): 297.

Fitzgerald, J. 2003. "A liberal dose of conservatism: The 'new consensus' on welfare and other strange strategies," In *Fundamental differences: Feminists talk back to social conservatives,* edited by C. Burack and J. Josephson, 95–112. New York: Rowman and Littlefield.

Florida Department of Health. 2007." It's Great to Wait: Program information." http://www.greattowait.com/program.html.

Forhan, S., S. Gottlieb, M. Sternberg, F. Xu, S. Datta, G. McQuillan, S. Berman, and L. Markowitz. 2009. "Prevalence of sexually transmitted infections among female adolescents aged 14 to 19 in the U.S." *Pediatrics* 124 (6): 1505.

Fortenberry, J. 2004. "The effects of stigma on genital herpes care-seeking behaviours." *Herpes* 11:8–11.

Fortenberry, J., M. McFarlane, A. Bleakley, S. Bull, M. Fishbein, D. Grimley, K. Malotte, and B. Stoner. 2002. "Relationships of stigma and shame to gonorrhea and HIV screening." *American Journal of Public Health* 92 (3): 378–81.

Fox, C. 1990. "Implementation research: Why and how to transcend positivist methodologies." In *Implementation and the policy process: Opening up the black box,* edited by D. Palumbo and D. Calista, 199–212.Westport, CT: Greenwood Press.

Frankenberger, K., and A. Sukhdial. 1994. "Segmenting teens for AIDS preventive behaviors with implications for marketing communications." *Journal of Public Policy and Marketing* 13:133–50.

Franklin, C., and J. Corcoran. 2000. "Preventing adolescent pregnancy: A review of programs and practices." *Social Work* 45 (1): 40–52.

Fraser, J. 1997. *Reading, writing, and justice: School reform as if democracy matters.* Albany: State University of New York Press.

Frost, J., and S. Oslak. 1999. *Teenagers' pregnancy intentions and decisions: A study of young women in California choosing to give birth.* Occasional Report 2. New York: AGI.

Furstenburg, F. 1991. "As the pendulum swings: Teenage childbearing and social concern." *Family Relations* 40 (2): 127–38.

Gallagher, S., and C. Smith. 1999. "Symbolic traditionalism and pragmatic egalitarianism." *Gender and Society* 13:221–33.

Gay, Lesbian and Straight Education Network (GLSEN). 1999. *Report on anti-gay school violence.* New York: GLSEN.

———. 2007. *Gay-straight alliances: Creating safer schools for LGBT students and their allies.* GLSEN Research Brief. New York: GLSEN.

Geronimus, A. 2003. "Damned if you do: Culture, identity, privilege, and teenage childbearing in the U.S." *Social Science and Medicine* 57 (5): 881–93.

Geronimus A. and J. Thompson. 2004. "To denigrate, ignore, or disrupt: The health impact of policy-induced breakdown of urban African American Communities of Support." *Du Bois Review* 1 (2): 247–79.

Gerson, K. 2009. *The unfinished revolution: How a new generation is reshaping, family, work, and gender in the U.S.* Oxford: Oxford University Press.

Gibson, J. 2005. *The war on Christmas: How the liberal plot to ban the sacred Christian holiday is worse than you thought.* New York: Sentinel.

Gilbert, J. 2004. "Between sexuality and narrative: On the language of sex education." In *Youth and sexualities: Pleasure, subversion and insubordination in and out of schools,* edited by M. Rasmussen, E. Rofes, and S. Talburt, 109–30. New York: Palgrave.

Glanz, K., B. Rimer, and K. Viswanath. 2008. *Health behavior and health education: Theory, research, and practice.* San Francisco: Jossey-Bass.

Goertz, M. 2005. "Implementing the No Child Left Behind Act: Challenges for the states." *Peabody Journal of Education* 80 (2): 73–89.

Goldhaber, D., and J. Hannaway. 2004. "Accountability with a kicker: Observations on the Florida A+ accountability plan." *Phi Delta Kappan* 85 (8): 598–605.

Gray, L., and S. Phelps. 2003. *Navigator* (Student workbook). Golf, IL: Project Reality.

Greenberg, M., R. Weissberg, M. O'Brien, J. Zins, L. Fredericks, H. Resnik, and M. Elias. 2003. "Enhancing school-based prevention and youth development through coordinated social, emotional, and academic learning." *American Psychologist* 58 (6/7): 466–74.

Gross, L. 2006. "Scientific illiteracy and the partisan takeover of biology." *PLoS Biology* 4 (5): e167.

Grudem, W. 2004. *Evangelical feminism and biblical truth.* Colorado Springs: Multnomah.

Guidotti, T., P. Deb, R. Bertera, and L. Ford. "The Fort McMurray Demonstration Project in social marketing: No demonstrable effect on already falling injury rates following intensive community and workplace intervention." *Journal of Community Health* 34 (5): 392–99.

Gutmann, A. 1987. *Democratic education.* Princeton, NJ: Princeton University Press.

———. 1995. Civic education and social diversity. *Ethics* 105 (3): 557–79.

Guttmacher Institute. "State Data Center." http://www.guttmacher.org/datacenter/profile.jsp.

Hanson, K., R. Nathan, T. Marchant, H. Mponda, C. Jones, J. Bruce, G. Stephen, J. Mulligan, H. Mshinda, and J. Armstrong Schellenberg. 2008. "Vouchers for scaling up insecticide treated nets in Tanzania: Methods for monitoring and evaluation of a national health system intervention." *BMC Public Health* 8:205.

Hart, G. 2002. *Disabling globalization: Places of power in post-apartheid South Africa*. Berkeley: University of California Press.

Haslam, N. 2002. "Kinds of kinds." *Philosophy, Psychiatry, and Psychology* 9: 203–17.

Hastings, G. 2003. "Relational paradigms in social marketing." *Journal of Macromarketing* 23 (1): 6–15.

Hedman, A., D. Larsen, and S. Bohnenblust. 2008. "Relationship between comprehensive sex education and teen pregnancy in Minnesota." *American Journal of Health Studies* 23 (4): 185–94.

Hendricks, K., P. Thickstun, A. Khurshid, S. Malhotra, and H. Thiele. 2006. "The attack on abstinence education: Fact or fallacy?" Technical paper. Austin, TX: Medical Institute for Sexual Health.

Hess, D. 2009. *Controversy in the classroom: The democratic power of discussion*. New York: Routledge.

Hess, D., and J. Posselt. 2002. "How high school students experience and learn from the discussion of controversial public issues." *Journal of Curriculum and Supervision* 17 (4): 283–314.

Hewett, P., B. Mensch, and A. Erulkar. 2004. "Consistency in the reporting of sexual behaviour by adolescent girls in Kenya: A comparison of interviewing methods." *British Medical Journal* 80, Supplement 2.

Hirsch, E., J. Kett, and J. Trefil. 1987. *Cultural literacy*. Boston: Houghton Mifflin.

Hokoda, A., D. Galván, V. Malcarne, D. Castañeda, and E. Ulloa. 2007. "An exploratory study examining teen dating violence, acculturation and acculturative stress in Mexican-American adolescents." *Journal of Aggression, Maltreatment & Trauma* 14 (3): 33–49.

Holland, J., C. Ramazanoglu, S. Sharpe, and R. Thompson. 1998. *The male in the head: Young people, heterosexuality, and power*. London: Tunfell Press.

hooks, b. 1992. *Black looks: Race and representations*. Toronto: Between the Lines Press.

———. 1994. *Teaching to transgress: Education as the practice of freedom*. London: Routledge.

Hunter, J. D. 1991. *Culture wars: The struggle to define America*. New York: Basic Books.

Hursh, D. 2003. "Discourse, power and resistance in New York: The rise of testing and accountability and the decline of teacher professionalism and local control." In *Discourse, power and resistance: Challenging the rhetoric of contemporary education*, edited by J. Satterthwaite, E. Atkinson, and K. Gale, 43–56. Stoke-on-Trent, UK: Trentham Books.

Hutchens, N. 2009. "Silence at the schoolhouse gate: The diminishing first amendment rights of public school employees." *Kentucky Law Journal* 97:37.

Irvine, J. 1994. *Sexual cultures and the construction of adolescent identities*. Philadelphia: Temple University Press.

———. 2002. *Talk about sex: The battles over sex education in the U.S*. Berkeley: University of California Press.

James, A., C. Jenks, and A. Prout. 1998. *Theorizing childhood*. Cambridge: Polity Press.

Jemmott, J., L. Jemmott, and G. Fong. 2010. "Efficacy of a theory-based abstinence-only intervention over 24 months." *Archives of Pediatrics and Adolescent Medicine* 164 (2): 152–59.

Jenks, C. 1996. *Childhood*. London: Routledge.

Jethani, S. 2009. *The divine commodity: Discovering a faith beyond consumer Christianity*. Grand Rapids, MI: Zondervan.

Kaiser Family Foundation. 2000. "Sex education in America: A view from inside the nation's classrooms." http://www.kff.org/youthhivstds/3048-index.com.

Kalina, L. 2011. *Florida's Youth*. Washington, DC: Advocates for Youth.

Kasl, E., and L. Yorks. 2002. "An extended epistemology for transformative learning theory and its application through collaborative inquiry." *Teachers College Record* Online. http://www.tcrecord.org/Content.asp?ContentID=10878.

Kehily, M. 2002a. "Sexing the subject: Teachers, pedagogies and sex education." *Sex Education* 2 (3): 215–31.

———. 2002b. *Sexuality, gender and schooling: Shifting agendas in social learning*. New York: Routledge.

Kendall, C., A. Afabel-Munsuz, I. Speizer, and A. Avery. 2005. "Understanding pregnancy in a population of inner-city women in New Orleans: Results of qualitative research." *Social Science and Medicine* 60:297–311.

Kendall, N. 2008a. "Sexuality education in an abstinence-only era: A comparative case study of two US states." *Sexuality Research and Social Policy* 5 (2): 23–44.

———. 2008b. "The state(s) of sexuality education in America." *Sexuality Research and Social Policy* 5 (2): 1–11.

———. 2010. "Student voice in school-based sex education research: National comparisons." Presented at the Annual Meeting of the American Educational Studies Association, October 2010, Denver, CO.

Kilbourne, J. 2000. *Can't buy my love: How advertising changes the way we think and feel*. New York: Simon and Schuster.

Kirby, D. 1985. "The effects of selected sexuality education programs: Toward a more realistic view." *Journal of Sex Education and Therapy* 11:28–37.

———. 1991. "School-based clinics: Research results and their implications for future research methods." *Evaluation and Program Planning* 14:35–47.

———. 1997. *No easy answers: Research findings on programs to reduce teen pregnancy*. Washington DC: National Campaign to Prevent Teen Pregnancy.

———. 2001. "Understanding what works and what doesn't in reducing adolescent sexual risk-taking." *Family Planning Perspectives* 33 (6): 276–81.

———. 2002. "The impact of schools and school programs upon adolescent sexual behavior." *Journal of Sex Research* 39 (1): 27–33.

———. 2007. *Emerging answers 2007: Research finding on programs to reduce teen pregnancy and sexually transmitted diseases*. Washington, DC: National Campaign to Prevent Teen and Unplanned Pregnancy.

Konner, M., and M. Shostak. 1986. "Adolescent childbearing and pregnancy: An anthropological perspective." In *School-age pregnancy and parenthood*, edited by J. Lancaster and B. Hamburg, 325–45. New York: Aldine De Gruyter.

Kotler, P., and G. Zaltman. 1971. "Social marketing: An approach to planned social change." *Journal of Marketing* 35:3–12.

Kreeft, P. 2002. *How to win the culture war: A Christian battle plan for a society in crisis*. Downers Grove, IL: InterVarsity Press.

Ladson-Billings, G. 1999. "Preparing teachers for diverse student populations: A critical race theory perspective." *Review of Research in Education* 24:211–47.

Landau, E. 2010. "$250 million for abstinence education not evidence-based, groups say." CNN. Retrieved from http://www.cnn.com.

Larner, W., and M. Butler. 2005. "Governmentalities of local partnerships : The rise of a 'partnering state' in New Zealand." *Studies in Political Economy* 75:79–101.

Lee, J., W. Donlan, and J. Paz. 2009. "Culturally competent HIV/AIDS prevention: Understanding program effects on adolescent beliefs, attitudes, and behaviors." *Journal of HIV/AIDS and Social Services* 8 (1): 57–79.

Lefebvre, R. 2011. "An integrative model for social marketing." *Journal of Social Marketing* 1 (1): 54–72.

Lefebvre, R., and J. Flora. 1988. "Social marketing and public health intervention." *Health Education Quarterly* 15:299–315.

Lehr, V. 2003. "'Family values': Social conservative power in diverse rhetoric." In *Fundamental differences: Feminists talk back to social conservatives*, edited by C. Burack and J. Josephson, 127–42. Lanham, MD: Rowman and Littlefield.

Levine, J., C. Emery, and H. Pollack. 2007. "The wellbeing of children born to teen mothers." *Journal of Marriage and Family* 69 (Feb.): 105–22.

Levy, A. 2005. *Female chauvinist pigs: Women and the rise of raunch culture.* New York: Free Press.

———. 2009. "Either/Or: Sports, sex and the case of Caster Semenya." *New Yorker.* http://www.newyorker.com/reporting/2009/11/30/091130fa_fact_levy.

Lieber, E., L. Li, Z. Wu, M. J. Rotheram-Borus, J. Guan, and the National Institute of Mental Health Collaborative HIV Prevention Trial Group. 2006. "HIV/STD stigmatization fears as health seeking barriers in China." *AIDS and Behavior* 10 (5): 463–71.

Liebman, R., and R. Wuthnow. 1983. *The new Christian right: Mobilization and legitimation.* New York: Aldine De Gruyter.

Lima, A. 2008. "Shedding first amendment rights at the classroom door: The effects of *Garcettia* and *Meyer* on education in public schools." *George Mason Law Review* 16 (1): 173–201.

Lipsky, M. 1980. *Street-level Bureaucracy: Dilemmas of the individual in public services.* New York: Russell Sage Foundation.

Lopez, N. 2003. *Hopeful girls, troubled boys: Race and gender disparity in urban education.* New York: Routledge.

Luker, K. 1997. *Dubious conceptions: The politics of teenage pregnancy.* Cambridge, MA: Harvard University Press.

———. 2006. *When sex goes to school: Warring views on sex—and sex education—since the sixties.* New York: W. W. Norton.

Mackey, E. 2008. *Street-level bureaucrats and the shaping of university housing policy.* Fayetteville: University of Arkansas Press.

Marcus, G. 1995. "Ethnography in/of the world system: The emergence of multi-sited ethnography." *Annual Review of Anthropology* 24 (1): 95–117.

Marcus, S. 2002. "Fighting bodies, fighting words: A theory and politics of rape prevention." In *Theorizing feminisms: A reader*, edited by E. Hackett and S. Haslanger, 385–403. New York: Oxford University Press.

Markowitz, G., and D. Rosner. 2003. "Politicizing science: The case of the Bush administration's influence on the lead advisory panel at the Centers for Disease Control." *Journal of Public Health Policy* 24 (2): 105–29.

Martin, C., and S. Parker. 1995. "Folk theories about sex and race differences." *Personality and Social Psychology Bulletin* 21 (1): 45.

Marx, R., and C. Harris. 2006. "No Child Left Behind and science education: Opportunities, challenges, and risks." *The Elementary School Journal* 106 (5): 467–78.

Massat, C. 1995. "Lifting the shadow: Race, gender and county of parents of children in foster care in Illinois. *Journal of Applied Social Sciences* 19: 121–8.

Mast, C. 2001. *The Option of True Sexual Freedom*. 4th ed. Lockport, IL: Respect, Inc.

Mather, M., and D. Adams. 2006. *The risk of negative child outcomes in low-income families*. Baltimore: Annie E. Casey Foundation and Population Reference Bureau.

Maynard-Moody, S., and M. C. Musheno. 2003. *Cops, teachers, counselors: Stories from the front lines of public service*. Ann Arbor: University of Michigan Press.

Mayo, C. 2006. Pushing the limits of liberalism: Queerness, children, and the future. *Educational Theory* 56 (4): 469–87.

Mays, V., and S. Cochran. 2001. "Mental health correlates of perceived discrimination among lesbian, gay, and bisexual adults in the United States." *American Journal of Public Health* 91 (11): 1869–76.

McClelland, S., and M. Fine. 2008. "Writing on cellophane: Studying teen women's sexual desires; inventing methodological release points." In *The methodological dilemma: Critical and creative approaches to qualitative research*, edited by K. Gallagher, 232–60. London: Routledge.

McCullum, D., and G. deLashmutt. 1996. *The myth of romance*. Minneapolis: Bethany House Publishers.

McDermott, J. 2000. "Social marketing: A tool for health education." *American Journal of Health Behavior* 24 (1): 6–10.

McKay, A. 1997. "Accommodating ideological pluralism in sexuality education." *Journal of Moral Education* 26 (3): 285–300.

———. 1998. *Sexual ideology and schooling: Towards democratic sexuality education*. Albany: State University of New York Press.

Meyer, J. 1980. "The world polity and the authority of the nation-state." In *Studies of the modern world-system*, edited by A. Bergsen, 109–37. New York: Academic Press.

Miller, K., D. Sabo, M. Farrell, G. Barnes, and M. Melnick. 1998. "Athletic participation and sexual behavior in adolescents: The different worlds of boys and girls." *Journal of Health and Social Behavior* 39 (2): 108–23.

Miller, M., and A. Summers. 2007. "Gender differences in video game characters' roles, appearances, and attire as portrayed in video game magazines." *Sex Roles* 57:733–42.

Miller, V. 2003. *Consuming religion: Christian faith and practice in a consumer culture*. New York: Continuum International Publishing Group.

Milner, M. 2004. *Freaks, geeks, and cool kids: American teenagers, schools, and the culture of consumption*. New York: Theatre Arts Books.

Mintzes, J, J. Wandersee, and J. Novak, eds. 1998. *Teaching science for understanding: A human constructivist view*. Maryland Heights, MO: Academic Press.

Mitchell, T. 2002. *Rule of experts: Egypt, techno-politics, modernity*. Berkeley: University of California Press.

Mollborn, S. 2007. "Making the best of a bad situation: Material resources and teenage parenthood." *Journal of Marriage and Family* 69 (Feb.): 92–104.

Mooney, C., and M. Lee. 1995. "Legislating morality in the American states: The case of pre-Roe abortion regulation reform." *American Journal of Political Science* 39:599–627.

Moore, J., M. Raymond, J. Mittelstaedt, and J. Tanner. 2002. "Age and consumer socialization agent influences on adolescents' sexual knowledge, attitudes, and behavior: Implications for social marketing initiatives and public policy." *Journal of Public Policy and Marketing* 21 (1): 37–52.

Moore, N., J. Davidson, and T. Fisher, eds. 2009. *Speaking of sexuality*. Oxford: Oxford Univeristy Press.

Moran, J. 2000. *Teaching sex: The shaping of adolescence in the 20th century*. Cambridge, MA: Harvard University Press.

Morris, R. 2005. "Research and evaluation in sexuality education: An allegorical exploration of complexities and possibilities." *Sex Education* 5 (4): 405–22.

Murcott, A. 1980. "The social construction of teenage pregnancy: A problem in the ideologies of childhood and reproduction." *Sociology of Health and Illness* 2 (1): 1–23.

Nahmod, H. 2008. "Academic freedom and the post-Garcetti blues." *First Amendment Law Review* 7:54–74.

National Abstinence Education Association. 2007. "Zogby International Poll: Parental Support for Abstinence Education. NAEA Executive Summary of Key Findings." http://www.abstinence association.org/newsroom/050307_zogby_key_findings.html.

National Committee for Responsible Philanthropy (NCRP). 2005. *Funding the culture wars: Philanthropy, church and state*. Washington DC: NCRP.

National Institute of Allergy and Infectious Diseases (NIAID). 1998. "Sexually transmitted diseases statistics," NIAID fact sheet. Washington, DC: NIAID.

National Public Radio, Kaiser Family Foundation, and Kennedy School of Governement. 2004. *Sex education in America: General public/parents survey*. Menlo Park, CA: Kaiser Family Foundation.

Oakley, A., D. Fullerton, J. Holland, S. Arnold, M. France-Dawson, P. Kelly, and S. McGrellis. 1995. "Sexual health interventions for young people: A methodological review." *British Medical Journal* 310:158–62.

Orr, D., J. Fortenberry, and M. Blythe. 1997. "Validity of self-reported sexual behaviors in adolescent women using biomarker outcomes." *Sexually Transmitted Diseases* 24 (5): 261.

Ott, M., N. Adler, S. Millstein, J. Tschann, and J. Ellen. 2002. "The trade-off between hormonal contraceptives and condoms among adolescents." *Perspectives on Sexual and Reproductive Health* 34 (1): 6–14.

Parker, W. C. 2006. "Public discourses in schools: Purposes, problems, possibilities." *Educational Researcher* 35 (8): 11–18.

Parkin, M., R. Bray, J. Ferlay, and P. Pisani. 2005. "Global cancer statistics." *CA: A Cancer Journal for Clinicians* 55:74–108.

Pascoe, C. 2007. *Dude, you're a fag: Masculinity and sexuality in high school*. Berkeley: University of California Press.

———. 2008. "The first year out: Understanding American teens after high school." *Contemporary Sociology: A Journal of Reviews* 37 (3): 239–40.

Patton, C. 1996. *Fatal advice: How safe-sex education went wrong*. Durham, NC: Duke University Press.

Paul, J. 2000. "Bisexuality: Reassessing our paradigms of sexuality." In *Bisexuality in the U.S.: A social science reader*, edited by P. Rust, 11–23. New York: Columbia University Press.

Pawlowski, N. 2011. "Public vs. private: An examination of sex educators' training, experiences, and challenges." Master's thesis, University of Wisconsin–Madison, Department of Educational Policy Studies.

Peacock, B. 1986. *The anthropological lens: Harsh light, soft focus*. New York: Cambridge University Press.

Pearson, J. 2006. "Personal control, self-efficacy in sexual negotiation, and contraceptive risk among adolescents: The role of gender." *Sex Roles* 54:615–25.

Peirce, K. 1993. "Socialization of teenage girls through teen-magazine fiction: The making of a new woman or an old lady?" *Sex Roles* 29 (1/2): 59–68.

Perrin, K., and S. DeJoy. 2003. "Abstinence-only education: How we got here and where we're going." *Journal of Public Health Policy* 24 (3/4): 445–59.

Pfeiffer, J. 2004. "Condom social marketing, Pentecostalism, and structural adjustment in Mozambique: A clash of AIDS prevention messages." *Medical Anthropology Quarterly* 18 (1): 77–103.

Phoenix, F. 1993. "The social construction of teenage motherhood: A Black and White issue?" In *The politics of pregnancy/adolescent sexuality and public policy*, edited by A. Lawson and D. Rhode, 74–100. New Haven, CT: Yale University Press.

Pillow, W. 2004. *Unfit subjects: Educational policy and the teen mother.* New York and London: RoutledgeFalmer.

Pithers, R., and R. Soden. 2000. "Critical thinking in education: A review." *Educational Researcher* 42 (3): 237–49.

Pollock, M. 2004. *Colormute: Race talk dilemmas in an American school.* Princeton, NJ: Princeton University Press.

Pope, D. 2003. *Doing school: How we are creating a generation of stressed out, materialistic, and miseducated students.* New Haven, CT: Yale University Press.

Price, C. 2010. "Can gays really change? A review of the Jones and Yarhouse study on ex-gays." Focus on the Family. http://www.citizenlink.com/2010/06/can-gays-really-change-a-review-of-the-jones-and-yarhouse-study-on-ex-gays/.

Prout, A., and A. James. 1990. *Constructing and reconstructing childhood: Contemporary issues in the sociological study of childhood.* London: Falmer Press.

Pruitt, B. 2007. "An abstinence education research agenda: What I really learned." *American Journal of Health Education* 38 (6): 25–258.

Quart, A. 2003. *Branded: The buying and selling of teenagers.* Cambridge, MA: Perseus.

Qvortrup, J. 1994. "Childhood matters: An introduction." In *Childhood Matters: Social Theory, Practices and Politics*, edited by J. Qvortrup, M. Bardy, G. Sgritta, and H. Wintersberger, 1–24. London: Ashgate Avebury.

Rasmussen, M., E. Rofes, and S. Talburt. 2004. *Youth and sexualities: Pleasure, subversion and insubordination in and out of schools.* New York: Palgrave.

Raymond, A. 2009. "Women aren't vending machines: How video games perpetuate the commodity model of sex." GameCritics.com. http://www.gamecritics.com/alex-raymond/women-arent-vending-machines-how-video-games-perpetuate-the-commodity-model-of-sex.

Raymond, M., L. Bogdanovich, D. Brahmi, L. Cardinal, G. Fager, L. Frattarelli, G. Hecker, E. Jarpe, A. Viera, and L. Kantor. 2008. "State refusal of federal funding for abstinence-only programs." *Sexuality Research and Social Policy* 5 (3): 44–55.

Rayner, S. 2003. "Democracy in the age of assessment: Reflections on the roles of expertise and democracy in public-sector decision making." *Science and Public Policy* 30 (3): 163–70.

Regnerus, M. D. 2007. *Forbidden fruit: Sex and religion in the lives of American teenagers.* New York: Oxford University Press.

———. 2009. "Mark Regnerus—Freedom to marry young." *Washington Post*, Op-Ed, Sunday, April 26.

Reinhold, S. 1994. "Local conflict and ideological struggle: 'Positive images' and Section 28." PhD diss., University of Sussex.

Reiss, I. 1992. *Sexual pluralism: Ending America's sexual crisis.* New York: Prometheus Books.

Remafedi, G. 1999a. "Sexual orientation and youth suicide." *Journal of the American Medical Association* 282:1291–92.

———. 1999b. "Suicide and sexual orientation: Nearing the end of controversy?" *Archives of General Psychiatry* 56: 885–86.

Rhoads, R., and S. Calderone. 2007. "Reconstituting the democratic subject: Sexuality, schooling, and citizenship." *Educational Theory* 57 (1): 105–21.

Rhoten, D. 1999. *Global-local conditions of possibility: The case of education decentralization in Argentina.* Phd diss., Stanford University.

Ridgeway, C. 2006. "Gender as an organizing force in social relations: Implications for the future of inequality." In *The declining significance of gender?,* edited by F. Balu, M. Brinton, and D. Grusky, 245–87. New York: Russell Sage Foundation.

Robertson, J. 2003. "Rape among incarcerated men: Sex, coercion and STDs." *AIDS Patient Care and STDs* 17 (8): 423–30.

Rose, P. 2005. "Privatisation and decentralisation of schooling in Malawi: Default or design?" *Compare* 35 (2): 153–65.

Rose, S. 1989. "Gender, education and the new Christian right." *Society* 26 (2): 59–66.

Rust, P. 2000. *Bisexuality in the U.S.: A social science reader.* New York: Columbia University Press.

Ryan, C., D. Huebner, R. Diaz, and J. Sanchez. 2009. "Family rejection as a predictor of negative health outcomes in White and Latino LGB young adults." *Pediatrics* 123:346–52.

Ryan, C., and I. Rivers. 2003. "Lesbian, gay, bisexual, and transgender youth: Victimization and its correlates in the USA and UK." *Culture, Health, and Sexuality* 5 (2): 103–19.

Sabatier, P. 1993. "Top down and bottom up approaches to implementation research." In *The policy process: A reader,* edited by M. Hill, 266–93. New York: Harvester Wheatsheaf.

Sadker, M., and D. Sadker. 1995. *Failing at fairness: How America's schools cheat girls.* New York: C. Scribner's Sons.

Sandler, J. 2008. "What works? Who decides? Scientific evidence, local governance, and the politics of knowledge in social and educational reform." PhD diss., University of Wisconsin–Madison.

Santelli, J., M. Ott, M. Lyon, J. Rogers, D. Summers, and R. Schleifer. 2006. "Abstinence and abstinence-only education: A review of US policies and programs." *Perspectives on Sexual and Reproductive Health* 38 (4): 182–89.

Sawyer, R., P. Pinciaro, and J. Jessell. 1998. "Effects of coercion and verbal consent on university students' perception of date rape." *American Journal of Health Behavior* 22 (1): 46–53.

Schaalma, H., C. Abraham, M. Gillmore, and G. Kok. 2004. "Sex education as health promotion: What does it take?" *Archives of Sexual Behavior* 33 (3): 259–69.

Schalet, A. 2004. Must we fear adolescent sexuality? *Medscape General Medicine* 6 (4): 44.

Schor, J. 2004. *Born to buy: The commercialized child and the new consumer culture.* New York: Scribner.

Schwalbe, M., S. Godwin, D. Holden, and D. Schrock. 2000. "Generic processes in the reproduction of inequality: An interactionist analysis." *Social Forces* 79 (2): 419–52.

Sears, J. 1992. *Sexuality and the curriculum: The politics and practices of sexuality education.* New York: Teachers College Press.

Segura, L. 2005. "Teaching sexuality." *The Nation.* http://www.thenation.com/article/teaching-sexuality.

Seidman, S. 1992. "An investigation of sex-role stereotyping in music videos." *Journal of Broadcasting and Electronic Media* 36 (2): 209–16.

Sewall, G. 2005. "Textbook publishing." *Phi Delta Kappan* 86 (7): 5.

Sex, Etc. "Sex in the States." http://www.sexetc.org/state.

SexEdLibrary. "Wyoming received no federal funding for abstinence-only-until-marriage programs in Fiscal Year 2007." http://www.sexedlibrary.com/index.cfm?pageId=868.

Sexuality Information and Education Council of the United States (SIECUS). 2008. *Choosing the Best Soul Mate Review.* Washington, DC: SIECUS.

———. 2009. "Sex education in the sunshine state: How abstinence-only-until-marriage programs are keeping Florida's youth in the dark." Report conducted with Healthy Teens Campaign. Washington, DC: SIECUS.

———. 2010. A History of Federal Abstinence-Only-Until-Marriage Funding FYIO. Washington, DC: SIECUS.

Sheffield, R. 2010. "Washington must face the facts of life: Parents and teens favor abstinence." The Heritage Foundation. http://blog.heritage.org/2010/08/26/washington-must-face-the-facts-of-life-parents-and-teens-favor-abstinence/.

Shive, S., and N. Morris. 2006. "Evaluation of the Energize Your Life! social marketing campaign pilot study to increase fruit intake among community college students." *Journal of American College Health* 55 (1): 33–40.

Shore, C., and S. Wright. 1997. *Anthropology of policy: Critical perspectives on governance and power.* New York: Routledge.

Siegel, D. 2007. *Sisterhood, interrupted: From radical women to grrls gone wild.* New York: Palgrave Macmillan.

Silva, M. 2002. "The effectiveness of school-based sex education programs in the promotion of abstinent behavior: A meta-analysis." *Health Education Research* 17 (4): 471–81.

Simkins, T. 2000. "Education reform and managerialism: Comparing the experience of schools and colleges." *Journal of Education Policy* 15 (3): 317–32.

Skinner, E., and M. Belmont. 1993. "Motivation in the classroom: Reciprocal effects of teacher behavior and student engagement across the school year." *Journal of Educational Psychology* 85:571–81.

Socarides, C. 1995. *Homosexuality: A freedom too far.* Phoenix: Adam Margrave Books.

Staiger, A. 2006. *Learning difference: Race and schooling in the multiracial metropolis.* Stanford, CA: Stanford University Press.

Stephens, D., and L. Phillips. 2003. "Freaks, gold diggers, divas, and dykes: The sociohistorical development of adolescent African-American women's sexual scripts." *Sexuality & Culture* 7 (Winter): 3–49.

Stephens, S. 1995. "Children and the politics of culture in 'late capitalism.'" In *Children and the politics of culture,* edited by S. Stephens, 3–50. Princeton, NJ: Princeton University Press.

Stone, D. 2001. *Policy paradox: The art of political decision making.* 3rd ed. New York: W.W. Norton and Co.

Strathern, M. 2000. *Audit cultures: Anthropological studies in accountability, ethics, and the academy.* New York: Routledge.

Struckman-Johnson, C., D. Struckman-Johnson, and P. B. Anderson. 2003. "Tactics of sexual coercion: When men and women won't take no for an answer." *Journal of Sex Research* 40 (1): 76–86.

Suellentrop, K. 2009. *What Works 2009: Curriculum-based programs that prevent teen pregnancy.* Washington, DC: National Campaign to Prevent Teen and Unplanned Pregnancy.

Sunderman, G. 2009. "The federal role in education: From the Reagan to the Obama administration." *Voices in Urban Education* 24 (Summer): 6–14.

Sutton, M., and B. Levinson. 2001. *Policy as practice: Toward a comparative sociocultural analysis of educational policy.* Westport, CT: Ablex Publishing.

Tadajewski, M., and D. Brownlie, eds. 2008. *Critical marketing: Issues in contemporary marketing.* New York: John Wiley and Sons Limited.

Tatalovich, R., and B. Daynes. 1998. "Social regulations and moral conduct." In *Moral controversies in American politics: Cases in social regulatory policy,* edited by R. Tatalovich and B. Daynes. Armonk, NY: M. E. Sharpe.

Taylor, C. 1994. *Multiculturalism: Examining the politics of recognition.* Princeton, NJ: Princeton University Press.

Tjaden, P., and N. Thoennes. 1998. *Stalking in America: Findings from the National Violence Against Women Survey, research in brief.* Washington, D.C.: U.S. Department of Justice, National Institute of Justice.

Tolman, D. 2002. *Dilemmas of desire.* Cambridge, MA: Harvard University Press.

Tolman, D., C. Hirschman, and E. Impett. 2005. There's more to the story: The place of qualitative research on female adolescent sexuality in policy making. *Sexuality Research and Policy Studies* (Special issue on Adolescent Sexuality). 2 (4): 4–20.

Tolman, D., M. Striepe, and T. Harmon. 2003. "Gender matters: Constructing a model of adolescent sexual health." *Journal of Sex Research* 40 (1): 4–12.

Trenholm, C., B. Devaney, K. Fortson, L. Quay, J. Wheeler, and M. Clark. 2007. *Impacts of four Title V, Section 510 abstinence education programs: Final report.* Princeton, NJ: Mathematica Policy Research, Inc.

Trinder, L., and S. Reynolds, eds. 2000. *Evidence-based practice: A critical appraisal.* Oxford: Blackwell Science.

Trudell, B. 1985. The first organized campaign for school sex education: A source of critical questions about current efforts. *Journal of Sex Education and Therapy* 11 (1): 10–15.

———. 1993. *Doing sex education: Gender politics and schooling.* New York: Routledge.

Trudell, B., and M. Whatley. 1991. "Sex Respect: A problematic public school sexuality curriculum." *Journal of Sex Education and Therapy* 17 (2): 125–40.

UNICEF. 2001. "A league table of teenage births in rich nations." http://www.unicef-icdc.org/publications/pdf/repcard3e.pdf. Florence: UNICEF Innocenti Research Centre.

United States House of Representatives, Committee on Government Reform—Minority Staff, Special Investigations Division. 2004. "The content of federally funded abstinence-only education programs."Accessed June 5, 2011: http://www.apha.org/apha/PDFs/HIV/The_Waxman_Report.pdf.

Valdes, F. 1995. "Queers, sissies, dykes, and tomboys: Deconstructing the conflation of 'sex,' 'gender,' and 'sexual orientation' in Euro-American law and society." *California Law Review* 83 (1): 1–377.

Varenne, H., and R. McDermott. 1999. *Successful failure: The school America builds.* Boulder, CO: Westview Press.

Vavrus, F., and L. Bartlett. 2006. "Comparatively knowing: Making a case for the vertical case study." *Current Issues in Comparative Education* 8 (2): 95–103.

Vinovskis, M. 1988. *An "epidemic" of adolescent pregnancy? Some historical and policy considerations.* New York: Oxford University Press.

Walkerdine, V. 1990. *Schoolgirl fictions.* New York: Verso.

Waxman, H. 2006. "Politics and science: Reproductive health." *Health Matrix* 16 (1): 5–25.

Weeks, J., and J. Holland, eds. 1996. *Sexual cultures: Communities, values and intimacy.* New York: Palgrave McMillan.

Weis, L., and D. Carbonell-Medina. 2000. "Learning to speak out in an abstinence based sex education group: Gender and race work in an urban magnet school." *Teachers College Record* 102 (3): 620–50.

Weis, L., and M. Fine. 1993. *Beyond silenced voices: Class, race, and gender in U.S. schools.* New York: State University of New York Press.

Whatley, M. 1988. "Photographic images of blacks in sexuality texts." *Curriculum Inquiry* 18 (2): 137–55.

———. 1991. "Images of gays and lesbians in sexuality texts." *Journal of Homosexuality* 22 (314): 197–211.

Whatley, M., and E. Henken. 2001. *Did you hear about the girl who—? Contemporary legends, folklore, and human sexuality.* New York: New York University Press.

Whatley, M., and B. Trudell. 1993. "Teen-aid: Another problematic sexuality curriculum." *Journal of Sex Education and Therapy* 19 (4): 251–71.

Whitehead, N. n.d. "Homosexuality and mental health problems." http://www.narth.com/docs/whitehead.html.

Whitty, G., S. Power, and D. Halpin. 1998. *Devolution and choice in education: The school, the state, and the market.* Buckingham: Open University Press.

Wight, D., and C. Abraham. 2000. "From psycho-social theory to sustainable classroom practice: Developing a research-based teacher-delivered sex education programme." *Health Education Research* 15:25–38.

Wilcox, W. 1998. "Conservative Protestant childrearing: Authoritarian or authoritative?" *American Sociological Review* 63 (6): 796–809.

Wiley, D., and K. Wilson. 2009. "Just say Don't Know: Sexuality education in public schools." Austin: Texas Freedom Network Education Fund.

Witt, S. 2000. "The influence of television on children's gender role socialization." *Childhood Education* 76 (5): 322–24.

Wyatt, G. 1997. *Stolen women: Reclaiming our sexuality, taking back our lives.* New York: Wiley and Sons.

Wyoming Department of Education. 1998. *HIV/AIDS model policy for Wyoming public schools.* Cheyenne, WY: Department of Education.

Young, I. 1997. "Difference as a resource for democratic communication." In *Deliberative democracy: Essays on reason and politics,* edited by J. Bohman and W. Rehg, 383–404. Cambridge, MA: MIT Press.

Zeichner, K. 1998. "Investigative trends in U.S. teacher education." *Revista Educação* (Brazil) 9:76–87.

Zimmerman, J. 2005. *Whose America? Culture wars in the public schools.* Cambridge, MA: Harvard University Press.

Zimmerman, R., P. Cupp, L. Donohew, C. Kristin Sionean, S. Feist-Price, and D. Helme. 2008. "Effects of a school-based, theory-driven HIV and pregnancy prevention curriculum." *Perspectives on Sexual and Reproductive Health* 40 (1): 42–51.

Index